Humerus

Other books in the Musculoskeletal Trauma Series:

Femur
Radius and ulna
Tibia and fibula

Series Editors:

Charles Court-Brown MD, FRCSEd (Orth)
Consultant Orthopaedic Surgeon
The Royal Infirmary of Edinburgh
Edinburgh, UK

D. Pennig
Abteilung für Unfallchirurgie, Hand- und
Wiederherstellungschirurgie
St Vinzenz Hospital
Köln, Germany

Musculoskeletal Trauma Series

Humerus

Edited by

Evan L. Flatow MD
Herbert Irving Associate Professor of Orthopedic Surgery;
and Associate Chief, The Shoulder Service
New York Orthopedic Hospital,
Columbia Presbyterian Medical Center
New York, USA

C. Ulrich MD
Professor for Traumatology Chief Surgeon
Trauma Department
Klinik am Eichert
Göppingen, Germany

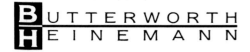

BUTTERWORTH
HEINEMANN

Butterworth-Heinemann
Linacre House, Jordan Hill, Oxford OX2 8DP
A division of Reed Educational and Professional Publishing Ltd

ℛ A member of the Reed Elsevier plc group

OXFORD BOSTON JOHANNESBURG
MELBOURNE NEW DELHI SINGAPORE SYDNEY

First published 1996

British Library Cataloguing in Publication Data
Humerus – (Musculoskeletal trauma series)
   1 Humerus – Fractures   2 Humerus – Surgery
   I Flatow, Evan L.   II Ulrich, C.
   617.1'57

ISBN 0 7506 0840 4

Library of Congress Cataloguing in Publication Data
Humerus/edited by Evan L. Flatow, C. Ulrich.
   p. cm. – (Musculoskeletal trauma series)
   Includes bibliographical references and index.
   ISBN 0 7506 0840 4
   1 Humerus – Fractures.   I Flatow, Evan L.   II Ulrich, C.   III Series.
   [DNLM: 1 Shoulder Fractures – surgery.   2 Humeral Fractures – surgery. WE 810 H922]
   RD557.H85.
   617.1'57–dc20

96–17376
CIP

Printed and bound in Great Britain by The Bath Press plc, Bath

Contents

Contributors

Louis U. Bigliani MD
Professor of Orthopedic Surgery and Chief
The Shoulder Service
New York Orthopedic Hospital
Columbia Presbyterian Medical Center
161 Fort Washington Avenue
New York NY 10032, USA

C.M. Court-Brown MD FRCS Ed (Orth)
Consultant Orthopaedic Surgeon
The Royal Infirmary of Edinburgh
Lauriston Place
Edinburgh EH3 9YW, UK

Frances Cuomo MD
Associate Chief, Shoulder Service
Hospital for Joint Diseases
301 East 17th Street
New York NY 10003, USA

Evan L. Flatow MD
Herbert Irving Associate Professor of Orthopedic
    Surgery and
Associate Chief, The Shoulder Service
New York Orthopedic Hospital
Columbia Presbyterian Medical Center
161 Fort Washington Avenue
New York NY 10032, USA

Richard J. Friedman MD FRCS(C)
Professor of Orthopedic Surgery
Medical University of South Carolina
171 Ashley Avenue
Charleston SC 29425, USA

Christian Gerber MD
Professor and Chairman
Department of Orthopaedic Surgery
University of Zurich
Balgrist
Forchstrasse 340
Zurich, Switzerland

Andrew Green MD
Assistant Professor
Department of Orthopedic Surgery
Brown University
2 Dudley Street, Suite 200
Providence RI 02903, USA

Richard J. Hawkins MD
Clinical Professor
Department of Orthopedics
University of Colorado
and
Steadman Hawkins Clinic
181 W. Meadow Drive, Suite 400
Vail, CO 81657, USA

Kenneth J. Koval MD
Chief, Fracture Service
Hospital for Joint Diseases
301 East 17th Street
New York NY 10003, USA

Christoph Lampert MD
Leiter der Abt
Kinderorthopädie
Kantonspital
CH-9000 St Gallen, Switzerland

Lutz von Laer MD
Professor
Leiter der traumat Abt
Baseler Kinderspital
CH-4005 Basel, Switzerland

Margaret McQueen MD FRCS Ed (Orth)
Consultant Orthopaedic Surgeon
The Royal Infirmary of Edinburgh
Lauriston Place
Edinburgh EH3 9YW, UK

Tom R. Norris MD
California-Pacific Medical Center
Suite 510
2351 Clay Street
San Francisco CA 94115, USA

Roger G. Pollock MD
Assistant Professor of Orthopedic Surgery
The Shoulder Service
New York Orthopedic Hospital
Columbia Presbyterian Medical Center
161 Fort Washington Avenue
New York NY 10032, USA

Stephen Ridgeway MD
Resident
Medical University of South Carolina
171 Ashley Avenue
Charleston SC 29425, USA

Mark W. Rodosky MD
The Shoulder Service
Minneapolis Sports Medicine Center
701 25th Avenue S.
#400 Minneapolis
MN 55454–1443, USA

P.M. Rommens MD PhD
Professor and Chairman
University Hospitals of the Johannes
    Gutenberg University
Langenbeckstraße 1
D-55131 Mainz, Germany

Theodore F. Schlegel MD
Associate, Steadman Hawkins Clinic
181 W. Meadow Drive, Suite 400
Vail, CO 81657, USA

Edward B. Self MD
The Shoulder Service
New York Orthopedic Hospital
Columbia Presbyterian Medical Center and the
    Valley Hospital
Ridgewood
New Jersey, USA

Michael L. Sidor MD
Assistant Professor
Department of Orthopedic Surgery
University of Pennsylvania and
Associate Director
PENN Sports Medicine Center
Weightman Hall
235 South 33rd St
Philadelphia PA 19104, USA

C. Ulrich MD
Professor of Traumatology
Chief Surgeon
Trauma Department
Klinik am Eichert
Postfach 660
D-73006 Göppingen, Germany

Jon J.P. Warner MD
Director, Shoulder Service
Department of Orthopedic Surgery
University of Pittsburgh
and The Center for Sports Medicine
Baum Blvd at Craig Street
Pittsburgh PA 15213, USA

Joseph D. Zuckerman MD
Chief, Shoulder Service
Hospital for Joint Diseases
301 East 17th Street
New York NY 10003, USA

Series Foreword

Surgeons who deal with musculoskeletal injuries tend, on the whole, to use the methods of treatment practised at the units where they trained and served their apprenticeships. The more adventurous and intellectual of them also study other methods, but they are inevitably influenced by their earlier experiences. Those who trained where operative fixation was the norm are inclined to look down on those whose first choice of treatment is conservative, and the latter may in turn feel (if only unconsciously) that the 'always operate' merchants do so because 'fixation is fun'. Indeed, who can deny the joy of using skilled hands effectively.

What trauma surgeons need is a balanced view and here, in this series, we have precisely that. I was tempted to apply the initials NATO meaning, in the present context, the North Atlantic Trauma Organization. Certainly the contents are a happy blend of North American and European views on fractures. Charles Court-Brown and Dietmar Pennig, the series editors, have earned great renown on both sides of the Atlantic for their work on the understanding and management of musculoskeletal trauma. They have collected a most distinguished set of authors and have been careful to ensure that the text does not read as if it was written by a committee; though it is clear that they have provided guidelines and minimized overlap,

they have wisely allowed each contributor to retain something of their national lingusitic flavour.

The series consists of four volumes, Court-Brown and Pennig have themselves edited the volume on the tibia and fibula; the other three volumes are on the humerus (edited by Evan L. Flatow and C. Ulrich), the radius and ulna (edited by M. McQueen and J. Jupiter), and the femur (edited by Charles Court-Brown and J. Chapman). Each volume provides a comprehensive description of all the injuries discussed. Epidemiology, classification and fractures of the shafts as well as the upper and lower ends of each bone are described in detail; management includes authorative accounts and clear illustrations of both operative and conservative treatment. Summaries of the literature are a notable feature of text, and the lists of references will satisfy even the greediest reader.

This is the work which every trauma surgeon has been waiting for, using it to revise their knowledge of a particular field or to give practical guidance in approaching the individual patient. I wish it had been available when I was in active practice. I would have treated my patients better and slept more soundly at night.

Alan Apley

Series Preface

Our aims in editing a series of four books dealing with limb fractures were twofold. There has been an explosion of interest in the management of fractures in the last decade with the result that the large textbooks dealing with the management of fractures have tended to become reference books and we believe that there is a need for a series of short concise texts describing the management of fractures in different bones. We have, therefore, been pleased to help with the production of four books detailing the epidemiology, classification, treatment and complications of fractures of the femur, tibia, humerus and forearm.

Our second goal was to try to combine the talents of North American and European editors and authors. Textbooks have tended to be based in one continent, often to their detriment. This collaboration has not always been easy or even possible but we are happy with the results of the enterprise and we are grateful to the volume editors and the individual authors for their contributions. We hope that the series will be of interest to all surgeons interested in musculoskeletal trauma.

C.M. Court-Brown and D. Pennig

Preface

As the ancient arts of bone setting and plaster immobilization gave way to modern internal fixation, many principles of operative treatment of fractures became widely accepted. The management of humeral fractures, however, remained a controversial and poorly understood area. The often soft, osteoporotic bone of the proximal humerus, combined with the need for preservation of the soft tissues and head vascularity, contributed to disappointing results with early efforts at plate and screw fixation. Furthermore, clearance of bulky implants under the coraco-acromial arch presented a unique anatomical challenge. Humeral shaft fractures have inspired debates over the relative merits of functional bracing and intramedullary fixation, a disagreement made more acute by recent advances in interlocking intramedullary technology. Finally, the complex geometry of the distal humerus, together with the need for anatomical fixation of intra-articular fractures, has been a constant challenge both as to optimum surgical exposure (and choice of approach) and to selection of fixation devices.

An explosion in interest in humeral fractures has brought new technology, fresh ideas and innovative operative approaches to bear on these difficult injuries. It is our great pleasure to have assembled in this volume representative contributions from the leaders in the field. They have shared their expertise with us, and given us experience of the cutting edge while still emphasizing practical, proven strategies for achieving good clinical results after these severe fractures.

E.L. Flatow and C. Ulrich

1

The evaluation and classification of proximal humeral fractures

Michael L. Sidor, Kenneth J. Koval and Joseph D. Zuckerman

Fractures of the proximal humerus are relatively common, especially in the elderly. They represent approximately 4–5% of all fractures[1–3], and occur twice as frequently in females[4,5]. Since proximal humeral fractures are considered osteoporosis-related fractures, their incidence increases with age, particularly after age 50[1,4–6].

Clinical evaluation

In eliciting a history from a patient who has sustained a proximal humeral fracture, determination of the mechanism of injury can be helpful. The mechanism may be direct, such as a blow to the lateral aspect of the shoulder. However, the indirect mechanism is much more common and generally involves a fall onto the outstretched arm which in younger patients may result in a dislocation but in the elderly most commonly results in a fracture. The indirect mechanism is usually associated with a greater degree of fracture displacement than the direct mechanism[7]. Other indirect causes of proximal humeral fractures are seizures or electroconvulsive therapy without the use of muscle relaxants; both are often associated with posterior dislocations.

The symptoms and signs associated with proximal humeral fractures can be quite variable; however they most often correlate with the degree of fracture displacement and comminution. Pain, especially with any attempts at shoulder motion, is almost always present. Inspection of the shoulder may reveal swelling and ecchymosis. The patient should be instructed that over the first 4–5 days following injury the ecchymosis may extend

distally into the arm and forearm, or even to the chest wall and breast area (Figure 1.1).

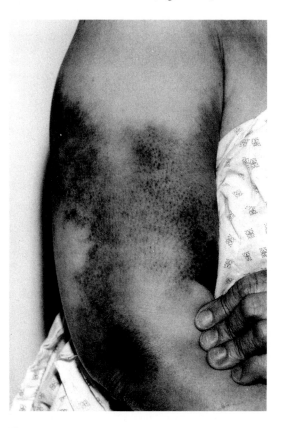

Figure 1.1 Following proximal humeral fractures, ecchymosis almost always develops and can extend distally beyond the elbow and frequently into the distal forearm. This elderly patient sustained a low-energy one-part fracture 5 days before. Ecchymosis is evident about the entire arm and beyond the elbow

Palpation of the shoulder will usually reveal tenderness about the proximal humerus. Crepitus may be evident with motion of the fracture fragments. The entire upper extremity should be examined. A fall on the outstretched arm can also result in a fracture of another area such as a distal radius fracture. The chest should also be examined, since rib fractures may also occur in association with the fall[8–11].

Assessment of fracture stability is an essential part of the examination. The humeral shaft should be gently rotated both internally and externally as the proximal portion of the humerus is palpated (Figure 1.2). If the proximal and distal portions move as a unit, the fracture is stable; however, motion or crepitus is consistent with an unstable or less stable fracture pattern. Essential to the clinical evaluation of the patient with a proximal humerus fracture is a complete neurovascular examination of the involved upper extremity. Associated axil-

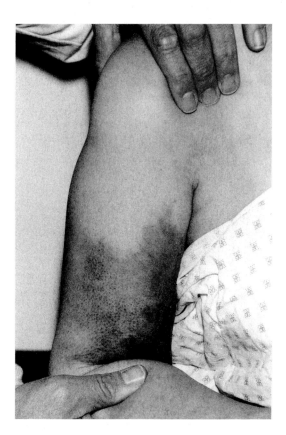

Figure 1.2 Stability of proximal humeral fractures can be determined by grasping the distal humerus with one hand and the proximal humerus with the other. Gentle rotation of the distal humerus will determine if the entire humerus moves as a unit. This is the definition of fracture stability

lary artery and brachial plexus injuries have been reported[12–16], especially with fracture fragments displaced medial to the coracoid process. A fracture-dislocation also increases the incidence of neurovascular injury[17]. The most commonly injured peripheral nerve is the axillary nerve[18], which should be differentiated from the more commonly encountered deltoid atony. Both conditions may demonstrate inferior humeral subluxation on anteroposterior radiographs.

Radiographic evaluation

One of the most important aspects in the evaluation of proximal humeral fracture is the determination of the position of the fracture fragments and the degree of displacement. Thus, an adequate radiographic evaluation is mandatory.

Trauma series

The cornerstone of the radiographic evaluation of proximal humeral fractures is the trauma series. The trauma series consists of anteroposterior (AP) and lateral views of the shoulder obtained in the plane of the scapula and an axillary view (Figure 1.3). Fracture classification and treatment decisions are generally based upon these three radiographic views. Each view contributes information obtained from three different perpendicular planes[2,18–21].

The scapular AP (Figure 1.3a) view offers a general overview of the fracture, and is usually evaluated first. This view should be made perpendicular to the scapular plane, which requires angling the X-ray beam approximately 40° from medial to lateral. This compensates for the position of the scapula on the chest wall. It will demonstrate the glenoid in profile, as well as the true glenohumeral joint space.

At least one view obtained 90° to the scapular AP is required for assessment of the proximal humeral fractures or fracture-dislocations[22]. Specifically, this orthogonal view provides information about angulation and displacement[18], as well as associated humeral head dislocations[23–26]. Both the scapular lateral and axillary views are oriented orthogonally to the scapular AP and fulfil the criteria for a second projection. However, the trauma series generally includes all three views.

The scapular lateral (Figure 1.3b), also known as the scapular 'Y', can provide important information not evident on the scapular AP

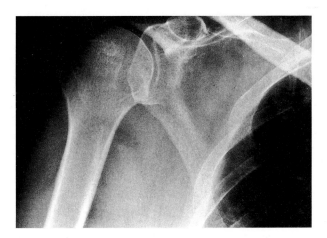

Figure 1.3 The trauma series consists of a scapular AP (a), a scapular lateral (b), and an axillary view (c)

(a)

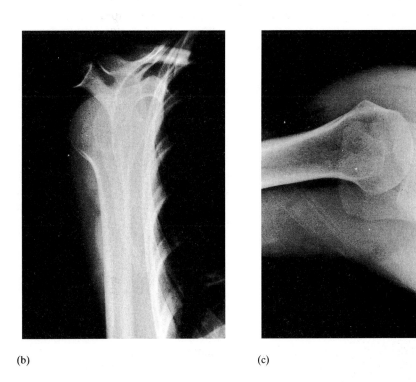

(b)

(c)

view[7,26–28]. This view is a true lateral of the scapula, with the X-ray beam passing parallel to the spine of the scapula. It can be obtained with the involved upper extremity immobilized in a sling and does not require any movement of the extremity and as such does not add to patient discomfort. The scapular lateral assists in delineating the position of the humeral head relative to the glenoid and is particularly useful in showing dislocations or posteriorly displaced fragments.

The axillary view (Figure 1.3c) also permits assessment of the glenohumeral relationship. This is generally obtained with the patient supine. The arm must be positioned in at least 30° abduction. In the acute setting this positioning is often performed by the physician. The X-ray plate is placed above the shoulder and the beam is directed to the plate from a caudad position. The axillary view can also be useful in identifying fractures of the glenoid rim and humeral head articular fractures[22,29–31].

The relative efficacy of these different views has not been studied extensively. Silfverskiold *et al.*[32] reported in their prospective study that the scapular lateral view was more sensitive than the axillary view in detecting shoulder dislocations. They did not study fractures specifically. In 92% of their 75 cases, however, the scapular lateral and axillary views resulted in the same diagnosis.

We recently published a study in which the trauma series radiographs of 50 proximal humeral fractures were used to assess the relative contribution of the scapular lateral and axillary radiographs to fracture classification using the Neer system[33]. The radiographs were reviewed by four different orthopaedic surgeons with varying levels of experience and expertise and one skeletal radiologist. In the first viewing, radiographs were reviewed and classified in the following sequence: (a) after scapula AP alone; (b) after review of scapular AP and lateral views; and (c) after review of scapular AP, lateral and axillary views. A second viewing of the same 50 cases was performed 6 months later in a changed sequence: (a) after scapular AP alone; (b) after review of scapular AP and axillary views; (c) after review of scapular AP, lateral and axillary views.

For the cumulative experience of these five observers, review of the scapular AP and axillary views achieved the final classification in 99% of cases. However, after review of the scapular AP and lateral views, the final classification was achieved in only 79% of cases ($p < 0.05$). These results indicate that when combined with the scapular AP radiograph, the axillary view contributes significantly more information leading to fracture classification than the scapular lateral radiograph.

Additional radiographic views

If any of the three views of the trauma series is inadequate, it should be repeated. Usually, the fracture can be evaluated and treated based upon this set of radiographs. Additional radiographic views may be helpful and have been advocated by others.

The apical oblique view[34] is taken by directing the X-ray beam through the glenohumeral joint at an angle of 45° to the plane of the chest wall and angled 45° caudally. When compared to the scapular lateral view, it has been shown to provide additional useful information in the evaluation of proximal humeral fractures and fracture-dislocations[35,36]. It is particularly useful in demonstrating dislocations and posterolateral humeral head compression fractures. However, it has not become as widely accepted as the scapular lateral view.

Modified axillary views such as the Velpeau axillary lateral[23], the Stripp axillary lateral[37] and the trauma axillary lateral[38] have been described. These views allow one to obtain an axillary lateral view without removing the injured arm from the sling, similar to obtaining the scapular AP and lateral views. The Velpeau axillary lateral view is probably the most commonly used, taken with the patient leaning backwards approximately 30° over the X-ray table. The X-ray cassette is placed beneath the shoulder on the table, and the X-ray beam passes vertically from superior to inferior through the shoulder joint. Although this view has the benefit of avoiding the need to position the injured extremity, we prefer the standard axillary view because it offers less distortion and bony overlap of the shoulder joint.

Other diagnostic modalities

Computed tomography (CT) scans of proximal humeral fractures and fracture-dislocations may be indicated when the trauma series radiographs are indeterminate. CT scans have been recommended to evaluate the degree of tuberosity displacement as well as articular impression fractures (Figure 1.4), head-splitting fractures and chronic fracture-dislocations[18,39–41]. Castagno *et al.*[39] reported a small series of 17 patients in whom CT scans of acute proximal humeral fractures demonstrated important information not evident on plain radiographs.

We recently completed a preliminary study on the effect of the CT scan on the inter-observer reliability of the Neer classification when combined with the standard trauma series. We compiled 10 trauma series, each with a CT scan. Each case was reviewed by five observers of varying experience and expertise who first classified the fracture after review of the trauma series and again following review of the CT scan. In this small series, the additional information provided by the CT scan did not improve the inter-observer reliability. We recognize that this data is preliminary and more data is needed to accurately determine what benefit, if any, can be obtained from CT scans of proximal humeral fractures. In our experience, CT

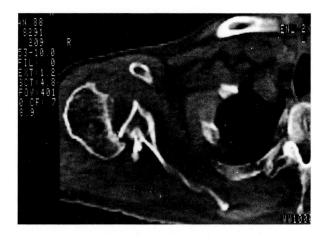

Figure 1.4 CT scans provide useful information about impression fractures associated with chronic dislocations

scans are most helpful in the evaluation of chronic fracture-dislocations specifically to identify the size and location of humeral head impression defects and the degree of secondary glenoid changes.

Other modalities to consider as a method of increasing the amount of information available are CT scanning with three-dimensional reconstructions or magnetic resonance imaging[42]. Magnetic resonance imaging could also demonstrate associated soft tissue lesions of the rotator cuff, biceps tendon and glenoid labrum which may be helpful in the management of these patients. However, cost-benefit issues have to be considered carefully when deciding to utilize a study of this type.

Proximal humeral fracture classification

Fracture classification systems play a key role in the practice of orthopaedic surgery. They provide a way of describing fractures and fracture-dislocations, which has a direct impact on the treatment approaches utilized. Classification systems are essential to the orthopaedic literature as a means of describing the results of a specific treatment method for injuries of comparable type.

A classification system for proximal humeral fractures should provide a comprehensive means of describing fracture fragment displacement and position, and the presence of dislocation. It should also assist in determining treatment and in predicting long-term clinical outcomes, as well as providing an acceptable level of inter- and intra-observer reliability. And finally, the classification should be based on a standard radiographic evalu-ation that is easily and reproducibly obtained in the clinical setting[43].

The evolution of proximal humeral fracture classification

Proximal humeral fracture classification has evolved over the past century as our understanding of proximal humerus fractures has also evolved. Major milestones in this evolution include Kocher's classification[44] which was based upon the different anatomical levels of fracture: anatomical neck, epiphyseal region and surgical neck. The disadvantages of this simplistic system include the lack of attention to important issues such as the presence of fractures at multiple levels, the degree of fracture displacement, the presence of dislocation or the mechanism of injury.

Recognizing that classification systems based solely on anatomical level of fracture did not provide information about mechanism of injury nor aid in the choice of treatment, Watson-Jones[45] proposed a different classification system. He divided proximal humeral fractures into three types: contusion crack fractures, impacted adduction fractures and impacted abduction fractures. He believed that each type was caused by a specific mechanism of injury and required a specific treatment approach. A major disadvantage of this system is that changes in humeral rotation alter the radiographic appearance of the fracture – specifically, the same fracture patterns could appear as an abduction- or adduction-type fracture depending on the rotational position of the humerus when the X-ray was obtained[2].

In 1934, Codman presented an analysis system based upon the epiphyseal regions of the proximal

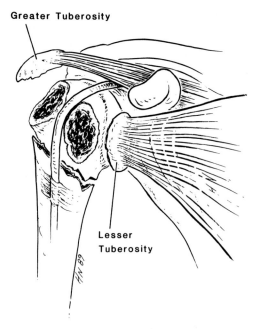

Greater Tuberosity

Lesser
Tuberosity

Figure 1.5   The understanding of proximal humeral fractures was significantly enhanced by the recognition by Codman that these fractures occurred along old epiphyseal lines resulting in the possibility of four fragments. This concept provided the background for the development of the Neer classification

Displaced Fractures

	2 PART	3 PART	4 PART	
Anatomical Neck				Minimal Displacement
Surgical Neck				
Greater Tuberosity				
Lesser Tuberosity				
Fracture-Dislocation	Anterior Posterior			Articular Surface

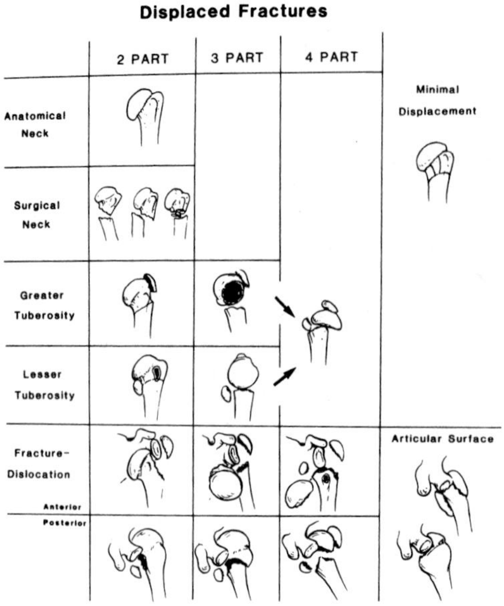

Figure 1.6   The Neer classification of proximal humeral fractures (see text)

humerus[46]. This description, which was an important precursor to the Neer classification, identifies four possible fracture fragments: greater tuberosity, lesser tuberosity, anatomical head and shaft (Figure 1.5). His appreciation that fractures occurred along the lines of the epiphyseal scars formed the basis for Neer's development of his classification system.

The Neer classification

Neer[2,47] proposed his classification of proximal humeral fractures in 1970, and since then it has become the most widely used system in clinical practice[18,21,48–50] (Figure 1.6). This system is based on the anatomical relationship of the four major anatomical segments: articular segment, greater tuberosity, lesser tuberosity and the proximal shaft beginning at the level of the surgical neck. Knowledge of the rotator cuff insertions and the effects of the muscular deforming forces on the four segments is essential to understanding this classification system. Fracture types are based upon the presence of displacement of one or more of the four segments. For a segment to be considered dis-

placed, it must be either greater than 1 cm displaced or angulated more than 45° from its anatomical position. The number of fracture lines is not important in this classification system. For example, one-part fractures, or minimally displaced fractures, are the most common type of proximal humeral fractures and account for up to 85% of all proximal humeral fractures[4,5,51]. Although these fractures may have multiple fracture lines, they are characterized by the fact that none of the four segments fulfils the criteria for displacement. Hence, they are considered one-part or minimally displaced.

Displaced fractures include two-part, three-part and four-part fractures. A two-part fracture is characterized by displacement of one of the four segments, with the remaining three segments either not fractured or not fulfilling the criteria for displacement. Four types of two-part fractures can be encountered (greater tuberosity, lesser tuberosity, anatomical neck and surgical neck). A three-part fracture is characterized by displacement of two of the segments from the remaining two non-displaced segments. Two types of three-part fracture patterns are encountered. The more common pattern is characterized by displacement of the greater tuberosity and the shaft from the lesser tuberosity which remains with the articular segment. The much less commonly encountered pattern is characterized by displacement of the lesser tuberosity and shaft from the greater tuberosity which remains with the articular segment. A four-part fracture is characterized by displacement of all four segments.

Neer also categorized fracture-dislocations which are displaced proximal humeral fractures – two-part, three-part or four-part – associated with either anterior or posterior dislocation of the articular segment. Therefore, six types of these fracture-dislocation patterns can occur. Neer also described articular surface fractures which were of two types: impression fractures or head-splitting fractures. Impression fractures of the articular surface most often occur in association with chronic dislocations. As such, they can be either anterior or posterior and involve variable amounts of the articular surface[18]. Head-splitting fractures are usually associated with other displaced fractures of the proximal humerus in which the disruption or 'splitting' of the articular surface is the most significant component.

Reliability of the Neer classification

The Neer classification is the most widely used classification system for proximal humeral fractures being used by the vast majority of orthopaedic surgeons and radiologists. This classification has a direct effect on the treatment decision-making process[2,21,48–50]. However, to our knowledge, there are only three reports in the orthopaedic literature that examine the reliability of the Neer classification[52,53,54].

Among four observers of varying expertise who evaluated a series of 100 proximal humeral fractures, Kristiansen *et al.*[52] found a low level of inter-observer reliability using a condensed Neer classification system. The level of expertise was noted to be an important factor in predicting inter-observer reliability. However, this study was limited by a number of factors. First, a complete trauma series was not used; rather, only AP and lateral radiographs were examined. Secondly, the condensed Neer classification used consisted of five categories (one-part fractures, two-part fractures, three-part fractures, four-part fractures, all other fractures and fracture-dislocations) which were somewhat disparate with respect to fracture type, treatment options and prognosis. And thirdly, intra-observer reliability (reproducibility) was not assessed.

We recently published a study to assess the inter- and intra-observer reliability of the Neer classification system using the radiographs of 50 proximal humeral fractures[53]. Trauma series radiographs were available for each fracture consisting of good-quality scapular AP, scapular lateral and axillary view. The radiographs were reviewed by an orthopaedic shoulder specialist, an orthopaedic traumatologist, skeletal radiologist, an orthopaedic resident in the fifth postgraduate year of training, and an orthopaedic resident in the second year of postgraduate training. The radiographs were reviewed on two different occasions, 6 months apart. Inter-observer reliability was assessed by comparing the fracture classification determined by the five observers. Intra-observer reliability was assessed by comparing the fracture classification determined by each observer for the first and second reviews. Kappa reliability coefficients (κ) were used to adjust the observed proportion of agreement between or among observers by correcting for the proportion of agreement that could have occurred by chance.

All five observers agreed on the final classification in 32% and 30% of cases for the first and second viewings, respectively. Paired comparisons between the five observers showed a mean corrected reliability coefficient[55,56] of 0.50 (range 0.37–0.62) for both testings which corresponds to a 'moderate' level of reliability. An 'excellent' level of reliability ($\kappa > 0.81$) was not obtained for any paired evaluation. Attending physicians demonstrated slightly higher inter-observer reliability than orthopaedic residents. Intra-observer reliability ranged from 0.83 (shoulder specialist) to 0.50 (skeletal radiologist) with a mean of 0.65 which corresponds to a 'substantial' level of agreement.

The relatively low level of inter-observer reliability found in these studies could be due to a variety of factors. The comminution and osteopenia often associated with proximal humeral fractures can make the precise delineation of fracture fragment difficult. In addition, the Neer displacement criteria can be difficult to measure accurately on radiographs. This is particularly true for the 45° angulation/rotation criteria. Relative inexperience and lack of expertise can also decrease inter-observer reliability. In the future, efforts could be directed towards improving the level of reliability of the Neer classification – either by increasing expertise or providing additional radiographic data – so that treatment choices and the interpretation of treatment results can be optimized.

The AO classification

The AO group has modified the Neer classification, placing more emphasis on the vascular

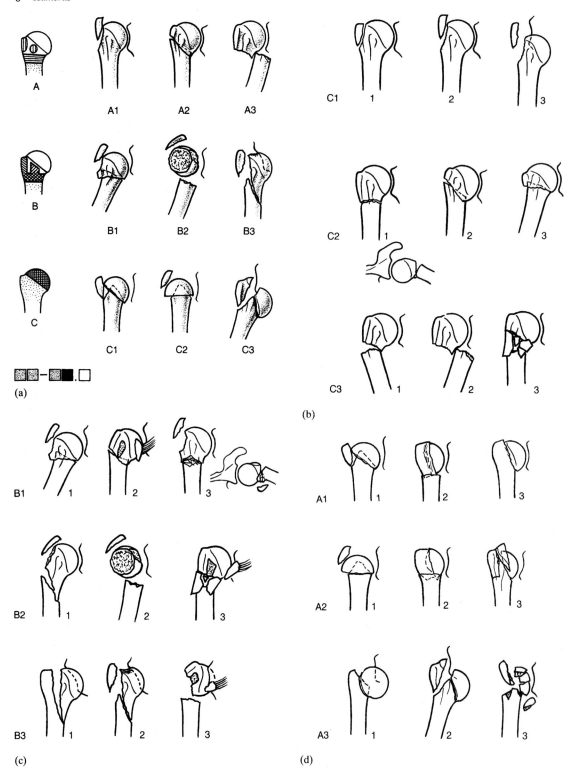

Figure 1.7(a–d)   The AO classification of proximal humeral fractures. Each major type (A, B, C) is divided into groups (A1, A2, A3, etc.); groups are further subdivided into a more detailed classification (A1.1, B2.2, C3.1, etc.)

supply to the articular segment of the proximal humerus[57,58] (Figure 1.7). The severity of the injury and risk of osteonecrosis forms the basis of the AO classification system. In this system, it is accepted that if either tuberosity and its attached rotator cuff remain in continuity with the articular segment, the vascular supply is probably adequate. Proximal humeral fractures are separated into three types: extra-articular unifocal, extra-articular bifocal and articular. Each of these types is further subdivided into different groups based on alignment, degree and direction of displacement, presence of impaction and associated dislocation.

Type A fractures are extra-articular and involve one of the tuberosities with or without a concomitant metaphyseal fracture. Group A1 are the extra-articular unifocal tuberosity fractures; group A2 are the extra-articular unifocal fractures with an impacted metaphyseal fracture; and group A3 are the extra-articular unifocal fractures with a non-impacted metaphyseal fracture. Osteonecrosis is unlikely in this type of fracture.

Type B fractures are also extra-articular but involve both tuberosities with a concomitant metaphyseal fracture or glenohumeral dislocation. Group B1 are the extra-articular bifocal fractures associated with an impacted metaphyseal fracture; group B2 fractures are the extra-articular bifocal fractures with a non-impacted metaphyseal fracture; and group B3 fractures are the extra-articular bifocal fractures with a glenohumeral dislocation. There is a low risk of osteonecrosis in this type.

Type C fractures are articular and involve vascular isolation of the articular segment. Group C1 are fractures with slight displacement; group C2 are impacted fractures with marked displacement; and group C3 fractures are associated with a glenohumeral dislocation. There is a high risk of osteonecrosis in this type.

This more complex classification system theoretically should allow for more detailed guidelines for treatment and prognosis. However, its complexity may actually preclude attaining the widespread utilization that the Neer classification currently commands. Thus far, clinical studies utilizing the AO classification have been quite limited. Recent assessment of its inter-observer reliability has not shown it to be significantly better than the Neer system[54]. No long-term results of treatments using the AO system of classification have been presented to date.

Conclusion

In the evaluation of proximal humeral fractures, a thorough history and complete physical examination of the involved extremity are required. One of the most important aspects of the examination is the determination of fracture stability. The three views of the trauma series – scapular AP, scapular lateral and axillary – are essential to understand the fracture pattern. Additional radiographic views such as the apical oblique or Velpeau axillary and other diagnostic modalities such as computed tomography may also be useful in certain situations.

The Neer classification of proximal humeral fractures is the most widely used system. It is based upon the presence of displacement of one or more of the four major anatomical segments: articular segment, greater tuberosity, lesser tuberosity and the proximal shaft beginning at the level of the surgical neck. The AO group has advocated a classification scheme which emphasizes the vascular supply to the articular segment of the proximal humerus. The severity of the injury and risk of osteonecrosis forms the basis of this system. By increasing our expertise and possibly by providing additional radiographic data, we may be able to increase the reliability of these classification systems.

References

1 Lind, T., Kroner, T.K. and Jensen, J. The epidemiology of fractures of the proximal humerus. *Arch. Orthop. Trauma Surg.* **108**, 285–287 (1989)

2. Neer, C.S. II. Displaced proximal humeral fractures Part I: Classification and evaluation. *J. Bone Joint Surg.,* **52A**, 1077–1089 (1970)

3. Stimson, B.B. *A Manual of Fractures and Dislocations,* 2nd edn, Lea and Febiger, Philadelphia (1947), pp. 241–260

4. Rose, S.H., Melton, L.J., Morrey, B.F., Ilstrup, D.M. and Riggs, L.B. Epidemiologic features of humeral fractures. *Clin. Orthop.,* **168**, 24–30 (1982)

5. Horak, J. and Nilsson, B. Epidemiology of fractures of the upper end of the humerus. *Clin. Orthop.,* **112**, 250–253 (1975)

6. Bengnér, U., Johnell, O. and Redlund-Johnell, I. Changes in the incidence of fracture of the upper end of the humerus during a three-year period. A study of 2125 fractures. *Clin. Orthop.,* **231**, 179–182 (1988)

7. McLaughlin H.L. Posterior dislocation of the shoulder. *J. Bone Joint Surg.,* **34A**, 584–590 (1952)

8. Glessner, J.R. Intrathoracic dislocation of the humeral head. *J. Bone Joint Surg.,* **43A**, 428–430 (1961)

9. Hardcastle, P.H. and Fisher, T.H. Intrathoracic displacement of the humeral head with fracture of the surgical neck. *Injury*, **12**, 313–315 (1981)

10. Patel, M.R. Pardee, M.L. and Singerman, R.C. Intrathoracic dislocation of the head of the humerus. *J. Bone Joint Surg.*, **45A**, 1712–1714 (1963)

11. West, E.F. Intrathoracic dislocation of the humerus. *J. Bone Joint Surg.*, **31B**, 61–62 (1949)

12. Hayes, M.J. and Van Winkle, N. Axillary artery injury with minimally displaced fracture of the neck of the humerus. *J. Trauma*, **23**, 431–433 (1983)

13. Smyth, E.H.J. Major arterial injury in a closed fracture of the neck of the humerus: report of a case. *J. Bone Joint Surg.*, **51B**, 508–510 (1969)

14. Lindholm, T.S. and Elmstedt, E. Bilateral posterior dislocation of the shoulder combined with fracture of the proximal humerus. *Acta Orthop. Scand.*, **51**, 485–488 (1980)

15. Stableforth, P.G. Four-part fractures of the neck of the humerus. *J. Bone Joint Surg.*, **66B**, 104–108 (1984)

16. Zuckerman, J.D., Flugstad, D.L., Teitz, C.C. and King, H.A. Axillary artery injury as a complication of proximal humeral fractures. *Clin. Orthop.*, **189**, 234–237 (1984)

17. Pasila, M., Jeroma, H., Kivilnoto, O. and Sundholm, A. Early complications of primary shoulder dislocations. *Acta Orthop. Scand.*, **49**, 260–263 (1978)

18. Bigliani, L.U. Fractures of the shoulder. Part I: Fractures of the proximal humerus. In *Fracture in Adults*, 3rd edn, (eds C.A. Rockwood, D.P. Green and R.W. Bucholz), J.B. Lippincott, Philadelphia (1991), pp. 871–882

19. Cofield, R.H. Comminuted fractures of the proximal humerus. *Clin. Orthop.*, **230** 49–57

20. Hawkins, R.J. and Angelo, R.L. Displaced proximal humeral fractures: selecting treatment, avoiding pitfalls. *Orthop Clin. N. Am.*, **18**, 421–431 (1987)

21. Seeman, W.R., Siebler, G. and Rupp, H.G. A new classification of proximal humeral fractures. *Eur. J. Radiol.*, **6**, 163–167 (1986)

22. Rockwood, C.A., Szaleay, E.A., Curtis, R.J., Young, D.C. and Kay, S.P. X-ray evaluation of shoulder problems. In *The Shoulder*, Vol. 1 (eds CA Rockwood and FA Matsen), W.B. Saunders, Philadelphia (1990), pp. 178–184

23. Bloom, M.H. and Obata, W.G. Diagnosis of posterior dislocation of the shoulder with use of Velpeau axillary and angle-up roentgenographic views. *J. Bone Joint Surg.*, **49A**, 943–949 (1967)

24. Brems-Dalgaard, E., Davidsen, E. and Sloth, C. Radiographic examination of the acute shoulder. *Eur. J. Radiol.*, **11**, 10–14 (1990)

25. McLaughlin, H.L. Posterior dislocation of the shoulder. *J. Bone Joint Surg.*, **34A**, 584–590 (1952)

26. Zuckerman, J.D. and Buchalter, J.S. Shoulder injuries. In *Comprehensive Care of Orthopaedic Injuries in the Elderly* (ed. J.D. Zuckerman), Baltimore, Urban and Schwarzenberg, Baltimore (1990), p. 307

27. DeSmet, A.A. Anterior oblique projection in radiography of the traumatized shoulder. *Am. J. Radiol.*, **134**, 515–518 (1980)

28. Rubin, S.A., Gray, R.L. and Green, W.R. The scapular 'Y': a diagnostic aid in shoulder trauma. *Radiology*, **110**, 725–726 (1974)

29. Neviaser, R.J. Radiologic assessment of the shoulder: plain and arthrographic. *Orthop. Clin. N. Am.*, **18**, 343–349 (1987)

30. Hawkins, R.J. and Angelo, R.L. Displaced proximal humeral fractures: selecting treatment, avoiding pitfalls. *Orthop. Clin. N. Am.*, **18**, 421–431 (1987)

31. Whiston, T.B. Fractures of the surgical neck of the humerus: a study in reduction. *J. Bone Joint Surg.*, **36B**, 423–427 (1954)

32. Silverskiold, J.P., Straehley, D.J. and Jones, W.W. Roentgenographic evaluation of suspected shoulder dislocations: a prospective study comparing the axillary view and the scapular 'Y' view. *Orthopedics*, **13**, 63–69 (1990)

33. Sidor, M.L., Zuckerman, J.D., Lyon, T., Koval, K. and Schoenberg, N. Classification of proximal humerus fractures: the contribution of the scapular lateral and axillary radiographs. *J. Shoulder Elbow Surg*, **3**, 24–27 (1994)

34. Garth, W.P. Jr, Slappey, C.E. and Ochs, C.W. Roentgenographic demonstration of instability of the shoulder: the apical oblique projection – a technical note. *J. Bone Joint Surg.*, **66A**, 1450–1453 (1984)

35. Korngluth, P.J. and Salazar, A.M. The apical oblique view of the shoulder: its usefulness in acute trauma. *Am. J. Radiol.*, **149**, 113–116 (1987)

36. Richardson, J.B., Ramay, A., Davidson, J.K. and Kelly, I.G. Radiographs in shoulder trauma. *J. Bone Joint Surg.* **70B**, 457–460 (1988)

37. Horsfield, D. and Jones, S.N. A useful projection in radiography of the shoulder. *J. Bone Joint Surg.*, **69B**, 338 (1987)

38. Tietge, R.A. and Cuiollo, J.V. C.A.M. axillary x-ray. Exhibit to the Academy meeting of the American Academy of Orthopaedic Surgeons. *Orthop. Trans.*, **6**, 451 (1982)

39. Castagno, A.A., Shuman, W.P., Kilcoyne, R.F., Haynor, D.R., Morris, M.E. and Matsen, F.A. Complex fractures of the proximal humerus: role of CT in treatment. *Radiology*, **165**, 759–762 (1987)

40. Kilcoyne, R.F., Shuman, W.P., Matsen, F.A. III, Morris, M. and Rockwood, C.A. The Neer classification of displaced proximal humeral fractures: spectrum of findings on plain radiographs and CT scans. *Am. J. Radiol.*, **154**, 1029–1033 (1990)

41. Morris, M.E., Kilcoyne, R.F., Shuman, W. and Matsen, F.A. III. Humeral tuberosity fractures: evaluation by CT scan and management of malunion. *Orthop. Trans.*, **11**, 242 (1987)

42. Kuhlman, J.E., Fishman, E.K., Ney, D.R. and Magid, D. Complex shoulder trauma: three-dimensional CT imaging. *Orthopedics*, **11**, 1561–1563 (1988)

43. Burstein, A.H. Fracture classification systems: do they work and are they useful? *J. Bone Joint Surg.*, **75A**, 1743–1744 (1993)

44. Kocher, T. *Bietrage zur Kenntnis einigir praktischi wichtiger Fracturen formen*, Carl Sallman Verlag, Basel (1896)

45. Watson-Jones, R. *Fractures and Joint Injuries*, 3rd edn. Williams and Wilkins, Baltimore (1943), pp. 438–445

46. Codman E.A. *The Shoulder*, Thomas Todd Co., Boston (1934)

47. Neer, C.S. II. Displaced proximal humeral fractures Part II: Treatment of three-part and four-part displacement. *J. Bone Joint Surg.*, **52A**(6), 1090–1103 (1970)

48. Habermeyer, P. and Schweiberer, L. Frakturen des proximalen humerus. *Orthopäde*, **18**, 200–227 (1989)

49. Kristiansen, B. and Christensen, S.W. Proximal humeral fractures. Late results in relation to classification and treatment. *Acta Orthop. Scand.*, **58**, 124–127 (1987)

50. Mills, H.J. and Horn, G. Fractures of the proximal humerus in adults. *J. Trauma*, **25**, 801–805 (1985)

51. Neer, C.S. and Rockwood, C.A. Jr. Fractures and dislocations of the shoulder. In *Fractures in Adults*, 2nd edn (eds C.A. Rockwood and D.P. Green), J.B. Lippincott, Philadelphia (1984), p. 675

52. Kristiansen, B., Andersen, V.L.S., Olsen, C.A. and Varmarken, J.E. The Neer classification of fractures of the proximal humerus. An assessment of interobserver variation. *Skeletal Radiol.*, **17**, 420–422 (1988)

53. Sidor, M.L., Zuckerman, J.D., Lyon, T., Koval, K., Cuomo, F. and Schoenberg, N. The Neer classification system for proximal humeral fractures: an assessment of interobserver reliability and intraobserver reliability. *J. Bone Joint Surg.*, **75A**, 1745–1750 (1993).

54. Siebenrock, K.A. and Gerber, C. The reproducibility of classification of fractures of the proximal end of the humerus. *J. Bone Joint Surg.*, **75A**, 1751–1755 (1993)

55. Fleiss, J.L. *Statistical Methods for Rates and Proportions*, 2nd edn, John Wiley and Sons, New York (1981), p. 217.

56. Landis, J.R. and Koch, G.G. The measurement of observer agreement for categorical data. *Biometrics*, **33**, 159–174 (1977)

57. Jakob, R.P., Kristiansen, T., Mayo, K., Ganz, R. and Muller, M.E. Classification and aspects of treatment of fractures of the proximal humerus. In *Surgery of the Shoulder* (eds J.E. Bateman and R.P. Welsh), B.C. Decker, Philadelphia (1984), pp. 330–343

58. Muller, M.E., Nazarian, S., Koch, P. *AO Fracture Classification*, Springer Verlag, New York (1987), pp. 54–63.

2

Minimally displaced fractures of the proximal humerus

Roger G. Pollock

Fractures of the proximal humerus are common, accounting for approximately 5% of all fractures[1]. They occur at almost 70% of the reported rate for hip fractures and thus are a frequent cause of morbidity, especially in the elderly population[2]. Moreover, recent studies have found an apparent increase in the incidence of these fractures over the past several decades[1,3]. Minimally or undisplaced fractures comprise 80–85% of proximal humeral fractures[2,4,5] and will form the subject of this chapter.

It is first necessary to define what is meant by a minimally displaced fracture of the proximal humerus. In the Neer classification system, the group with minimal displacement consists of fractures in which no segment (the anatomical head, the greater tuberosity, the lesser tuberosity and the shaft) is displaced more than 1.0 cm or is angulated more than 45°, regardless of the number or orientation of the fracture lines[5]. In the AO system for fracture classification, minimally displaced proximal humeral fractures are subgrouped with the type A fractures, which are the least severe[6]. Undisplaced fractures are classified as A1.1 (surgical neck), A1.2 (tuberosity) or A1.3 (surgical neck and tuberosity). For the purposes of this chapter we shall include, in our discussion of minimally displaced fractures, those in which no segment is displaced more than 1 cm or angulated more than 45° (Neer's definition).

Diagnosis

Most minimally displaced fractures of the proximal humerus occur as a result of a fall onto the outstretched extremity or directly onto the upper arm. In the elderly or osteoporotic patient, they usually result from relatively low energy trauma, such as a fall on level ground. In younger patients, they may be associated with motor vehicle accidents or falls from a height or during athletic pursuits, such as skiing. The patient will typically present with pain localized to the upper arm (shoulder and deltoid regions) and an inability or unwillingness to raise the arm.

On physical examination, the signs of fracture are few and non-specific, especially in the case of minimally displaced fractures. The proximal humerus is well invested with soft tissues, and deformity is not usually appreciable. There is usually some degree of soft tissue swelling, which may extend down the entire extremity. Ecchymosis appears within a few days of injury and is seen on the medial aspect of the arm (often as far distally as the elbow) and on the chest wall. There is tenderness over the proximal humerus in the region of the fracture.

In cases of suspected fracture, the shoulder is immobilized in a sling until radiographs are obtained. The shoulder is not taken through a range of motion either actively or passively, in order to prevent possible displacement of the fragments. However, a careful neurological examination is performed upon presentation to rule out any associated neurological injury. In particular, sensation over the lateral deltoid is assessed and the patient is asked to set each of the three parts of the deltoid. This will yield information about the status of the axillary nerve, the most frequently injured neuromuscular structure in fractures and dislocations of the proximal humerus. Pain inhibi-

(a)

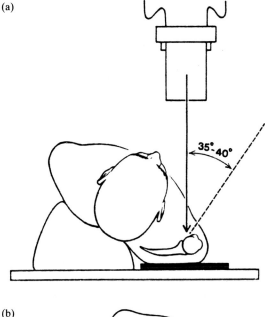

(b)

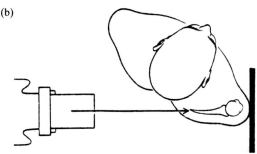

Figure 2.1 Two views of the shoulder and proximal humerus are initially obtained with the arm immobilized in a sling: an anteroposterior view (a) and a lateral view (b) in the plane of the scapula. Accurate views are essential for proper classification of fractures of the proximal humerus

tion may make it difficult to assess deltoid function acutely, especially that of the anterior and middle parts. Biceps function is also tested, as is the status of the more distal neuromuscular units. The distal pulses are also assessed and compared to those of the contralateral extremity. In cases of non-displaced fractures of the proximal humerus, neurovascular complications are exceedingly rare. However, the extent of the bony injury is not apparent on physical examination because of the soft tissue investment. Thus, protective splinting and a careful neurological and vascular examination should be carried out during triage of all suspected proximal humerus fractures.

The diagnosis of a minimally displaced fracture

of the proximal humerus is made on the basis of the radiographic configuration, using Neer's criteria (i.e. displacement of no segment greater than 1 cm and no angulation greater than 45°). Neer and others have pointed out that the use of his classification system requires that accurate radiographs of the glenohumeral joint and proximal humerus be obtained[7–9]. Two views of the shoulder and proximal end of the humerus, which are taken at right angles to each other, are initially obtained. These are taken with the arm immobilized in a sling in planes parallel to and perpendicular to the scapula (Figure 2.1). They may be taken with the patient sitting, standing or lying supine. These views are supplemented with an axillary view, which allows evaluation of the fracture in a third orthogonal plane. The Velpeau axillary view, in which the patient leans backward 45° with the arm immobilized in the sling, and the X-ray beam projects downward onto the plate, is the preferred view[10] (Figure 2.2). The Velpeau view adds important information about the relationship between the articular surfaces and about tuberosity displacement, without moving the injured extremity. However, in elderly patients and in those with

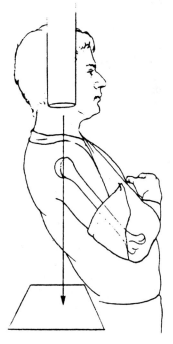

Figure 2.2 The Velpeau axillary view allows evaluation of the fracture in a third orthogonal plane and completes the trauma series. It is preferred because it adds information about the relationship between the articular surfaces and about tuberosity displacement, without moving the injured extremity

multiple injuries, it may not be possible to obtain this view. In these cases, the standard supine axillary view may be obtained with a physician carefully positioning the shoulder in mild abduction so as not to displace the fracture and directing the beam into the axilla. Other views, such as the transthoracic lateral view and rotation views, have been described for evaluating proximal humeral fractures. Computed tomography scans are helpful in appreciating head-splitting elements and in determining the size of articular defects in fracture-dislocations. However, for classifying most fractures of the proximal humerus, the three orthogonal plain radiographs are sufficient.

Treatment

The treatment of minimally displaced fractures of the proximal humerus generally involves an initial brief period of immobilization in a sling followed by gradual progressive mobilization of the shoulder. The aim of treatment is to prevent the development of adhesions and to maintain or restore the shoulder's almost global range of motion while the fracture is uniting. Codman pointed out that in these fractures, the rotator cuff and the periosteum of the proximal humerus hold the fragments together 'in a jumbled mass'[11]. He advocated early 'stooping exercises with the arm released . . . to make sure that adhesions in the bursa do not take place'[11]. These passive circumduction exercises comprise the initial step in many of the rehabilitative programmes reported for proximal humerus fractures[12–17]. It was Codman's opinion that most of these fractures should have fairly good motion at six weeks, allowing return to work certainly by six months.

In a review of the proximal humeral fractures treated at the Massachusetts General Hospital in the 1930s, Roberts pointed out 'a definite trend of treatment away from apparatus and prolonged immobilization toward the simpler forms of fixation and early active motion'[18]. In those fractures that were comminuted but not displaced, early active motion was usually started within a few days. Airplane splints and plaster were largely replaced by the sling and swathe. A very high percentage were found to have good anatomical and functional results,[18]. Alldredge and Knight also pointed out 'that greater care must be exercised in the treatment of any fracture, dislocation, injury, disease about the shoulder joint than in any other joint', since the shoulder tends to lose abduction

and rotation after injury[12]. They urged against the use of the body spica with the shoulder in abduction and traction splints and emphasized that the objective of treatment should be the early restoration of function. Massage and relaxed circumduction are advocated by those authors, based on the method described by Lindsay and Brown[12]. After two or three weeks, active motion is begun, and the sling is discarded. Brostrom reported success using a similar programme of early mobilization for proximal humeral fractures[13]. In this series, which included all fractures of the proximal humerus, relative immobilization was achieved between exercise sessions using a collar and cuff with a swathe. Passive circumduction exercises and massage were begun 4 days after injury, and active motion was allowed after 5–7 days. The bandage was used for 3–4 weeks, after which active motion of the shoulder was encouraged. Good or excellent results were achieved in 72% of patients treated by this method[13].

Even more aggressive treatment has been recommended by others for these non-displaced fractures. In Watson-Jones' classification, these fractures are referred to as 'contusion crack fractures of the neck of the humerus'[19]. He stated that it was unnecessary to immobilize the limb and that early exercises should be started to minimize adhesions. Wentworth, too, reported that many of the fractures of the surgical neck and greater tuberosity in the aged showed only insignificant displacement and were stable. He added that patients with this fracture 'need scarcely any more protection after reduction than carrying the hand in the side pocket part of the time'[17]. Others have reported on the use of procaine injections and immediate mobilization of proximal humeral fractures, finding superior results in patients treated in this manner, as compared with those treated with bandage immobilization for 2 weeks followed by physiotherapy[15]. They believed that procaine injection and immediate mobilization led to restoring a normal range of motion more quickly, to shortening the period of absence from work and even to accelerating the formation of callus[15].

Neer has pointed out that although the fragments in minimally displaced fractures are usually held together by the rotator cuff and periosteum, occasionally one of the fragments may be disimpacted: the fragments do not then move together, as one piece, and 'false motion' is present[8]. When this situation pertains, initial immobilization with a sling and swathe is necessary to allow sufficient clinical healing to occur, so that the head and shaft will rotate together before exercises are started. The absence of false motion can be assessed by palpating the proximal humerus, while gently rotating the arm at the side. When the fragments move as a unit, the sling and swathe can be safely removed to allow pendulum exercises, which are then progressed to other passive and assistive exercises, so that motion may be regained. This simple manoeuvre to test for early clinical union prior to initiating exercises can prevent displacement of one or more of the fragments, which could result in malunion of the fracture.

Another issue concerning minimally displaced fractures of the proximal humerus is whether formal physiotherapy is necessary, or whether the patients can perform the exercises independently. There are not many studies which deal with this issue. Lundberg and associates have reported on 42 patients with minimally displaced proximal humeral fractures by Neer's criteria, who were randomly assigned to two groups: one group received formal physiotherapy once or twice each week for 2–3 months, while the other group performed the same exercises independently[20]. Each group began active movements of the shoulder and arm after 1 week of immobilization in a sling. No differences appeared between the two groups with respect to pain or motion at early follow-up (1 and 3 months after fracture) or at later follow-up (1 year after injury)[20]. Interestingly, avulsion of the greater tuberosity occurred in both groups: in 6 cases with formal physiotherapy and in 7 cases with home exercises. The authors concluded that economy can be achieved without harm to the patients by instructing them in independent exer-

cises. Bertoft and associates carried out a similar study in 20 patients with minimally displaced proximal humeral fractures[21]. In this randomized and blind trial, again no significant differences were seen between the patients with formal physiotherapy and those with the self-assisted home programme. The greatest improvement in function was made in both groups between 3 and 8 weeks after injury. The rehabilitation then proceeded at a slower rate until 6 months to 1 year after injury[21].

Author's recommended treatment

Minimally displaced proximal humeral fractures are initially treated with a sling and swathe at our institution. As discussed above, obtaining well-positioned radiographs in at least two, but preferably three different planes is crucial to classifying the fracture correctly as minimally displaced. The swathe is added for patient comfort and can usually be discontinued after several days. At approximately 10 days after injury, the patient is re-examined for signs of early clinical healing. The physician stands at the patient's side, supporting the injured extremity at the elbow with one hand. The other hand is placed over the proximal humerus, palpating the biceps groove and lesser tuberosity. The arm is then gently rotated while palpating the movement of the proximal humerus. If the arm (distal fragment) and the biceps groove and lesser tuberosity (proximal fragment) move 'as a unit', the fracture is considered stable and demonstrating signs of early union (Figure 2.3). Radio-

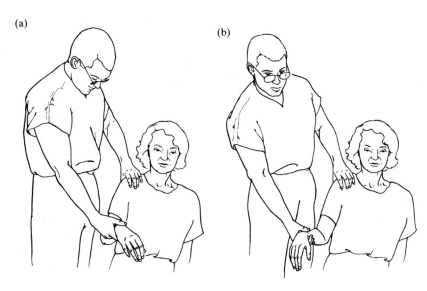

(a)

(b)

Figure 2.3 To assess early clinical healing, the physician assesses whether the fragments move together 'as a unit'. The injured extremity is supported at the elbow by the physician. The physician's other hand is placed over the proximal fragment, palpating the tuberosity and bicipital groove (a). The arm is gently rotated (b). If the fragments move 'as a unit', the fracture is considered to be stable and exhibiting signs of early healing

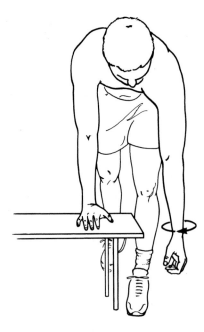

Figure 2.4 The pendulum exercise is demonstrated. It is usually the first of the passive exercises initiated after early fracture healing has occurred. It can be performed independently by the patient, after appropriate instruction by the physician or therapist

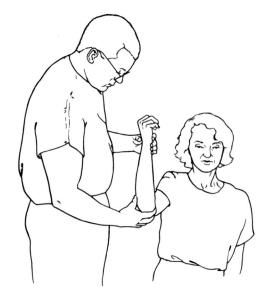

Figure 2.5 As early healing progresses, further passive exercises can be added to the therapy regimen. This figure demonstrates passive elevation of the shoulder in the scapular plane. Usually, passive elevation is limited initially to 90° and then is advanced as healing progresses. Limited passive external rotation exercises are also initiated at this point

graphs of the proximal humerus are obtained again at this visit to demonstrate that satisfactory alignment has been maintained and that none of the fragments have displaced. If the fracture alignment has not shifted significantly and the fragments appear to move together, early passive range of motion exercises are begun. On the other hand, if motion between the fragments is still present, which would be unusual for this group of fractures, exercises would be deferred for a slightly longer period, until sufficient clinical union had occurred.

The rehabilitation protocol that continues to be used at our institution is the three-phase programme devised by Neer[22,23]. The earliest phase consists of passive exercises performed by the patient in conjunction with a physiotherapist or family member. The pendulum exercise (Codman's stooping exercises) can be performed independently by the patient (Figure 2.4). The patient may also actively flex and extend the elbow to avoid stiffness at this joint. Active movement of the wrist and fingers is also encouraged to avoid secondary stiffness distally in the extremity. Limited passive elevation in the scapular plane (initially 90°) (Figure 2.5) and external rotation

(initially to neutral or 20°) exercises are performed by the therapist or instructed family member. These exercises are advanced to allow greater degrees of motion as healing progresses. The use of a self-assistive pulley is usually deferred during the early healing period, as incorrect use of this device (i.e. active muscle contraction by the injured shoulder) can result in displacement of the fragments, particularly the greater tuberosity.

Use of the sling is usually continued for approximately 6 weeks, not to strictly immobilize the shoulder, but rather to discourage active use during early fracture healing. These fractures are in the cancellous bone of the proximal humerus and tend to heal in 6–8 weeks. One study reported that callus was usually evident by radiographs at 3 weeks, though complete radiographic consolidation took 7–9 months[24]. After clinical union has occurred, the sling is discarded and the exercise regimen is advanced. More aggressive stretching exercises, such as stretching in a doorway or sliding up a wall, are employed to regain motion and prevent soft tissue contracture. Active functional use of the extremity is also allowed at this point. The focus of rehabilitation, however, during this early period (i.e. the first 2–3 months after injury) should remain the restoration of full motion.

Active and resistive exercises to restore strength (phases II and III of the Neer protocol) are deferred until fracture healing is advanced and good motion passively has been restored. It is a fruitless pursuit to attempt to strengthen a stiff shoulder. The best opportunity for regaining motion is in the first few months after the injury. Too early emphasis on strengthening can distract the patient from this goal and lead to frustration. After motion has been restored, the patient and therapist can then work on strengthening the shoulder to allow resumption of satisfactory shoulder function. Motivated patients who are diligent in performing the exercise protocols will usually regain full or nearly full motion and excellent function, though this may take up to six or seven months after injury.

Complications

Stiffness

Though most patients with minimally displaced fractures of the proximal humerus will achieve a satisfactory range of motion after union has occurred, some will have persistent stiffness. This will occur especially if an excessive period of strict immobilization has been employed or if there has been inadequate effort at rehabilitation. The stiffness may result in pain and limitation of function, similar to that seen with adhesive capsulitis. This is a problem that is best avoided by timely institution and progression of early range of motion exercises, as soon as the fracture fragments move 'as a unit'. When post-traumatic stiffness is encountered, it can often be treated successfully with a programme of stretching exercises. This is often initiated under the supervision of a physical therapist, who can assist and encourage the patient with the exercises.

Occasionally, the stiffness will be resistant to physical therapy and the disability will warrant further intervention. We recommend against manipulation under anaesthesia as a means of regaining motion after a fracture of the proximal humerus. The healing bone may yield before the stiff soft tissues, and this would result in re-fracture of the humerus. Instead, when post-fracture stiffness is sufficiently disabling and has been resistant to a programme of stretching exercises (usually of at least 6 months to 1 year in duration), we would perform an open release of the soft tissues to regain shoulder motion. Lysis of adhesions in the subacromial space, as well as

the release of the contracted inferior glenohumeral joint capsule, allow restoration of flexion and abduction. Furthermore, release of the coracohumeral ligament assists in restoring external rotation[23]. Postoperatively, these patients are immediately started with an aggressive programme of strengthening exercises in order to maintain the motion that has been achieved by the surgical release of contractures.

Pseudosubluxation

Downward or inferior subluxation of the humeral head with respect to the glenoid has long been recognized after proximal humeral fractures[25-27]. Cotton believed that this occurred due to 'gradual exhaustion of the muscles', particularly of the deltoid[25]. Fairbank found an incidence of 10% of downward subluxation in proximal humeral fractures[26]. He observed that the subluxation often disappears spontaneously and probably results from lack of tone in the scapulohumeral muscles supporting the weight of the limb. A sling to support the arm, rather than a collar and cuff, was the advocated treatment. Neer pointed out that the ligaments and capsule of the glenohumeral joint are normally loose enough to permit inferior subluxation when the deltoid and rotator cuff muscles became atonic[8]. Perhaps traumatic disruption of the normal negative intra-articular pressure contributes to this phenomenon of 'pseudosubluxation'[28]. This subluxation, however, is usually transitory and spontaneously resolves over a period of several weeks (Figure 2.6). When it fails to resolve, and there is clinical evidence of persistent deltoid dysfunction, an electromyographic (EMG) study is warranted. In most cases, treatment consists merely of supporting the weight of the arm with a sling to minimize stretching out the static stabilizers until the deltoid regains its tone.

Malunion

By definition, the fractures under consideration here are minimally displaced. As long as displacement during the early healing period does not occur, then significant malunion is not usually a problem in this group of fractures. However, two caveats should be given concerning 'minimally displaced' fractures of the greater tuberosity. Several authors have demonstrated that anteroposterior and lateral radiographs may underestimate the amount of posterior retraction of the greater tuberosity[29,30]. Axillary radiographs or computed

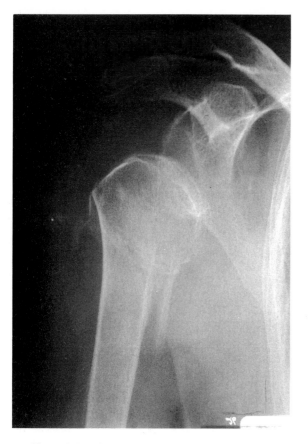

Figure 2.6 Inferior subluxation ('pseudosubluxation') of the humeral head with respect to the glenoid may occur after proximal humerus fractures. This is usually transitory and spontaneously resolves over several weeks

tomographic scans more accurately demonstrate this displacement. Thus, it is possible to classify incorrectly a greater tuberosity fragment as 'minimally displaced' if radiographs are inadequate. Such a fracture may conceivably go on to a symptomatic malunion. McLaughlin reviewed greater tuberosity fractures that occurred in association with shoulder dislocations and found that a prolonged convalescence was the rule, even with small residual displacement of the tuberosity fragment[24]. When the displacement was more than 0.5 cm but less than 1.0 cm, the convalescence was often greater than 6 months, and there was some permanent pain and disability (Figure 2.7). In 20% of these cases, persistent symptoms made late surgical treatment necessary[24]. More recently, Duralde and associates reported on a series of patients treated operatively for malunions of proximal humerus fractures[31]. In this series, preoperative superior displacement of the greater tuberosity averaged 8 mm, again demonstrating that displacement of this fragment less than 1 cm can lead to significant pain and dysfunction. Surgical treatment was designed to restore clearance of the greater tuberosity under the coraco-acromial arch and included release of adhesions, anterior acromioplasty, and osteotomy or ostectomy of the tuberosity, depending on the degree of malunion[31]. In cases of symptomatic malunion, where the greater tuberosity displacement is of a lesser degree, we generally perform an anterior acromioplasty combined with release of soft tissue adhesions and ostectomy of the prominent 'bump'. Osteotomy of

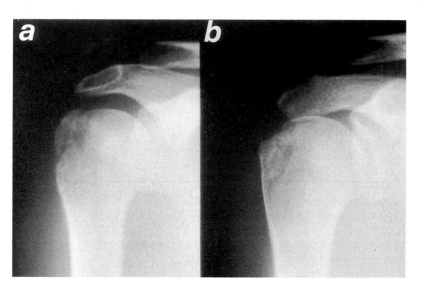

Figure 2.7 Symptomatic malunion of the greater tuberosity fragment may occur even when the initial superior displacement is less than 1.0 cm (a). Treatment options include acromioplasty and exostectomy of the prominent fragment versus osteotomy and repositioning of the tuberosity (b)

the malunited tuberosity and transposition to a more anatomical position are reserved for cases with greater deformity.

Delayed union/non-union

Delayed union or non-union of a minimally displaced fracture of the proximal humerus is a rare complication. This complication is more often seen in displaced fractures of the surgical neck of the humerus. In a minimally displaced fracture, the cancellous bone of the proximal humerus usually heals within 6–8 weeks. Progression to overly aggressive stretching or active use of the shoulder in the period immediately following fracture may allow subsequent disimpaction of the fragments and displacement of the fracture, increasing the chance of complications such as non-union. Verification that the fracture has undergone early healing and 'moves as a unit' before physiotherapy is begun can virtually eliminate this complication.

Avascular necrosis

Avascular necrosis of the humeral head is a rare complication after a minimally displaced proximal humerus fracture. It may occur, however, even two or three years after the initial injury. When collapse of the humeral head is symptomatic, prosthetic replacement of the humeral head is a good treatment for eliminating pain and restoring function of the shoulder. Neer pointed out that prosthetic replacement in this setting is straightforward, as the bony anatomy of the tuberosities and the rotator cuff are preserved[23]. However, the soft tissues around the shoulder may be quite contracted in these cases, as the spacer effect of the humeral head has been lost. Thus, careful attention must be paid to release of contractures and balancing the soft tissues when performing the prosthetic replacement. Occasionally, the glenoid will have become arthritic, secondary to long-standing articulation with a collapsed humeral head, and total shoulder arthroplasty will be necessary.

Axillary artery injury

Injury of the axillary artery with a minimally displaced fracture of the proximal humerus has been reported[32], though this is a rare complication. The possible mechanisms for this complication include direct injury from a sharp bony fragment, overstretching of the artery (especially in the setting of atheromatous plaques) or intimal disruption and thrombosis. Loss of palpable pulses may occur, but distal paraesthesiae are more commonly the presenting symptoms[33]. When this injury is suspected, angiography should be performed, followed by exploration and repair.

Conclusion

Minimally displaced fractures comprise 80–85% of proximal humeral fractures, and their incidence continues to rise, making these a common cause of morbidity. By definition, a proximal humeral fracture is one in which none of the four major segments is displaced more than 1 cm or angulated greater than 45°. As the proximal humerus is well invested with soft tissues, deformity after fracture is not readily apparent and signs of injury are limited to soft tissue swelling, ecchymosis which may extend down the arm or along the chest wall, and tenderness at the fracture site. Diagnosis and classification of the fracture pattern require that accurate radiographs of the glenohumeral joint and proximal humerus be obtained. Three orthogonal plain radiographs (anteroposterior and lateral views in the scapular plane and an axillary view) allow accurate classification of these fractures in most cases, while computed tomography scans are occasionally helpful in measuring tuberosity displacement.

Treatment of minimally displaced fractures of the proximal humerus consists of protection in a sling during the early healing period and gradual mobilization to prevent soft tissue adhesions and contractures. To prevent disimpaction and displacement of one or more of the segments, it is necessary to verify that early healing has occurred – that the entire proximal humerus 'moves as a unit' – before beginning physical therapy. Early therapy consists of pendulum and limited passive range of motion exercises. As healing continues, these are progressed to allow self-assistive and then advanced stretching exercises. Bony healing usually occurs by 6–8 weeks, and the sling is discarded. The earliest phases of physiotherapy are directed at maintaining and restoring motion, and stretching exercises take precedence over strengthening during this period. As motion normalizes, resistive exercises are then added to allow the shoulder to resume normal function. Though the bony injury heals relatively quickly, full restoration of motion, strength and function may take 6 months or longer.

Complications after minimally displaced fractures of the proximal humerus are uncommon. Some patients will have persistent stiffness, resembling a frozen shoulder. If the shoulder fails to respond to a supervised programme of therapy and remains symptomatic, open release of adhesions may be considered. Manipulation under anaesthesia is generally not advised after fractures, as the risk of re-fracture is too high. Pseudosubluxation is occasionally seen after fracture and usually resolves spontaneously, as tone returns to the deltoid. Symptomatic malunion, usually involving displacement of the greater tuberosity, may occur in this group of fractures. Accurate radiographs must be carefully addressed at the time of injury to avoid undercalculating greater tuberosity displacement, especially that in a posterior direction. Occasionally, these malunions will require later surgery, consisting either of soft tissue release combined with anterior acromioplasty and ostectomy, or osteotomy of the tuberosity, in cases with more severe displacement. Devastating complications, such as injury to the axillary artery, are exceedingly rare with minimally displaced fractures.

References

1 Lind, T., Kroner, K. and Jensen, J. The epidemiology of fractures of the proximal humerus. *Arch. Orthop. Trauma Surg.*, **108**, 285–287 (1989)

2. Rose, S.H., Melton, L.J. III, Morrey, B.F., Ilstrup, D.M. and Riggs, B.L. Epidemiologic features of humeral fractures. *Clin. Orthop.*, **168**, 24–30 (1982)

3. Horak, J. and Nilsson, B.E. Epidemiology of fractures of the upper end of the humerus. *Clin. Orthop.*, **112**, 250–252 (1975)

4. Moriber, L.A. and Patterson, R.L. Jr. Fractures of the proximal end of the humerus. *J. Bone Joint Surg.*, **49A**, 1–18 (1967)

5. Neer, C.S. II. Displaced proximal humerus fractures. Part I. Classification and evaluation. *J. Bone Joint Surg.*, **52A**, 1077–1089 (1970).

6. Jakob, R.P., Kristiansen, T., Mayo, K., Ganz, R. and Muller, M.E. Classification and aspects of treatment of fractures of the proximal humerus. In *Surgery of the Shoulder* (eds J.E. Bateman and R.P. Welsh), Decker, Philadelphia (1984)

7. Bigliani, L.U. Fractures of the proximal humerus. In *The Shoulder* (eds C.A. Rockwood Jr and F.A. Matsen III), W.B. Saunders, Philadelphia (1990)

8. Neer, C.S. II. Four segment classification of displaced proximal humerus fractures. *Instruct. Course Lect.*, **24**, 160–168, American Academy of Orthopedic Surgeons, Park Ridge, Illinois (1975)

9. Norris, T.R. Fractures of the proximal humerus and dislocations of the shoulder. In *Skeletal Trauma* (eds B.D. Browner, J.B. Jupiter, A.M. Levine and P.G. Tratton), W.B. Saunders, Philadelphia (1992)

10. Bloom, M.H. and Obata, W. Diagnosis of posterior dislocation of the shoulder with use of a Velpeau axillary and angle-up roentgenographic views. *J. Bone Joint Surg.* **49A**, 943–949 (1967)

11. Codman, E.A. *The Shoulder*, Robert E. Krieger, Malabar, FL (1984)

12. Alldredge, R.H. and Knight, M.P. Fractures of the upper end of the humerus treated by early relaxed motion and massage. *New Orleans Med. Surg. J.*, **92**, 519–524 (1994)

13. Brostrom, F. Early mobilization of fractures of the upper end of the humerus. *Arch. Surg.* **46**, 614–615 (1943)

14. DePalma, A.F. and Cautilli, R.A. Fractures of the upper end of the humerus. *Clin. Orthop.*, **20**, 73–93 (1961)

15. Ekstrom, T., Lagergren, C. and vonSchreeb, T. Procaine injections and early mobilization for fractures of the neck of the humerus. *Acta Chir. Scand.*, **130**, 18–24 (1965)

16. Garceau, G.J. and Cogland, S. Early physical therapy in the treatment of fractures of the surgical neck of the humerus. *J. Indiana Med. Ass.* **34**, 293–295 (1941)

17. Wentworth, E.T. Fractures involving the shoulder joint. *N.Y. State J. Med.*, **40**, 1282–1288 (1940)

18. Roberts, S.M. Fractures of the upper end of the humerus. An end result study which shows the advantage of early active motion. *J. Am. Med. Ass.*, **98**, 367–372 (1932).

19. Watson-Jones, R. *Fractures and Joint Injuries*, 4th edn, Baltimore, Williams and Wilkins (1955)

20. Lundberg, B.J., Svenungson-Hartwig, E. and Wilkmark, R. Independent exercises versus physiotherapy in non displaced proximal humerus fractures. *Scand. J. Rehab. Med.*, **111**, 133–136 (1979)

21. Bertoft, E.S., Lundh, I. and Ringqvist I., Physiotherapy after fracture of the proximal humerus. *Scand. J. Rehab. Med.* **16**, 11–16 (1984)

22. Hughes, M. and Neer, C.S. Glenohumeral joint replacement and postoperative rehabilitation. *Phys. Ther.*, **55**, 850–858 (1975)

23. Neer, C.S. II. *Shoulder Reconstruction*, W.B. Saunders, Philadelpia (1990)

24. McLaughlin, H.L. Dislocation of the shoulder with tuberosity fracture. *Surg. Clin. N. Am.*, **43**, 1615–1620 (1963)

25. Cotton, F.J. Subluxation of the shoulder downward. *Boston Med. Surg. J.*, **185**, 405–407 (1921)

26. Fairbank, T.J. Fracture-subluxations of the shoulder. *J. Bone Joint Surg.* **30B**, 454–460 (1948)

27. Thompson, F.R. and Winant, E.M. Unusual fracture-subluxations of the shoulder joint. *J. Bone Joint Surg.*, **32A**, 575–582 (1960)

28. Kumar, V.P. and Balasubramaniam, P. The role of atmospheric pressure in stabilizing the shoulder. An experimental study. *J. Bone Joint Surg* **67B**, 719–721 (1985)

29. Flatow, E.L., Cuomo, F., Maday, M.G., Miller, S.R., McIlveen, S.J. and Bigliani, L.U. Open reduction and internal fixation of two-part displaced fractures of the greater tuberosity of the proximal part of the humerus. *J. Bone Joint Surg.*, **73A**, 1213–1218 (1991)

30. Morris, M.E., Kilcoyne, R.F., Shuman, W. and Matsen,

F.A. III. Humeral tuberosity fractures: evaluation by CT scan and management of malunion. *Orthop. Trans.*, **11**, 242 (1987)

31. Duralde, X.A., Rodosky, M.W. and Flatow, E.L. Operative treatment of malunions of proximal humerus fractures. Presented at the American Shoulder and Elbow Surgeons 10th Open Meeting, New Orleans, LA (February 1994)

32. Neer, C.S. II, Satterlee, C.C., Dalsey, R.M. and Flatow, E.L. The anatomy and potential effects of contracture of the coracohumeral ligament. *Clin. Orthop.*, **280**, 15–16 (1992)

33. Hayes, J.M. and Van Winkle, G.N. Axillary artery injury with minimally displaced fracture of the neck of the humerus. *J. Trauma*, **23**, 431–433 (1983)

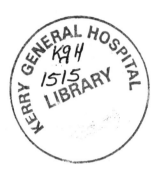

3

Two-part displaced tuberosity fractures of the proximal humerus

Frances Cuomo

Two-part displaced tuberosity fractures of the proximal humerus are rare injuries, representing only 3% of proximal humeral fractures reported[1]. Greater tuberosity fractures are the majority of cases within this group, with only 16 isolated lesser tuberosity fractures cited since 1895. On the basis of their infrequent occurrence alone, these injuries represent an intriguing and complex problem with regard to diagnosis and treatment. Unfortunately, few reports are available which adequately review methods and results of treatment regimens regarding these fractures[1,2].

Accurate diagnosis is essential in order to develop a proper treatment plan and is directly related to obtaining adequate radiographs and a sound knowledge of the complex anatomy of the shoulder. Radiographic findings in displaced tuberosity fractures may be subtle due to the possibility of small fracture fragment size, superimposition of the displaced fragment over the humeral head or glenoid, and incomplete imaging[1,3]. In addition, these small fragments may be confused with calcific tendinitis involving the rotator cuff tendons[4-7]. For these reasons, it has been suggested that the two-part displaced tuberosity fracture may be underdiagnosed[2,6].

Timely and proper treatment of these injuries is crucial as malunion and rotator cuff dysfunction may lead to pain, loss of motion and subsequent disability, especially with regard to the displaced greater tuberosity[5,8,13]. Clearly this dysfunction is compounded when there is an associated glenohumeral dislocation which eludes early identification.

Anatomical considerations

As the glenohumeral joint has more motion than any other joint in the human body, balance between the soft tissues and osseous structures is crucial to obtain stability and optimum function. This requires knowledge of the osseous, tendinous and neurovascular components surrounding the glenohumeral joint.

The humeral head, greater and lesser tuberosities and humeral shaft compose the bony constituents of the proximal humerus and are divided by their epiphyseal lines. The humeral head is retroverted 35–40° to articulate with the scapula, which is important during imaging as this joint is not directly situated in the coronal or sagittal plane. Also of note is that the articular surface of the humeral head is slightly higher than the greater tuberosity. Failure to appreciate this after a displaced greater tuberosity fracture may result in malunion and pain due to atypical impingement. The bicipital groove separating the greater and lesser tuberosities is also reported to be an important source of discomfort if its surface is disrupted along with the greater tuberosity at the time of fracture[14].

The tendinous insertions onto three of the four segments of the proximal humerus are intimately related to the displacement and fracture patterns seen. The articular surface, which is that portion of the head superior to the tuberosities and separated from the tuberosities by the anatomical neck, has no muscular attachments. This is in contrast to the humeral shaft which is inferior to the tuberosities and serves as the insertion for the pectoralis major. The most intricate tendinous anatomy surrounds the tuberosities, as all four rotator cuff tendons insert into them, and the biceps tendon lies in the groove between them. The superior, middle and inferior facets of the greater tuberosity allow for the insertion of the supraspinatus, infraspinatus and teres minor, respectively. As these muscles function in abduction and external rotation, the fragment is pulled superiorly and posteriorly to various degrees depending upon which facets are involved in the fracture. Due to the unopposed pull of the subscapularis tendon upon the lesser tuberosity, this fragment is pulled medially when the lesser tuberosity is fractured. Lastly, the biceps tendon, although not part of the rotator cuff, serves as a head depressor and surgical landmark dividing the lesser tuberosity medially from the greater tuberosity laterally. It has also been implicated in the inability to obtain reduction of two-part greater tuberosity fracture-dislocations as it may become entrapped within the glenohumeral joint[14] or under the tuberosity[15] and block reduction.

The importance of the vascular supply to the proximal humerus needs obvious emphasis. The tuberosities play a major role in the transmission of vasculature to the articular surface. The majority of direct blood supply is via the anterior humeral circumflex artery[16–18]. This artery gives rise to the ascending branch which continues as the arcuate artery and enters the humeral head through the superior portion of the bicipital groove and both tuberosities[16]. To a lesser extent, the articular surface also receives contributions from the rotator cuff tendinous insertions upon the tuberosities and the posterior circumflex artery.

The proximity of the brachial plexus makes all of these structures vulnerable to injury with displaced fractures, especially when associated with glenohumeral dislocations. This is particularly important as 15–30% of anterior dislocations are associated with greater tuberosity fractures[19,20]. The axillary nerve is the most commonly injured nerve as it traverses along the anterior aspect of the subscapularis and then along the inferior capsule. Owing to its relative fixation at the posterior cord and the deltoid, any abnormal downward motion of the proximal humerus can result in traction injury to this nerve[21]. Although the axillary nerve is the most frequently injured, any portion of the plexus including suprascapular and musculocutaneous nerves may be involved.

Classification

The classification system employed plays a major role in consistently and accurately diagnosing displaced tuberosity fractures. Prior to Codman's significant contribution identifying four basic fracture fragments formed by division along the epiphyseal lines of the proximal humerus in 1934, varied classification systems were presented based on mechanism of injury, vascular status of the articular surface, anatomical level and fracture displacement[1,20,22–24]. Subsequently, Neer developed a comprehensive yet concise classification system integrating these four osseous segments, local soft tissue anatomy, fracture mechanics and displacement which was to become the most useful and commonly used system in the orthopaedic literature.[25]

The cornerstone of Neer's classification is based upon the anatomical division of the articular surface, humeral shaft, greater and lesser tuberosities, and the degree of displacement of each fragment with respect to the others. The tendinous anatomy is also accounted for and noted to be responsible for the displacement forces, thereby making fracture patterns predictable. A fracture is considered displaced when any of the four major segments is displaced more than 1 cm or angulated greater than 45°[5,25]. Therefore two-part, three-part, and four-part fractures have been described.

When one fragment is displaced in reference to the other three, it is termed a two-part fracture. Therefore, by definition, a two-part displaced greater tuberosity fracture is one in which one or more of its facets is retracted more than 1.0 cm by the pull of its attached tendons (Figure 3.1). This separation is pathognomonic for a rotator cuff tear, most often found as a longitudinal tear in the rotator interval. If only the posterior portion of the tuberosity is displaced, the tear may be found posterior to the interval and between the supraspinatus and infraspinatus[1,25]. The articular segment remains in its normal relationship with the shaft, leaving a good portion of its blood supply. Likewise a two-part lesser tuberosity fracture is defined as 1.0 cm or more displacement of this fragment by the pull of the subscapularis tendon (Figure 3.2). The displacement of this fragment may spread the anterior fibres at the rotator interval, producing a bony prominence, but does not appear to have as clinically significant implications as its greater tuberosity counterpart.

Fracture-dislocations are also included in Neer's classification and are described as those injuries

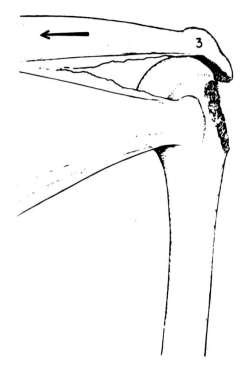

Figure 3.1 Two-part greater tuberosity fracture. Rotator cuff insertions onto superior, middle and inferior facets pull fragment superiorly and posteriorly. Note interval rotator cuff tear (From Neer[77], by permission)

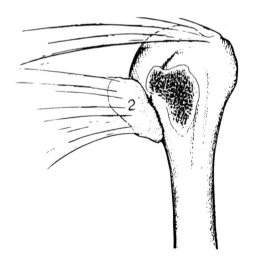

Figure 3.2 Two-part lesser tuberosity displacement. Medial and anterior displacement is noted due to pull of subscapularis tendon (From Neer[77], by permission)

where the head is completely displaced outside the joint. They may be anterior or posterior dislocations and can be classified as two-, three-, or four-part fracture-dislocations. By far the most common direction of dislocation is anterior with this group, including at least 95% of dislocations. Fifteen to 30% of anterior dislocations are associated with greater tuberosity fractures[5,19,20,26,27], and are therefore termed two-part greater tuberosity anterior fracture-dislocations. Posterior dislocations are rare and represent only 1.5–4.3% of all glenohumeral dislocation.[28–32] They are often associated with lesser tuberosity fractures (14%).

Mechanism of injury

The most commonly reported mechanism of injury for all proximal humeral fractures is a fall onto an outstretched, pronated upper extremity. Isolated greater tuberosity fractures, especially if seen with comminution, may be the result of a direct blow to the lateral aspect of the shoulder[20]. Although the exact mechanism of injury for tuberosity fractures is unknown, underlying osteoporosis and weak trabecular bone are thought to play a major role in their pathogenesis[33,34]. The cancellous bone in the greater tuberosity decreases in quantity, producing cavitation within a thin shell of cortical bone. Some authors have suggested that with abduction and external rotation, an anterior dislocation might produce a greater tuberosity fracture rather than a Hill–Sachs lesion if the pull of the external rotators propagates the impression fracture into an avulsion fracture of the tuberosity by a shearing mechanism against the glenoid[1,35] (Figure 3.3). The rotator interval and coracohumeral ligament between the supraspinatus and subscapularis have been implicated as stabilizing features which aid in the prevention of lesser tuberosity and subscapularis tendon involvement[36]. Avulsion by the pull of the external rotators alone has also been a hypothesized fracture mechanism[35].

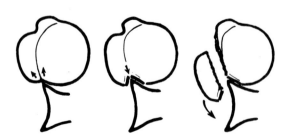

Figure 3.3 With abduction and external rotation, concomitant pull of the external rotators may cause a mere Hill–Sachs lesion to propagate into an avulsion fracture of the greater tuberosity (From Jakob *et al.*[1], by permission)

Lesser tuberosity fractures very rarely occur as isolated injuries. More often they are seen in conjunction with posterior dislocation. Jakob identified only two fractures of this type after reviewing 730 displaced proximal humeral fractures (0.3%)[1]. This may be due to the fact that the lesser tuberosity is protected from direct injury by its small size and its location on the medial side of the humeral head[37]. The reported mechanism of injury in most cases has been a strong external rotatory force applied while the arm is at maximum external rotation and at about 60° of abduction, as this is the position the subscapularis is at maximum stretch[38–42]. Resisted internal rotation has also been implicated as a possible mechanism. Just as the greater tuberosity is subject to avulsion with anterior dislocation[12,26,43], the lesser is susceptible to fracture, most likely due to similar shearing forces, with posterior dislocation. Indirect force causing a combination of internal rotation, adduction and forward elevation is the most common cause of traumatic posterior dislocations. This situation is most commonly seen with electrical shock and convulsive seizures as the unbalanced stimulation of internal rotators overpower the weaker external rotators[5,36,45–48].

Clinical presentation

In the acute situation, although isolated displaced tuberosity fractures commonly present with pain, swelling and either diffuse or localized tenderness about the tuberosities, the generous soft tissue covering about the shoulder may make the diagnosis obscure. Crepitus, ecchymosis and alteration of the bony contour at best are only suggestive of fracture. Humeral rotation is often painful and limited with resisted internal and external rotatory manoeuvres eliciting discomfort with lesser and greater tuberosity fractures, respectively.

Associated neurovascular injury is not uncommon and must be aggressively searched for at initial presentation. As the axillary nerve is the most common nerve injury seen, deltoid activity should be closely assessed as merely testing its sensory distribution is unreliable[49]. Pseudosubluxation may be noted in the early fracture period, at which time the more common cause of deltoid atony must be differentiated from axillary nerve injury[22,50,51]. Axillary artery injury has been reported in association with fractures and fracture-dislocations but most often includes fracture of the surgical neck[52,53]. No major artery injury has been reported

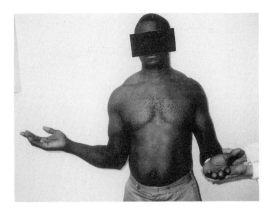

Figure 3.4 Left locked posterior glenohumeral dislocation. Note internally rotated extremity with inability to abduct and loss of normal shoulder contour

with an isolated tuberosity fracture. With prolonged time until reduction of dislocation, one could surmise that the incidence of axillary artery thrombosis might very well increase. Therefore, palpation of distal pulses pre- and post-reduction is essential.

Fracture-dislocations present an even more difficult diagnostic dilemma clinically[48,54,55]. This becomes more significant when one specifically examines posterior fracture-dislocations, with up to 80% reported having been missed at the time of injury[5,28,30–32,36,48,55,56]. Loss of the bony contour is often seen with an anterior or posterior bulge caused by the humeral head in the same direction as the dislocation. Posterior dislocations also exhibit a prominent coracoid anteriorly, a posteriorly directed acromiohumeral axis and loss of abduction and external rotation as shown by an adducted and internally rotated extremity (Figure 3.4). As previously stated, one should be alerted by a history of electroshock therapy or seizure disorder in which anterior and posterior dislocation may be encountered and easily overlooked in the patient with shoulder pain.

Diagnosis/radiographs

The need for multiple and precise radiographs cannot be overemphasized, both for diagnosis and treatment. Inadequate imaging may fail to identify small greater and lesser tuberosity fragments or those fragments which overlie the humeral head or inferior glenoid on simple anteroposterior views[3,57]. Any and all injuries about the proximal

(a)

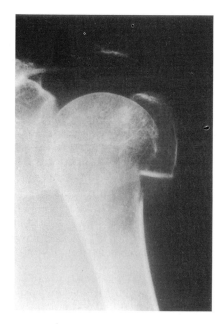

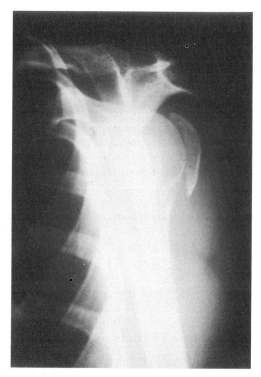

(b)

(c)

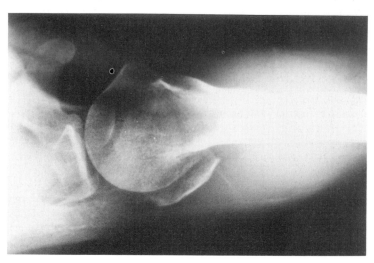

Figure 3.5 Trauma series set of radiographs of a two-part greater tuberosity fracture: (a) scapular AP showing superior displacement of greater tuberosity fragment; (b) scapular lateral reveals posterior retraction of fragment; (c) axillary view displays overlap of fragment onto articular surface

humerus are best initially evaluated with a trauma series set of radiographs in three perpendicular planes. As the glenohumeral joint does not lie in either the sagittal or coronal plane due to the obliquity of the scapula on the chest wall, anteroposterior and lateral scapular views are taken in addi-

tion to an axillary view. These scapular views allow for true anteroposterior and lateral projections and decrease the possibility of superimposition which may obscure bony detail (Figure 3.5).

Superior displacement of greater tuberosity fractures can be well delineated on the AP and scapu-

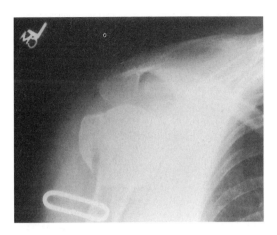

Figure 3.6(a) Although displacement of the distal spike of the greater tuberosity fragment from the shaft is noted on this Velpeau axillary view displacement proximal to the articular surface was minimal. This was therefore deemed a one-part fracture

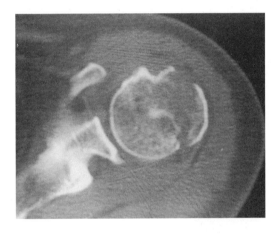

Figure 3.6(b) Confirmation of minimal superior tuberosity displacement from the articular surface as shown by CT scan

lar lateral views by assessing the distance of the fragment proximal to the insertion point of the rotator cuff just lateral to the articular surface, rather than by measuring the displacement of a distal bony spike of the tuberosity from the shaft[2] (Figures 3.6a,b). Appreciating the possibility of the greater tuberosity fragment being hidden by superimposition of the head, Phemister recom-

mended rotational anteroposterior radiographs for better visualization of these fractures[58]. Morris also noted that superior displacement of the greater tuberosity was adequately identified on plain radiographs but identification of its posterior displacement was misleading and he found that computed tomography better delineated location of both tuberosities. These findings were supported by Flatow *et al.*[2], who reported that 33% of a series of patients with displaced greater tuberosity fractures had *less* than 1 cm of superior displacement of the fragment on anteroposterior views, but all had more than 1 cm of posterior displacement on axillary radiographs. Ahovuo *et al.*[3] stated that displacement of both the lesser and greater tuberosities seemed to be more readily imaged with tangential intertubercular groove radiographs than with more conventional techniques. Three patients of 15 in this series were found to have tuberosity fragments displaced enough, as seen on this view, to require surgical treatment, which otherwise would not have been identified.

The axillary view not only allows for the evaluation of posterior displacement of the greater tuberosity, but also gives the best assessment of the glenohumeral articulation when determining anterior and posterior dislocations. Anteroposterior views of posterior dislocations provide only subtle findings of an internally rotated humeral head with the greater tuberosity superimposed over the humeral head, thus giving the appearance of a light-bulb. The overlap of the humeral head with the glenoid is missing, leaving an 'empty glenoid', which is suggestive of a posterior dislocation. The axillary view is therefore necessary to make the definitive diagnosis (Figures 2.7a,b). It is also quite valuable in identifying lesser tuberosity displacement, as the fragment is pulled medially by the subscapularis and often overlies the glenoid on anteroposterior films. This may often be misinterpreted as calcific tendinitis. The importance of this view has been stressed throughout the literature[26,32,59,60] and is best performed in the supine position with the arm held in only enough abduction so as to allow the beam to clear the body. If the patient is unable to co-operate, the Velpeau axillary is quite helpful and does not even require removal of the sling[61]. Computed tomography also plays a valuable role in assessing the degree of articular involvement in dislocations with impression fractures, articular surface defects and head-splitting fractures.

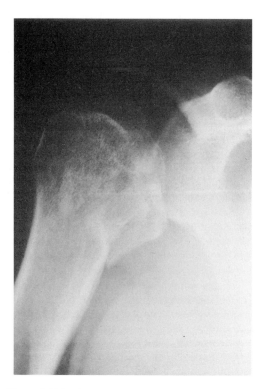

Figure 3.7(a)   Anteroposterior view showing an internally rotated humeral head, an empty glenoid in addition to a lesser tuberosity fracture

Treatment

Isolated greater tuberosity fractures

Various methods of treatment of two-part displaced greater tuberosity fractures have been recommended, from abduction splinting and sling immobilization[14,62–65] to fairly elaborate forms of open reduction and internal fixation[1,11,66–69]. Closed reduction is difficult to obtain and maintain due to posterior and superior displacement from the pull of the rotator cuff. DePalma[14] reviewed the results of 14 greater tuberosity fractures of uncertain degrees of displacement and reported that 12 of the 14 achieved good results with sling immobilization, although he did acknowledge that if the tuberosity was pulled under the acromion this would block abduction and compromise function. He implicated the biceps tendon and fracture of its groove as principal factors responsible for pain and dysfunction following fractures of the greater tuberosity, as did Ahovuo *et al.*[3].

Olivier *et al.*[11] reported on the non-operative results of 79 displaced and non-displaced greater tuberosity fractures, with only 69% rated as satisfactory. The fractures were separated according to tendon insertion sites and direction of displacement. These authors found that the worst results were in those fractures which were most displaced and involved the whole tuberosity. These displaced fractures were felt to be analogous with rotator cuff tears, and therefore the authors recommended open reduction and fixation with cerclage techniques rather than by screws.

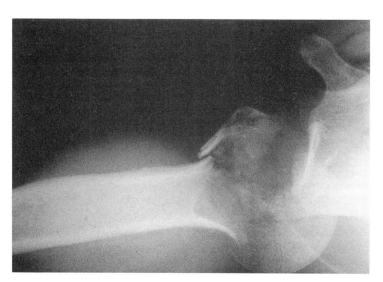

Figure 3.7(b)   Axillary view fully delineating a two-part posterior fracture dislocation

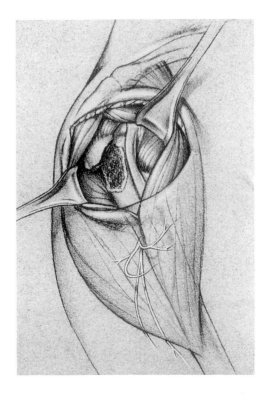

Figure 3.8 An oblique incision is made in Langer's lines 4–5 cm in length. The deltoid is then split, leaving its origin intact, from the anterolateral corner of the acromion to a point approximately 4 cm distally. In order to avoid injury to the axillary nerve, a stay suture is placed. (From Bigliani[21], by permission)

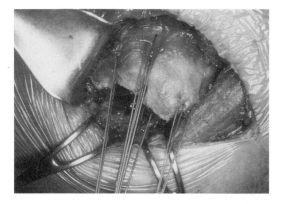

Figure 3.9 Mobilization of greater tuberosity with multiple heavy, non-absorbable sutures at the strong tendon–bone interface rather than through the osteoporotic tuberosity bone

In 1925, McWhorter reported on two cases of displaced greater tuberosity fractures treated by excision of the fragment and tendon repair as an alternative to non-operative management, but minimal data is available on this technique[4]. Open reduction and internal fixation appear to have been first described in the acute setting by Keen in 1907. Internal fixation has been achieved with screws[68,69], pins[66,67] and cerclage wiring[5,11].

It is now generally agreed that open reduction and internal fixation is the treatment of choice for fractures displaced 1.0 cm or more. McLaughlin reported that when displacement was less than 0.5 cm, a prolonged convalescence may be anticipated with an acceptable outcome without surgery. When the displacement was more than 0.5 cm but less than 1.0 cm, convalescence was usually in excess of 6 months, some permanent pain and disability were the rule and in about 20% of cases subsequent surgical intervention was mandated for late open reduction and internal fixation. Late

operations were difficult and were less satisfactory. He therefore advised whenever residual displacement *approached* 1.0 cm, early repair should receive serious consideration[55].

Most fractures can be adequately exposed by a superior approach which is made in Langer's lines just lateral to the anterolateral corner of the acromion. The deltoid is then split after placing a stay suture approximately 4 cm distal to the acromion in order to avoid injury to the axillary nerve which may be stretched with overzealous retraction (Figure 3.8). The fragment is then identified and mobilized with multiple heavy non-absorbable sutures inserted at the tendon–bone interface (Figure 3.9). This area is often stronger and holds sutures more securely than placing them through osteoporotic tuberosity bone where they may easily pull out. Once adequately mobilized, the fracture site is debrided and the fragment is returned to its bed (Figures 3.10a,b). The author prefers to stabilize the fragment with heavy, non-absorbable suture through drill holes in the shaft and bed. If the fragment is large it may require removal of a portion of the cancellous bone to be reduced. It is important to appreciate the presence of the three facets serving as insertions for the supraspinatus, infraspinatus and teres minor. Based on this anatomy, the fragment may be pulled superiorly and/or posteriorly depending upon the site of fracture within the tuberosity. Therefore, sutures need to be placed in such a fashion so as to bring the superior facet downward and the inferior facet of the teres minor forward in order to overcome the displacement forces. By definition, there is an associated rotator cuff tear

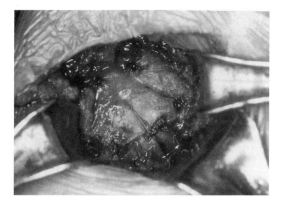

Figure 3.10(a)   Intraoperative photograph with tuberosity securely sutured through drill holes into its anatomical bed

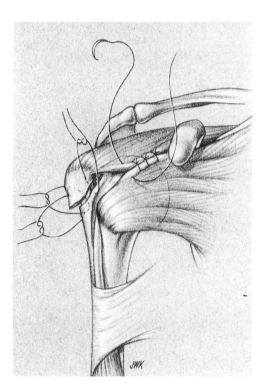

Figure 3.10(b)   Schematic drawing of tuberosity suture fixation to the head and shaft with repair of rotator cuff tear. (From Bigliani[21], by permission)

either in the rotator interval between the supraspinatus and subscapularis or posteriorly between the supraspinatus and infraspinatus which must be repaired. This is best repaired prior to suturing the greater tuberosity into its bed, as it will decrease the tension at the fracture site. The tuberosity is

then anatomically reduced and securely sutured to the shaft through drill holes. Early passive range of motion is then begun on the first postoperative day including pendulums, passive forward elevation, supine external rotation with a stick, and pulleys. Internal rotation and active motion are held for 6 weeks or until tuberosity and cuff healing have occurred. Advanced stretching and gentle strengthening exercises are then begun. We found good to excellent results in 12/12 patients treated in this manner, with average active forward elevation to 170° at an average of 5 years' follow-up[2].

Two-part anterior fracture-dislocation

These injuries should initially be treated by gentle atraumatic closed reduction if an associated surgical neck fracture can be reliably excluded by careful radiographs. In most instances, the ligaments and capsule will usually cause the fragment to reduce into good position after reduction of the dislocation[5,70,71] (Figures 3.11a, b). Prior to reduction manoeuvres, thorough neurovascular evaluation is warranted, as injuries to these structures are not uncommon. Reduction is performed with traction, abduction and gradual adduction and internal rotation after the head has reduced into the joint. The arm is then immobilized in a sling and swathe and repeat neurological exam performed. At times, the greater tuberosity will

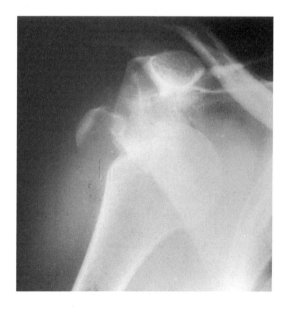

Figure 3.11(a)   Two-part anterior fracture-dislocation with displaced greater tuberosity fragment

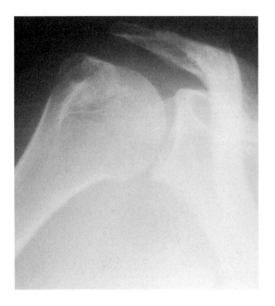

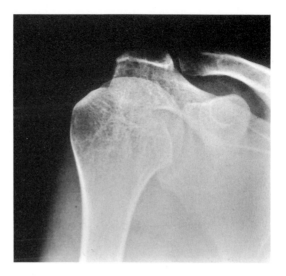

Figure 3.12(a)   Anteroposterior view of lesser tuberosity fracture. The fragment is obscured by superimposition over the humeral head.

Figure 3.11(b)   After closed reduction of the glenohumeral joint, the tuberosity fragment has reduced into its bed

remain displaced greater than 1.0 cm at which time it is treated as a two-part displaced fracture and open reduction should be performed. If the fragment reduces spontaneously with reduction of the joint, it must be followed closely radiographically as there is a tendency for these to redisplace in the early post-reduction period[55]. The prognosis is generally good as these cases have a lower redislocation rate secondary to the fact that the anterior ligaments have not been torn and, once greater tuberosity healing occurs, stability of the joint is restored[5]. There is a significant tendency toward stiffness; therefore, rehabilitation of this injury includes sling wear for not longer than 7–10 days at which time pendulum exercises are instituted. At 3 weeks, passive forward elevation and external rotation are added, with passive internal rotation and active forward elevation delayed for 6 weeks.

Two-part lesser tuberosity fractures

The rarity of the isolated lesser tuberosity fracture makes it difficult to be dogmatic about its treatment, as broad clinical experience is not reported. Most would agree that if the fragment is small and does not block medial rotation, successful outcome may be obtained by closed reduction and sling immobilization with early range of motion[1,5,21] (Figures 3.12a, b). Neer and others maintained that although the displacement produced spreading of

the anterior cuff fibres, neither of these defects was clinically significant unless a portion of the articular surface was broken off with the lesser tuberosity and/or a significant block to internal rotation developed[1,5,7,38,41,72]. In this latter case, open reduction and internal fixation are warranted in a manner similar to that described for greater tuberosity fractures, although exposure is better afforded by a deltopectoral or anterior axillary approach, preserving the deltoid origin. The subscapularis and attached lesser tuberosity are mobilized with stay sutures and returned to the freshened bed with sutures through drillholes in bone. Some authors have advised excision of the fragment by shelling it out of the subscapularis and anterior capsule with their subsequent repair[73]. Early passive motion is instituted on the first postoperative day, limiting external rotation to a point determined at surgery which will not place undue tension on the repair. Active motion is again held for 6 weeks or until adequate tuberosity healing has occurred.

Two-part posterior fracture-dislocations

The most important factor in obtaining a successful outcome with these injuries is to accurately identify the lesion at the initial presentation. Once identified, these injuries are best treated by closed reduction as long as the articular involvement is minimal. This may be performed gently with trac-

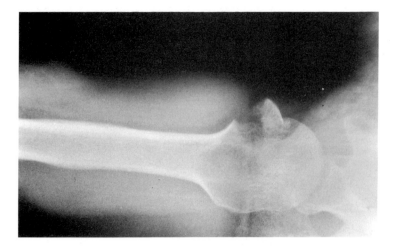

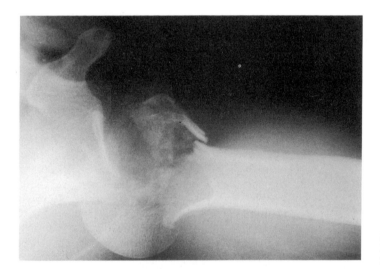

Figure 3.12(b) Axillary view identifies the small anteromedially displaced lesser tuberosity fragment. This fracture was successfully treated by non-operative measures

Figure 3.13(a) Two-part posterior fracture-dislocation prior to closed reduction

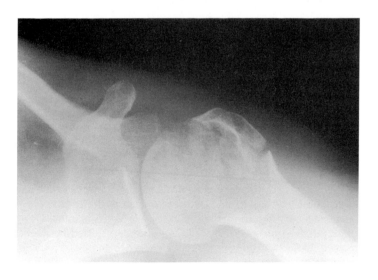

Figure 3.13(b) Post-reduction axillary reveals reduction of both glenohumeral joint and lesser tuberosity fracture

tion on the arm at 90° of forward flexion with gradual adduction, unlocking the head from behind the glenoid. The head may then be lifted into the joint by applying pressure posteriorly on the humeral head. This usually reduces both the joint and the tuberosity to an acceptable position (Figures 3.13a,b). The arm is then held in neutral to 10° of external rotation in a spica cast or splint for 6 weeks, with subsequent passive and active range of motion. DeMarquis reported a series of 13 posterior fracture-dislocations and recommended open treatment if significant displacement of the tuberosity persisted, as did Jakob and co-workers[1]. An osteochondral articular surface fracture may be associated with this injury which, if not reduced, may result in instability and joint incongruity thereby warranting open reduction[56]. Surgical reconstruction is best performed through an anterior deltopectoral approach with fixation as previously described using either heavy non-absorbable sutures or screw fixation. Open reduction is also indicated in those cases in which diagnosis has been delayed and the dislocation is irreducible by closed means. These cases are also best approached anteriorly, both for reduction of the joint and fixation of the fracture.

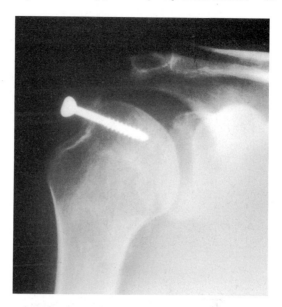

Figure 3.14 Loss of screw fixation into osteoporotic tuberosity bone leads to malunion with secondary impingement

Complications

Numerous complications specific to closed and open treatment of displaced tuberosity fractures and fracture-dislocations have been described, including malunion, adhesions, neurovascular injury, myositis ossificans and loss of fixation following repair[2,3,10,11,14,25,55,67,74]. Malunion is reported to be a primary cause of disability after greater tuberosity fracture[5,9–11,74,75]. Loss of fixation with resultant tuberosity malunion can result in bony impingement[14,43,74] and rotator cuff dysfunction[21,25,75,76] (Figure 3.14). Fixed retraction of the greater tuberosity superiorly may result in blockage of abduction, while a posteriorly displaced fragment can block external rotation by impinging against the posterior glenoid[25] (Figures 3.15a,b). As the arm is elevated this becomes accentuated and is often associated with pain. Malunion of fracture fragments involving the intertubercular groove has also been implicated as a source of pain, creating a potential disturbance in the gliding mechanism of the biceps tendon[3,14]. Associated rotator cuff dysfunction occurs due to shortening and/or loss of continuity, resulting in weakness and limited active abduction (if supra-

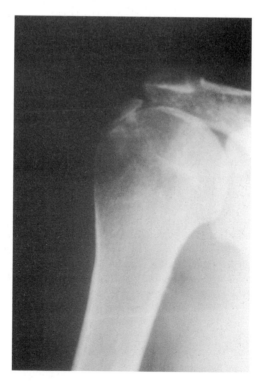

Figure 3.15(a) Fixed superior retraction of the greater tuberosity blocks abduction and forward elevation

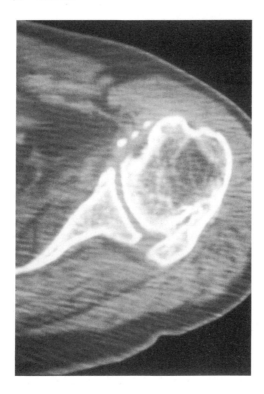

Figure 3.15(b) CT scan depicting greater tuberosity malunion with posterior retraction blocking external rotation as fragment impinges on posterior glenoid

spinatus is involved) and external rotation (infraspinatus and teres minor)[14,43,67,74]. Malunion of the lesser tuberosity fragment, although some spreading the anterior cuff fibres occurs, is usually not clinically significant unless the fragment is large enough to block internal rotation.

Joint stiffness with pain at the extremes may complicate the postoperative or post-fracture course if bursal and capsular adhesions are allowed to form. A conscientiously employed exercise programme can limit this problem if initiated early.

Neurovascular injuries, although less rare than in surgical neck fractures, occur primarily when tuberosity fractures are seen associated with dislocations. The axillary nerve is most commonly involved, but usually responds to watchful waiting. Follow-up care with EMGs to document progression of recovery or lack thereof is helpful to guide an appropriate treatment regimen.

References

1. Jakob, R.P., Kristiansen, T., Mayo, K. *et al.* Classification and aspects of treatment of fractures of the proximal humerus. In *Surgery of the Shoulder* (eds J.E. Bateman and R.P. Welsh), C.V. Mosby, St Louis (1984), pp. 330–343
2. Flatow, E.L., Cuomo, F., Maday, M.G. *et al.* Open reduction and internal fixation of two-part displaced fractures of the greater tuberosity of the proximal part of the humerus. *J. Bone Joint Surg.*, **73A**, 1213–1218 (1991)
3. Ahovuo, J., Paavolainen, P. and Björkenheim, J.M. Fractures of the proximal humerus involving the intertubercular groove. *Acta Radiol.*, **30**, 373–374 (1989)
4. McWhorter, G.L. Fracture of the greater tuberosity of the humerus with displacement. Report of two cases with author's technique of shoulder incision. *Surg. Clin. N. Am.*, **5**, 1005–1017 (1925)
5. Neer, C.S. II. Fractures about the shoulder. In *Fractures in Adults*, 2nd edn (eds C.A. Rockwood and D.P. Green), J.B. Lippincott, Philadelphia (1984), pp. 675–721
6. Ross, G.J. and Love, M.B. Isolated avulsion fracture of the humerus: report of two cases. *Radiology*, **172**, 833–834 (1989)
7. LaBriola, J.H. and Mahaghigh, H.A. Isolated avulsion fracture of the lesser tuberosity of the humerus: a case report and review of the literature. *J. Bone Joint Surg.* **57**, 1011 (1975)
8. Keene, J.S., Huizenga, R.E., Engber, W.D. *et al.* Proximal humerus fractures. A correlation of residual deformity with long-term function. *Orthopedics*, **6**, 173–178 (1983)
9. McLaughlin, H.L. Dislocation of the shoulder with tuberosity fracture. *Surg. Clin. N. Am.*, **43**, 1615–1620 (1963)
10. Morris, M.E., Kilcoyne, R.F., Shuman, W. *et al.* Humeral tuberosity fractures: evaluation by CT scan and management of malunion. *Orthop. Trans.*, **11**, 242 (1987)
11. Olivier, H., Duparc, J. and Romain, F. Fractures of the greater tuberosity of the humerus. *Orthop. Trans.*, **10**, 223 (1986)
12. Schlaepfer, K. Uncomplicated dislocation of the shoulder: Their rational treatment and late results. *Am. J. Med. Sci.*, **167**, 244–255 (1924)
13. Stevens, J.H. The action of the short rotators on the normal abduction of the arm, with a consideration of their action in some cases of subacromial bursitis and allied conditions. *Am. J. Med. Sci.*, **138**, 870–884 (1909)
14. DePalma, A.F. and Cautilli, R.A. Fractures of the upper end of the humerus. *Clin. Orthopaed. Rel Res.*, **20**, 73–93 (1961)
15. Henderson, R.S. Fracture-dislocation of the shoulder with interposition of the long head of the biceps. Report of a case. *J. Bone Joint Surg.*, **34B**, 240–241 (1952)
16. Laing, P.G. The arterial supply of the adult humerus. *J. Bone Joint Surg.*, **38A**, 1105–1116 (1956)
17. Moseley, H.F. and Goldie, I. The arterial pattern of the rotator cuff on the shoulder. *J. Bone Joint Surg.*, **45B**, 780–789 (1963)
18. Rothman, R.H. and Park, W.W. The vascular anatomy of the rotator cuff. *Clin. Orthopaed. Rel. Res.*, **41**, 176–186 (1965)

19. Tondeur, G. Les fractures récentes de l'epaule. *Acta Orthopaed. Belg.*, **30**, 1–144 (1964)

20. Watson-Jones, R. *Fractures and Joint Injuries*, 4th edn, Williams and Wilkins, Baltimore (1955)

21. Bigliani, L.U. Fractures of the proximal humerus. In *The Shoulder*, Vol. 1 (eds C.A. Rockwood, Jr and F.A. Matsen, III), W.B. Saunders, Philadelphia (1990), pp. 277–334

22. Dehne, E. Fractures at the upper end of the humerus. *Surg. Clin. N. Am.*, **25**, 28–47 (1945)

23. Drapanas, T., McDonald, J. and Hale, H.W. Jr. A rational approach to classification and treatment of fractures of the surgical neck of the humerus. *Am. J. Surg.*, **99**, 617–624 (1960)

24. Knight, R.A. and Mayne, J.A. Comminuted fractures and fracture-dislocations involving the articular surface of the humeral head. *J. Bone Joint Surg.*, **39A**, 1343–1355 (1957)

25. Neer, C.S. II. Displaced proximal humerus fractures. Part I. Classification and evaluation. *J. Bone Joint Surg.*, **52A**, 1077–1089 (1970)

26. Meyerding, H.W. Fracture-dislocation of the shoulder. *Minn. Med.*, **20**, 717–726 (1937)

27. Milch, H. The treatment of recent dislocations and fracture-dislocations of the shoulder. *J. Bone Joint Surg.*, **31A**, 173–180 (1949)

28. Dimon, J.H. III. Posterior dislocation and posterior fracture-dislocation. A report of 25 cases. *South. Med. J.*, **60**, 661 (1967)

29. Dorgan, J.A. Posterior dislocation of the shoulder. *Am. J. Surg.*, **89**, 890–895 (1955)

30. McLaughlin, H.L. Posterior dislocation of the shoulder. *J. Bone Joint Surg.*, **34A**, 584–588 (1952)

31. Rowe, C.R. Prognosis in dislocation of the shoulder. *J. Bone Joint Surg.*, **38A**, 957 (1956)

32. Wilson, J.C. and McKeever, F.M. Traumatic posterior dislocation of the humerus. *J. Bone Joint Surg.*, **31A**, 160–167 (1949)

33. Hall, M.C. and Rosser, M. The structure of the upper end of the humerus with reference to osteoporotic changes in senescence leading to fractures. *Can. Med. Ass.*, **88**, 290–294 (1963)

34. Horak, J. and Nilsson, B.E. Epidemiology of fractures of the upper end of the humerus. *Clin. Orthop. Rel. Res.*, **112**, 250–253 (1975)

35. Gibbons, A.P. Fracture of the tuberosity of the humerus by muscular violence. *Br. Med. J.*, **7**, 1674–1679 (1909)

36. Arndt, J.H. and Sears, A.D. Posterior dislocation of the shoulder. *Am. J. Roentgenol.*, **94**, 639–645 (1965)

37. Cocchi, U. Zur frage der epiphysenossifikation des humeruskopfes das tuberculum minus. *Radiol. Clin.*, **19**, 18–23 (1950)

38. Andreasen, A.T. Avulsion fracture of the lesser tuberosity of the humerus. *Lancet*, **1**, 750 (1941)

39. Earwaker, J. Isolated avulsion fracture of the lesser tuberosity of the humerus. *Skelet. Radiol.*, **19**, 121–125 (1990)

40. Shibuya, S. and Ogawa, K. Isolated avulsion fracture of the lesser tuberosity of the humerus: a case report. *Clin. Orthopaed. Rel. Res.*, **211**, 215–218 (1986)

41. Haas, S.L. Fractures of the lesser tuberosity of the humerus. *Am. J. Surg.*, **63**, 252 (1944)

42. Stangl, F.H. Isolated fracture of the lesser tuberosity of the humerus. *Minn. Med.*, **16**, 435–437 (1933)

43. Codman, E.A. The shoulder rupture of the supraspinatus tendon and other lesions in or about the subacromial bursa. Boston, privately printed (1934)

44. Ahlgren, O., Larentzon, R. and Larsson, S.E. Posterior dislocation of the shoulder associated with general seizures. *Acta Orthopaed. Scand.*, **52**, 694–695 (1981)

45. Carew-McColl, M. Bilateral shoulder dislocation caused by electric shock. *Br. J. Clin. Pract.*, **34**, 251–254 (1980)

46. Fipp, G.J. Simultaneous posterior dislocation of both shoulders. *Clin. Orthopaed. Rel. Res.*, **44**, 191–195 (1966)

47. Mills, K.L.G. Simultaneous bilateral posterior fracture-dislocation of the shoulder. *Injury*, **6**, 39–41 (1974–75)

48. Hawkins, R.J., Neer, C.S., Pianta, R.M., and Mendoza, F.X. Locked posterior dislocations of the shoulder. *J. Bone Joint Surg.*, **69A**, 9–18 (1987)

49. Cofield, R.H. Comminuted fractures of the proximal humerus. *Clin. Orthopaed. Rel. Res.*, **230**, 49–57 (1988)

50. Cotton, F.J. Subluxation of the shoulder downward. *Boston Med. Surg. J.*, **185**, 405–407 (1970)

51. Thompson, F.E. and Winant, E.M. Comminuted fracture of the humeral head with subluxation. *Clin. Orthopaed. Rel. Res.*, **20**, 94–97 (1961)

52. Zuckerman, J.D., Flugstad, D.L., Teitz, C.C. *et al.* Axillary artery injury as a complication of proximal humerus fractures. *Clin. Orthopaed. Rel. Res.*, **189**, 234–237 (1984)

53. Smyth, E.H.J. Major arterial injury in closed fractures of the neck of the humerus: report of a case. *J. Bone Joint Surg.*, **51**, 508 (1969)

54. Hawkins, R.J. Unrecognized dislocations of the shoulder. *Instruct. Course Lect.*, **34**, 258–263 (1985)

55. McLaughlin, H.L. Locked posterior subluxation of the shoulder. Diagnosis and treatment. *Surg. Clin. N. Am.*, **43**, 1621–1622 (1963)

56. Blasier, R.B. and Burkus, J.K. Management of posterior fracture-dislocations of the shoulder. *Clin. Orthopaed. Rel. Res.*, **232**, 197–204 (1988)

57. Ross, G.J. and Love, M.B. Isolated avulsion fracture of the humerus: report of two cases. *Radiology*, **172**, 833–834 (1989)

58. Phemister, D.B. Fractures of the greater tuberosity of the humerus. With an operative procedure for fixation. *Ann. Surg.*, **56**, 440–449 (1912)

59. Funsten, R.V. and Kinser, P. Fractures and dislocations about the shoulder. *J. Bone Joint Surg.*, **18**, 191–198 (1936)

60. Neer, C.S. II Displaced proximal humeral fractures. Part II. Treatment of three- and four-part displacement. *J. Bone Joint Surg.*, **52A**, 1090–1103 (1970)

61. Bloom, M.H. and Obata, W.G. Diagnosis of posterior dislocation of the shoulder with use of Velpeau axillary and angle-up roentgenographic views. *J Bone Joint Surg.*, **49**, 943–949 (1967)

62. Greeley, P.W. and Magnusson, P.B. Dislocation of the shoulder accompanied by fracture of the greater tuberosity and complicated by spinatus injury. *J. Am. Med. Ass.*, **102**, 1835–1838 (1934)

63. Sever, J.W. Fracture of the head of the humerus. Treatment and results. *New Engl. J. Med.*, **216**, 1100–1107 (1937)

64. Taylor, H.L. Isolated fracture of the greater tuberosity of the humerus. *Ann. Surg.*, **47**, 10–12 (1908)

65. Mills, H.J. and Horne, G. Fractures of the proximal humerus in adults. *Journal of Trauma*, **25**, 801–805 (1985)

66. Lovett, R.W. The diagnosis and treatment of some common injuries of the shoulder joint. *Surg. Gynecol. Obstet.*, **34**, 437–444 (1922)

67. Stevens, J.H. Fractures of the upper end of the humerus. *Ann. Surg.*, **69**, 147–160 (1919)

68. Müller, M.E., Allgöwer, M. and Willenegger, H. *Manual of Internal Fixation. Technique Recommended by the AO Group*, Springer, New York (1970)

69. Paavolainen, P., Bjorkenheim, J.M., Slätis, P. *et al.* Operative treatment of severe proximal humerus fractures. *Acta Orthopaed. Scand.*, **54**, 374–379 (1983)

70. Gratz, C.M. Anterior subglenoid dislocation with fracture of the greater tuberosity of the humerus. *Surg. Clin. N. Am.*, **10**, 549–551 (1930)

71. Roberts, S.M. Fractures of the upper end of the humerus. An end-result study which shows the advantage of early active motion. *J. Am. Med. Ass.*, **98**, 367–373 (1932)

72. McGuinness, J.P. Isolated avulsion fracture of the lesser tuberosity of the humerus. *Lancet*, **1**, 508 (1939)

73. Kunkel, S.S. and Monesmith, E.A. Isolated avulsion fracture of the lesser tuberosity of the humerus: a case report. *J. Shoulder Elbow Surg.*, **2**, 43–46 (1993)

74. Neviaser, J.S. Complicated fractures and dislocations about the shoulder joint. *J. Bone Joint Surg.*, **44**, 984–998 (1962)

75. Santee, H.E. Fractures about the upper end of the humerus. *Ann. Surg.*, **80**, 103–114 (1924)

76. Bigliani, L.U. Treatment of two- and three-part fractures of the proximal humerus. *Instruct. Course Lect.*, **38**, 231–244, American Academy of Orthopaedic Surgeons, Park Ridge, Illinois (1989)

77. Neer, C.S. II. Fractures. In *Shoulder Reconstruction*, W.B. Saunders, Philadelphia (1990), pp. 363–420

4

Two-part displaced surgical neck fractures

Mark W. Rodosky and Evan L. Flatow

Proximal humeral fractures are common, with the majority occurring in elderly patients, often women, as the result of a fall on level ground[1–3]. Nearly half of all proximal humeral fractures occur at the surgical neck[1,3,4]. Most of these are minimally displaced and stable, and may be treated nonsurgically[3,5–7]. By definition, the greater and lesser tuberosities remain attached to the humeral head in displaced two-part surgical neck fractures. For this reason, the head usually remains viable with a very low risk for the future development of avascular necrosis[8].

By strict criteria, surgical neck fractures are considered displaced when the measured angulation exceeds 45° and the displacement is more than 1 cm[9]. Although these criteria serve as a theoretical indication for the need of a closed or open reduction, in practice, more angulation and displacement may be tolerated, and is dependent on the functional demands of the individual patient[10,11]. Since the majority of these fractures occur in a population of elderly patients with lower functional demands, larger degrees of angulation and displacement are usually accepted. In these patients, surgery is most often contemplated when the fractures are non-impacted with minimal or no bony contact present between the humeral head and shaft.

Surgical treatment of displaced surgical neck fractures has involved a variety of techniques including skeletal traction, suture material, wire, screws, plates and screws, external fixators, pins and various types of intramedullary fixation.

Results of these various treatment types have been difficult to interpret because of variable preoperative indications, follow-up and methods of postoperative evaluation. Shoulder surgeons have been moving towards methods with more emphasis on soft tissue management including less stripping of fracture fragments as well as more incorporation of strong cuff tendons in osteoporotic patients with weak bone.

Indications for surgical treatment

In general, closed reduction should be considered when a surgical neck fracture is angulated more than 45°[12]. Larger amounts of angulation will have a negative influence on range of motion, especially elevation. However, in an elderly individual with a relatively low demand for normal shoulder range of motion, a stable impacted fracture with more than 45° of angulation may be acceptable. In contrast, a young athletic patient with very high demands for shoulder function and range of motion may require treatment when less than 45° of angulation is present.

In cases where a closed reduction is readily achieved but cannot be reliably maintained, percutaneous pin fixation may be useful[12–15]. However, if the closed reduction is unsuccessful, open reduction and internal fixation (ORIF) is indicated.

Closed reduction

In healthy patients who can be safely sedated, a closed reduction may be attempted in the emergency room. However, the most reliable way to perform a closed reduction is with general or regional (interscalene block) anaesthesia and image intensification, such as can be provided in the operating room. The possible need to proceed to open reduction if closed manoeuvres are unsuccessful must be discussed with the patient or their advocate when obtaining operative consent. They must understand the risk that a previously non-displaced tuberosity component might displace during manipulation and require a humeral head replacement. An explicit plan whether or not to proceed with open treatment must be formulated in order to prepare the operating room and staff for all possibilities.

In most displaced surgical neck fractures, the shaft is displaced anteriorly and medially by the pectoralis major (Figure 4.1). The close proximity of the medial neurovascular structures mandates the need for cautious and gentle reduction manoeuvres, especially when the shaft contains a spike. Abduction is to be avoided as it may increase the pull of the pectoralis major and further displace the shaft medially. The manoeuvre begins with the arm at the side in a relaxed neutral position. Gentle axial traction is applied in order to disimpact the malaligned fragments. The fragments are then realigned and impacted. Since the shaft is anterior and medial, the direct application of manual posterior and lateral pressure on the shaft should allow the fragments to realign. With axial compression in the realigned position, the fracture may be impacted in a satisfactory position. The next step is to test fracture stability by moving the arm in a limited arc such as would be allowed in a sling. This step may be carried out with the use of the image intensifier. If the reduction is obtained but unstable, pins may be introduced percutaneously across the fracture site to allow for interim stability in anticipation of early bone healing and removal of the pins at 4–6 weeks. If an adequate reduction is not obtained, or the pins cannot be placed in satisfactory position, open reduction must be considered.

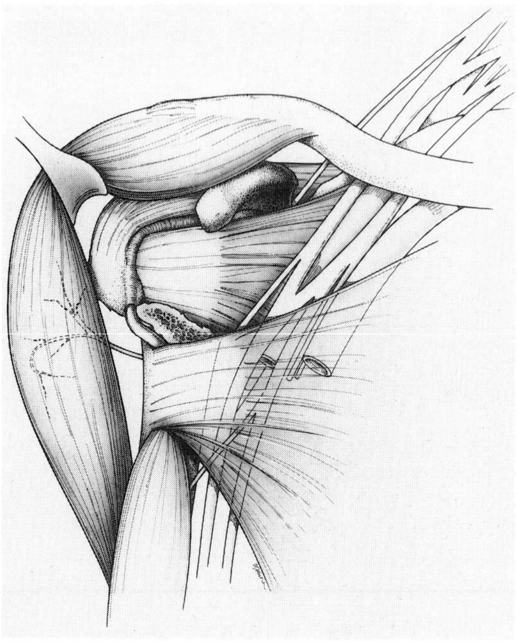

Figure 4.1   In displaced surgical neck fractures, the shaft is generally displaced anteriorly and medially by the pectoralis major. The medial spike of the proximal shaft may be in close proximity to the neurovascular pedicle

Open reduction and internal fixation

Many techniques of ORIF have been proposed for unstable surgical neck fractures. These have included skeletal traction[16], external fixation[17–19], staples[20], plates and screws[21–31], percutaneous pins[13–15], wire or suture loops[32–39], multiple small pins or screws and tension-band wiring[27,40–45], intramedullary devices[46–58], and tension-band intramedullary nail and wire constructs[5,12,59–64]. In the early 1970s, plate fixation was popularized by the AO group[25], but has become less desirable as surgeons have recently noted many problems with this technique, including avascular necrosis[22], loss of fixation in osteoporotic bone[15,26,45,65,66] and plate impingement on the surrounding tissues and acromion[26].

More recently, wire-loop or heavy suture fixation has been shown to be very advantageous as it allows incorporation of the strong rotator cuff tendons (often stronger than the surrounding osteoporotic bone) and minimizes soft tissue stripping[5,12,38,59,61,67,68]. This tension-band construct can be combined with intramedullary fixation in cases with bone loss or metaphyseal comminution, to achieve reliable longitudinal fixation[6].

Authors' preferred method of internal fixation

We employ a long deltopectoral approach, preserving the deltoid origin and insertion. A triangular portion of the leading edge of the coracoacromial ligament is resected for exposure. Partial release of the pectoralis major is often helpful in achieving reduction. To avoid injury to the brachial plexus and axillary artery, the shaft is carefully mobilized under direct vision.

Once adequate exposure is achieved, heavy non-absorbable sutures or wire incorporating the rotator cuff tendons are used to provide internal fixation (Figure 4.2). Sutures through the strong rotator cuff tendon insertion are usually more secure than other types of fixation in soft osteoporotic bone[61]. Wires provide greater immediate stability, but are often problematic as they may become an irritant in the subacromial space and may also break and migrate. When bone loss or comminution is encountered, wire or suture fixation alone may be inadequate[69], and longitudinal fixation is therefore supplemented with intramedullary rods or nails placed in the non-articular surface just inside the greater or lesser tuberosities. These devices do little damage to the rotator cuff as they are inserted through small longitudinal incisions in the cuff tendons. They augment longitudinal and rotational stability and enhance the rigidity of the fixation. Originally we used Rush pins, but they often migrated superiorly, impinging against the acromial undersurface, and afforded little rotational stability. Our recent experience is with Ender nails which are superior to straight rods since they provide three-point fixation[60,62]. The figure-of-eight wire or suture is then passed through the eyelets of the nails helping to prevent superior migration. However, the slot is long and an appreciable amount of metal can still protrude proximally (Figure 4.3). We have recently modified the Ender nail with an additional hole above this slot for suture or wire incorporation (Figure 4.4). With this addition, the nail can be inserted deeper into the head, so that its proximal tip is well below the surface of the cuff tendons[61]. The suture or wire is passed deep to the tendon, preventing proximal migration of the nail. We have had one patient fracture at the tip of two Ender

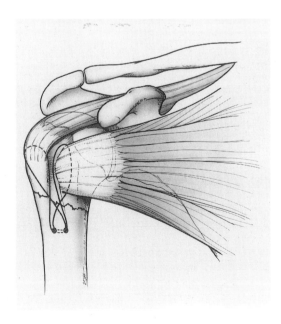

Figure 4.2 Heavy non-absorbable sutures or wire are used for fixation. They incorporate the rotator cuff tendon, which is generally stronger than the soft, osteoporotic bone (From Cuomo *et al.*[61], by permission)

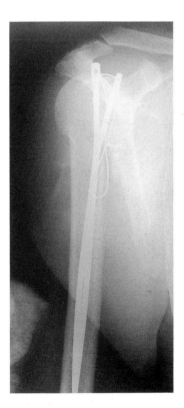

Figure 4.3 Tension-band construct using wire through the eyelet of the Ender nail. Because the slot is long, an appreciable amount of metal may protrude proximally

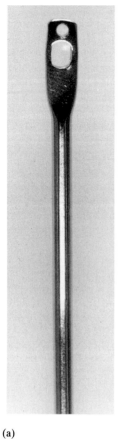

(a)

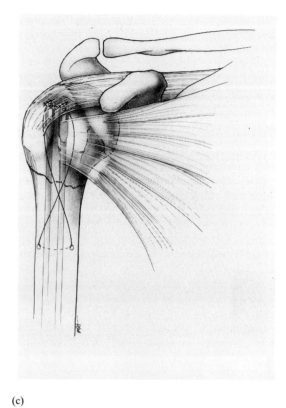

(c)

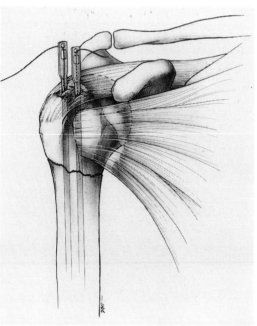

(b)

Figure 4.4 Use of Ender nail for fixation: (a) modified
Ender nail with added hole above slot; (b) the nails are
introduced through small (1 cm) longitudinal incisions in the
rotator cuff insertion, and the suture or wire is brought
through the proximal holes and under the intervening cuff
tendon; (c) the nails are driven distally until just the hole
protrudes above the cortex, which leaves the proximal end of
the nail below the surface of the rotator cuff tendon; the
suture is passed figure-of-eight through drill holes in the
shaft. (From Cuomo *et al.*[61], by permission)

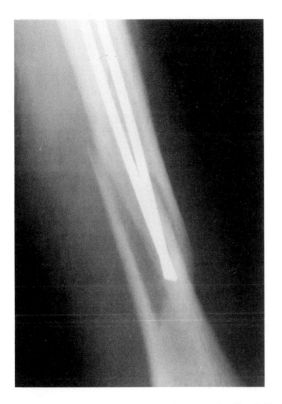

Figure 4.5 This patient fell onto his arm, and suffered this fracture of the humeral shaft at the level of the distal ends of the Ender rods

nails of the same length (Figure 4.5); using nails of different lengths may help to reduce the risk of stress concentration.

After the fixation is employed, the shoulder is put through a range of motion and the stability of the fixation assessed. The rotator cuff incisions, deltopectoral interval and skin are closed. Suction drains are used to avoid haematoma formation. On the first or second postoperative day, passive elevation in the plane of the scapula and pendulum exercises are generally begun. Depending on the stability observed at surgery, gentle assistive exercises may also be introduced, including pulley elevation and external rotation with a stick. Active motion is begun after bone and tendon healing, generally at 6 weeks, and resistive exercises are added later.

Results of ORIF

Our results with this technique have been recently reported[61]. Ten of 14 (71%) two-part displaced surgical neck fractures achieved good or excellent results (Figure 4.6). The average range of motion in these patients at an average follow-up of 3.3 years was 145° of elevation, 43° of external rotation, and internal rotation with the hand able to reach the level of the 11th thoracic vertebra posteriorly. All fractures healed. One patient had partial loss of fixation with wire-loop fixation. The fracture shortened, but maintained an acceptable reduction and final result. Serial radiographs revealed maintenance of reduction in all other cases. No heterotopic bone was encountered.

Prior to the use of the modified Ender nails, two patients required removal of Ender nails when they were noted to be prominent after fracture healing. No infections or non-unions were noted. One patient, as mentioned above (see Figure 4.5), fell onto the arm and suffered a humeral shaft fracture at the level of the tips of the two Ender rods. This eventually healed with non-operative management.

Conclusion

The use of heavy non-absorbable sutures incorporating the rotator cuff tendons, tuberosities and shaft of the humerus in a tension-band construct is a reliable method of fixation for unstable two-part displaced surgical neck fractures. In cases of bone loss or comminution, this type of tension-band construct can be augmented with intramedullary Ender rods for added longitudinal and rotational stability. The secure fixation provided with these techniques allows for early rehabilitation.

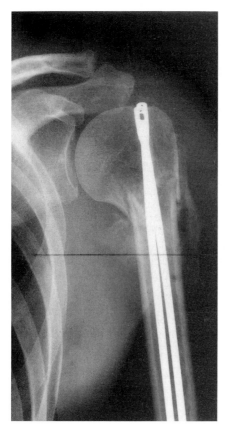

(a)

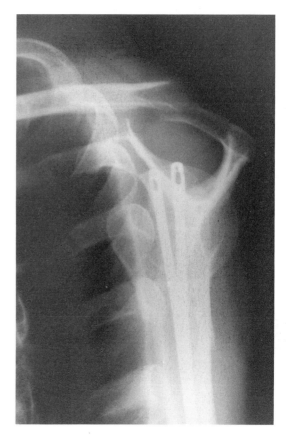

(b)

(c)

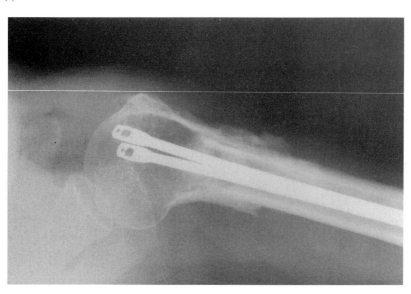

Figure 4.6 Results of ORIF: (a) AP radiograph 2 years after open reduction and internal fixation utilizing heavy sutures and Ender nails; (b) lateral radiograph at 2 years; (c) axillary radiograph at 2 years; (d) active elevation at 2 years; (e) active external rotation with the arms at the side at 2 years; (f) external rotation with the arms at 90° elevation at 2 years; (g) internal rotation at 2 years

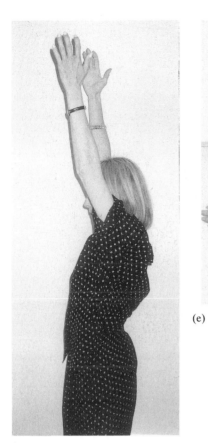

(d)

Figure 4.6 *cont.*

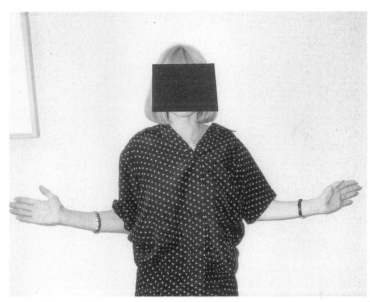

(e)

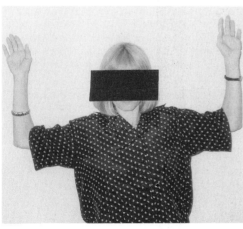

(f)

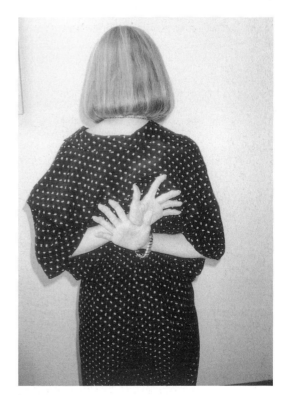

(g)

References

1. Horak, J. and Nilsson, B.E. Epidemiology of fracture of the upper end of the humerus. *Clin. Orthop.*, **112**, 250–253 (1975)
2. Kristiansen, B., Barford, G., Bredesen, J., Erin-Madsen, J., Grum, B., Horsnaes, M.W. and Aalberg, J.R. Epidemiology of proximal humeral fractures. *Acta Orthop. Scand.*, **58**, 75–77 (1987)
3. Lind, T., Kroner, K. and Jensen, J. The epidemiology of fractures of the proximal humerus. *Arch. Orthop. Trauma Surg.*, **108**, 285–287 (1989)
4. Rose, S.H., Melton, L.J., Morrey, B.F., Ilstrup, D.M. and Riggs, B.L. Epidemiologic features of humeral fractures. *Clin. Orthop.*, **168**, 24–30 (1982)
5. Bigliani, L.U. Shoulder trauma. In *Orthopaedic Knowledge Update 2* American Academy of Orthopaedic Surgeons, Park Ridge, Illinois (1987)
6. Cofield, R.H. Comminuted fractures of the proximal humerus. *Clin. Orthop.*, **230**, 49 (1988)
7. Razemon, J.P. and Baux, S. Les Fractures et les Fractures-Luxations de L'Extrémité Supérieure de L'Humérus. *Rev. Chir. Orthop.*, **55**, 387 (1969)
8. Laing, P.G. The arterial supply of the adult humerus. *J. Bone Joint Surg.*, **38A**, 1105–1116 (1956)
9. Neer, C.S. II. Displaced proximal humeral fractures. Part I. Classification and evaluation. *J. Bone Joint Surg.*, **52A**, 1077 (1970)
10. Kristiansen, B., Angerman, P. and Larsen, T.K. Functional results following fractures of the proximal humerus. A controlled clinical study comparing two periods of immobilization. *Arch. Orthop. Trauma Surg.*, **108**, 339–351 (1989)
11. Rasmussen, S., Hvass, I., Dalsgaard, J., Christensen, B.S. and Holstad, E. Displaced proximal humeral fractures: results of conservative treatment. *Injury*, **23**(1), 41–43 (1992)
12. Bigliani, L.U. Fractures of the proximal humerus. In: *The Shoulder* (eds C.A. Rockwood Jr. and F.A. Matsen III), W.B. Saunders, Philadelphia (1990)
13. Bohler, J. Les fractures recentes de l'epaule. *Acta Orthop. Belg.*, **30**, 235 (1964)
14. Jaberg, H., Warner, J.J.P. and Jakob, R.P. Percutaneous stabilization of unstable fractures of the humerus. *J. Bone Joint Surg.*, **74A**, 508–515 (1992)
15. Jakob, R.P., Kristiansen, T., Mayo, K., Ganz, R. and Muller, M.E. Classification and aspects of treatment of fractures of the proximal humerus. In *Surgery of the Shoulder* (eds J.E. Bateman and R.P. Welsh), C.V. Mosby, St Louis (1984), pp. 330–343
16. Caldwell, J.A. and Smith, J. Unimpacted fractures of the surgical neck of the humerus. *Am. J. Surg.*, **31**, 141 (1936)
17. Kristiansen, B. and Borgwardt, A. Fracture healing monitored with strain gauges. External fixation of 7 humeral neck fractures. *Acta Orthop. Scand.*, **63**(6), 612–614 (1992)
18. Kristiansen, B. External fixation of proximal humerus fracture. Clinical and cadaver study of pinning technique. *Acta Orthop. Scand.*, **58**, 645 (1987)
19. Kristiansen, B. and Kofoed, H. Transcutaneous reduction and external fixation of displaced fractures of the proximal humerus. A controlled clinical trial. *J. Bone Joint Surg.*, **70B**, 821 (1988)
20. Lorenzo, F.T. Osteosynthesis with Blount's staples in fractures of the proximal end of the humerus. A preliminary report. *J. Bone Joint Surg.*, **37A**, 45 (1955)
21. Bandi, W. Zur operative Therapie der Humeruskopf- und -halsfrakturen. *Hefte Unfallheilk.* **126**, 38 (1975)
22. Kristiansen, B. and Christensen, S.W. Proximal humeral fractures. Late results in relation to classification and treatment. *Acta Orthop. Scand.*, **58**, 124 (1987)
23. Kristiansen, B. and Christensen, S.W. Plate fixation of proximal humeral fractures. *Acta Orthop. Scand.*, **57**, 320 (1986)
24. Moda, S.K., Chadha, N.S., Sangwan, S.S., Khurana, D.K., Dahiya, A.S. and Siwach, R.C. Open reduction and fixation of proximal humeral fractures and fracture-dislocations. *J. Bone Joint Surg.*, **72B**, 1050 (1990)
25. Muller, M.E., Allgower, M. and Willenegger, H., *Manual of Internal Fixation*, Springer-Verlag, New York (1970), pp. 118–119
26. Paavolainen, P., Bjorkenheim, J-M., Slatis, P. and Paukku, P. Operative treatment of severe proximal humeral fractures. *Acta Orthop. Scand.*, **54**, 374 (1983)
27. Saitoh, S., Latta, L. and Milne, E. Osteoporosis of proximal humerus. 36th Annual Meeting, *Trans. Orthop. Res. Soc.*, **36**, 192 (1990)
28. Savoie, F.H., Geissler, W.B. and Vander Griend, R.A. Open reduction and internal fixation of three-part fractures of the proximal humerus. *Orthopaedics*, **12**, 65 (1989)
29. Sehr, J.R. and Szabo, R.M. Semitubular blade plate for fixation in the proximal humerus. *J. Orthop. Trauma*, **2**, 327 (1989).
30. Weise, K., Meeder, P.J. and Wentzensen, A. Indikation und Operationstechnik bei der Osteosynthese von Oberarmkopfluxationsfrakturen des Erwachsenen. *Langenbecks Arch. Chir.*, **351**, 91 (1980)
31. Yamano, Y. Comminuted fractures of the proximal humerus treated with hook plate. *Arch. Orthop. Trauma Surg.*, **105**, 359 (1986)
32. Dehne, E. Fractures at the upper end of the humerus. A classification based on the etiology of the trauma. *Surg. Clin. N. Am.*, **25**, 28 (1945)
33. Drapanas, T., McDonald, J. and Hale, H.W. Jr. A rational approach to the classification and treatment of fractures of the surgical neck of the humerus. *Am. J. Surg.*, **99**, 617 (1970)
34. Howard, N.J. and Eloesser, L. Treatment of fractures of the upper end of the humerus. An experimental and clinical study. *J. Bone Joint Surg.*, **32**, 1 (1934)
35. Mason, J.M. The treatment of dislocation of the shoulder-joint complicated by fracture of the upper extremity of the humerus, with an analysis of sixty-three cases with fracture at the neck of the humerus and twenty-one cases with fracture of the greater tuberosity reported since 1894. *Ann. Surg.* **47**, 672 (1908)
36. McBurney, C. and Dowd, C.N. Dislocation of the humerus complicated by fracture at or near the surgical neck, with a new method of reduction. *Ann. Surg.*, **19**, 399 (1894)

37. Meyerding, H.W. Fracture-dislocation of the shoulder. *Minnesota Med.*, **20**, 717 (1937)

38. Neer, C.S. II. Displaced proximal humeral fractures. Part II. Treatment of three-part and four-part displacement. *J. Bone Joint Surg.*, **52A**, 1090 (1970)

39. Worsdorfer, O. and Magerl, F. Operative Behandlung der Proximalen Humerusfrakturen. *Hefte Unfallheilkd.*, **160**, 136 (1982)

40. Lim, T.E., Ochsner, P.E., Marti, R.K. and Holscher, A.A. The results of treatment of comminuted fractures and fracture dislocations of the proximal humerus. *Nether. J. Surg.*, **35**, 139 (1983)

41. Magerl, F. Osteosynthesen im Bereich der Schulter pertuberkulare Humerusfrakturen, Skapulahalsfrakturen. *Helv. Chir. Acta*, **41**, 225 (1974)

42. Rosen, H. Tension band wiring for fracture dislocations of the shoulder. In *Proceedings of the International Society of Orthopaedic Surgery and Traumatology* (eds J. Delchef, R. DeMarneffe and V. Elst), Tel Aviv, Israel (9–12 October 1972)

43. Ruedi, T. The treatment of displaced metaphyseal fractures with screws and wiring systems. *Orthopaedics*, **12**, 55 (1989)

44. Siebler, G., Walz, H. and Kuner, E.H. Minimalosteosynthese von Oberarmkopffrakturen. Indikation, Technik, Ergebnisse. *Unfallchirurg.*, **92**, 169 (1989)

45. Sturzenegger, M., Fornaro, E. and Jakob, R.P. Results of surgical treatment of multifragmented fractures of the humeral head. *Arch. Orthop. Trauma Surg.*, **100**, 249 (1982)

46. Haas, K. Displaced proximal humeral fractures operated by Rush pin technique. *Opuscula Medica*, **23**, 100 (1978)

47. Hermann, O.J. Fractures of the shoulder joint with special reference to correction of defects. *Instruct. Course Lect.*, **2**, 359, American Academy of Orthopaedic Surgeons, Park Ridge, Illinois (1944)

48. Johansson, O. Complications and failures of surgery in various fractures of the humerus. *Acta Chir. Scand.*, **120**, 469–478 (1961)

49. Lentz, W. and Meuser, P. The treatment of fractures of the proximal humerus. *Arch. Orthop. Traumat. Surg.*, **96**, 283 (1980)

50. Mazet, R. Intramedullary nailing in the arm and the forearm. *Clin. Orthop.*, **2**, 75 (1953)

51. Mestdagh, H., Butruille, Y., Tillie, B. and Bocquet, F. Resultats du traitement des fractures de l'extrémité supérieure de l'humérus par embrochage pércutane. *Ann. Chir.*, **38**, 5 (1984)

52. Mouradian, W.H. Displaced proximal humeral fractures. Seven years' experience with a modified Zickel supracondylar device. *Clin. Orthop.*, **212**, 209 (1986)

53. Poilleux, F. and Courtois-Suffit, M. Des Fractures du Col Chirurgical de L'Humerus. *Rev. Chir.*, **75**, 133–158 (1954)

54. Seidel, H. Humeral locking nail: a preliminary report. *Orthopaedics*, **12**, 219 (1989)

55. Svend-Hansen, H. Displaced proximal humeral fractures. A review of 49 patients. *Acta Orthop. Scand.*, **45**, 359–364 (1974)

56. Weseley, M.S., Barenfeld, P.A. and Eisenstein, A.L. Rush pin intramedullary fixation for fractures of the proximal humerus. *J. Trauma*, **17**, 29 (1977)

57. Widen, A. Fractures of the upper end of humerus with great displacement treated by marrow nailing. *Acta Chir. Scand.*, **97**, 439 (1949)

58. Yano, S., Takamura, S. and Kobayashi, I. Use of the spiral pin for fracture of the humeral neck. *J. Jap. Orthop. Ass.*, **55**, 1607 (1981)

59. Bigliani, L.U. Treatment of two- and three-part fractures of the proximal humerus. *Instruct. Course Lect.*, **38**, 231, American Academy of Orthopaedic Surgeons, Park Ridge, Illinois (1989)

60. Contreras, D., Day, L., Bovill, D. and Appleton, A. Combined Enders rods and tension banding for humeral neck fractures. Poster, 57th Annual Meeting, American Academy of Orthopaedic Surgeons, New Orleans, Louisiana (9 February 1990)

61. Cuomo, F., Flatow, E.L., Maday, M.G., Miller, S.R. McIlveen, S.J. and Bigliani, L.U. Open reduction and internal fixation of two- and three-part displaced surgical neck fractures of the proximal humerus fractures. *J. Shoulder Elbow Surg.*, **1**, 287–295 (1992)

62. Day, L. My indications for closed versus open versus prosthesis. My technique for 2-part. Presented at Symposium: Update on Treatment of Displaced Proximal Humeral Fractures, 4th Open Meeting, American Shoulder and Elbow Surgeons, Atlanta, Georgia (7 February 1988)

63. Norris, T.R. Fractures of the proximal humerus and dislocations of the shoulder. In *Skeletal Trauma* (eds B.D. Browner, J.B. Jupiter, A.M. Levine, and P.G. Trafton), Philadelphia, W.B. Saunders (1992), pp. 1201–1290

64. Watson, K.C. Modification of Rush pin fixation for fractures of the proximal humerus. Presented at the American Shoulder and Elbow Surgeons Annual Meeting, Santa Fe, New Mexico (November 1988)

65. Hall, M.C. and Rosser, M. The structure of the upper end of the humerus with reference to osteoporotic changes in senescence leading to fractures. *Can. Med. Ass. J.*, **88**, 290 (1963)

66. Rappaport, J.R., Morris, S., Brennan, M.J. and Day, L.J. Two part humeral surgical neck fractures – outcome of treatment. *Orthop. Trans.*, **11**, 242 (1987)

67. Neer, C.S. II. *Shoulder Reconstruction*, Saunders, Philadelphia (1990), pp. 373–375

68. Szyszkowitz, R., Seggl, W., Schleifer, P. and Cundy, P.J. Proximal humeral fractures. Management techniques and expected results. *Clin. Orthop.*, **292**, 13–25 (1993)

69. Koval, K.J., Sanders, R., Zuckerman, J.D., Helfet, D.L., Kummer, F. and DiPasquale, T. Modified-tension band wiring of displaced surgical neck fractures of the humerus. *J. Shoulder Elbow Surg.*, **2**, 85–92 (1993)

70. Keene, J.S., Huizenga, R.E., Engber, W.D. and Rogers, S.C. Proximal humeral fractures. A correlation of residual deformity with long-term function. *Orthopedics*, **6**, 173 (1983)

71. Mills, H.J. and Horne, G. Fractures of the proximal humerus in adults. *J. Trauma*, **25**, 801–805 (1985)

5

Treatment of three-part displaced fractures of the proximal humerus

Theodore F. Schlegel and Richard J. Hawkins

Displaced three-part proximal humeral fractures remain a challenging problem for the orthopaedic surgeon. Neer's experience with proximal humeral fractures has greatly facilitated a rational guideline for their treatment based on a well-designed classification scheme[1]. Successful treatment relies on the surgeon's ability to make an accurate diagnosis, which requires a thorough understanding of the complex shoulder anatomy coupled with a precise radiographic examination. Appropriate and realistic goals need to be established in all cases. The patient's general medical health, physiological age and ability to co-operate with intense and prolonged rehabilitation will need to be considered when deciding on treatment.

This chapter reviews the pertinent anatomy, radiographic views and classification scheme necessary for understanding the treatment rationale of displaced three-part proximal humeral fractures. Treatment options along with potential complications are discussed, and a detailed description of the rehabilitation programme is outlined.

Anatomy

Bony architecture

The proximal humerus consists of four well-defined parts which include the humeral head, the lesser and greater tuberosities and the proximal humeral shaft. There exists a well-defined relationship between these parts, with the neck shaft inclination angle measuring an average of 145° in relationship to the shaft and retroverted on average

30°. The proximal humerus develops from three distinct ossification centres, including one for the humeral head and one each for the lesser and greater tuberosities. The humeral head ossification centre usually appears between the fourth and sixth month of life. The ossification centre of the greater tuberosity arises during the third year of life and the lesser tuberosity during the fifth year of life. The tuberosities fuse together by the fifth year of life and, in turn, fuse with the humeral head during the seventh year of life. Usually by the age of 19 the head and shaft have fused together. The fusion of the ossification centres creates a weakened area in the construct, known as the epiphyseal scar, making these regions of the proximal humerus susceptible to fracture.

The rotator cuff and girdle muscles

The rotator cuff and shoulder girdle muscles create forces on the proximal humerus as a result of their inherent pull. This balance is disrupted when one or several of the parts of the proximal humerus are fractured. Understanding these deforming forces will facilitate treatment.

The pectoralis major and deltoid are most influential on the shaft, or the distal fracture segment. The pectoralis major inserts along the lateral lip of the proximal bicipital groove, having the greatest effect on the humeral shaft, displacing it anterior and medial. The deltoid, with its more distal insertion on the humeral shaft, is a less deforming force on the distal fracture segment.

The proximal fragments, consisting of the articular head segment as well as the lesser and greater tuberosities, are most influenced by the rotator cuff musculature. Three of the four rotator cuff muscles, including the supraspinatus, infraspinatus and teres minor, insert onto the greater tuberosity, creating an outward rotational force on the humeral head. This is opposed by the remaining rotator cuff muscle, the subscapularis, which inserts on the lesser tuberosity, producing an inward rotational force on the head. In the uninjured state, a dynamic balance of these two forces exists. When there is a disruption of these forces, as in the case of a fracture of one of the tuberosity segments, a predictable rotatory deformity of the head occurs.

If the greater tuberosity is fractured, the attached cuff muscles will tend to pull the tuberosity superiorly and posteriorly into an externally rotated position, while the humeral head tends to rotate medially, secondary to the unopposed pull of the subscapularis. In cases in which the lesser tuberosity is fractured, the subscapularis will pull the detached tuberosity medially, while the humeral head will rotate posteriorly and externally as a result of the unopposed pull by the supraspinatus, infraspinatus and teres minor. Understanding the deformities created by the shoulder girdle and rotator cuff muscle will assist in both the classification and treatment of these fractures.

Arterial contributions

Disruption of the arterial blood supply to the proximal humerus from trauma or surgical intervention can result in avascular necrosis of the humeral head. There are three main arterial contributions to the proximal humerus[2–5]. The major arterial contribution to the humeral head segment is the anterior humeral circumflex artery (Figure 5.1). This usually lies anterior to the humeral shaft, travelling medial to lateral to anastomose with the posterior humeral circumflex. During its course it gives off an anterolateral ascending branch. This ascending branch runs parallel to the lateral aspect of the long head of the biceps tendon and enters the humeral head where the proximal end of the intertrabecular groove meets the greater tuberosity. The terminal portion of this vessel, the arcuate artery, is interosseous in nature and perfuses the entire epiphysis[2,3]. Laing was first to identify this vessel and document its importance in the vascularity of the humeral head. Gerber confirmed its significance in a cadaveric study, demonstrating that the vessel was responsible for perfusing the entire epiphysis, and that if this vessel were

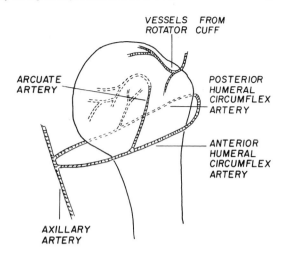

Figure 5.1 Blood supply of the proximal humerus

injured, only an anastomosis distal to the lesion could compensate for the resulting loss of blood supply.

Less significant blood supply to the humeral head is delivered by a branch of the posterior humeral circumflex artery, as well as the small vessels entering through the rotator cuff insertions. The posterior humeral circumflex artery, which penetrates the posteromedial cortex of the humeral head, is felt to supply only a small portion of the posterior inferior part of the articular surface of the humerus. The vessels that enter the epiphysis via the rotator cuff insertions are also felt to be inconsequential as well as inconsistent in their vascular supply to the humeral head when compared to the arcuate artery.

Classification

In order for a classification system to be functional, it must be designed to provide a means for an accurate reproducible diagnosis, allow for ease of communication, and direct treatment and effect prognosis. The system must be comprehensive enough to encompass all factors, yet specific enough to allow for an accurate diagnosis and treatment[6]. Over the years, a wide array of classification systems have been proposed. In the past, they have been based on the anatomical level of location of the fracture, mechanism of injury, amount of contact by fracture fragments, degree of displacement and vascular status of the articular segment[7–10]. These systems have failed in their ability to provide a functional classification system with an inability to reproduce diagnosis and treat these complex injuries.

Codman[1] was the first to propose that fractures of the proximal humerus occurred in four parts: the greater tuberosity, the lesser tuberosity, the head and the shaft. He appreciated that the fracture lines followed the old healed epiphyseal plates, delineating the tuberosities and anatomical head from the diaphysis. This was a significant advancement in the understanding of proximal humeral fractures and their treatment.

In 1970, Neer[1,12] described a classification based on the displacement of these four segments. Later, he eliminated numbered groups and detailed the application of the simplified version, referring only to the segments involved. A segment is considered to be displaced if it is separated from its neighbouring segment by more than 1 cm or angulated more than 45°. The fracture pattern refers to the number of displaced parts (segments – e.g. two-part, three-part or four-part). Comminutions in a number of fracture fragments or lines are irrelevant unless they fit into a previously described classification. Unfortunately, Neer's system does not consider all the various sub-patterns that affect treatment, but it is the accepted standardized classification, at least in North America.

It is important to appreciate that the terminology used to identify proximal humeral fractures denotes first the 'pattern of displacement' and secondly the 'key segment' displaced. Thus in the three-part pattern, a displaced tuberosity is always considered the 'key segment' even though a displaced shaft segment is also present (e.g. three-part greater tuberosity displacement). With fracture-dislocations, the fracture pattern is again identified first, but the direction of the dislocation replaces the key segment in the description. A fractured tuberosity segment is always displaced in the direction opposite the dislocation. Therefore, a three-part anterior fracture-dislocation would refer to anterior dislocation of the head and attached lesser tuberosity and posterior displacement of the greater tuberosity. The position of the associated displaced shaft segment is variable.

Radiographic evaluation

An accurate diagnosis is essential for the proper treatment of proximal humeral fractures. Three radiographic views are required in any shoulder injury to ensure consistent identification of fracture types (Figure 5.2a–c). Radiographs of the injured shoulder are taken first, perpendicular to, and second, parallel to, the scapular plane[12]. Although fracture fragments may be shifted with any movement of the patient's arm, it is nevertheless important to consider the axillary view in 20–40 degrees of abduction essential as a third view, for three reasons. First, it contributes valuable additional information regarding the fracture configuration, since it is orientated at right angles to the two previous views. Secondly, it is the most reliable means of detecting a locked posterior dislocation with an impression fracture. Thirdly, it provides assessment of the glenoid margins. Each of these views may be obtained with the patient in a standing, sitting or supine position. These three plain radiographs are sufficient to make an accurate diagnosis. On occasion, computed axial tomography will be helpful in further defining the magnitude of humeral head defects and assessing glenoid pathologies.

Treatment rationale

The treatment of displaced three-part proximal humeral fractures is based on proper classification of the fracture type, appreciation of the patient's activity level, and experience of the treating surgeon. Appropriate and realistic goals need to be established. The patient's general medical health, physiological age and ability to co-operate with an intense and prolonged rehabilitation should be considered. Based on these features, some patients should not be exposed to operative intervention. It is imperative that there is a full appreciation of the fracture pattern, bone quality and associated injuries when deciding on the method of treatment. Finally, a self-appraisal with regards to knowledge and expertise must be made by the treating surgeon. These complex proximal humeral fractures can challenge even the most experienced shoulder surgeons.

Non-operative management

In selected cases, accepting the deformity of the displaced three-part proximal humeral fracture is an option. In those patients who are medically unfit or are unable to participate in the intense rehabilitation programme surgical intervention may not be warranted. Non-operative treatment, by simply accepting the deformity, may often result in malunion with pain and stiffness of the shoulder[1,13,14]. Attempts to improve the deformity

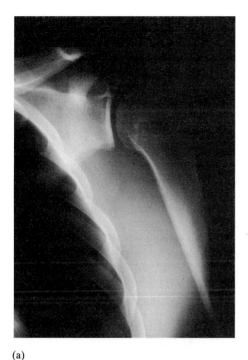

(a)

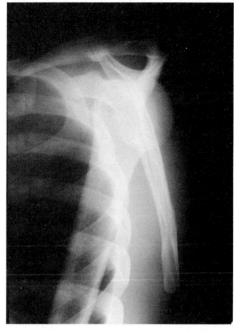

(b)

Figure 5.2 (a–c) Standard radiographic examination of the shoulder: three required views

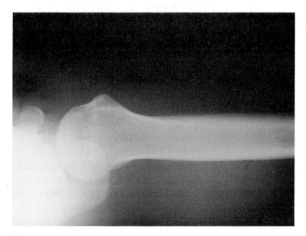

(c)

through closed reduction are often difficult. Even if the fracture reduction is obtained, it is even more difficult to maintain the reduction through closed means. Non-operative treatment should be reserved for sedentary patients, patients with medical problems, or those with limited expectations.

Closed reduction and percutaneous pinning

This method of treatment has been proposed as a means of achieving acceptable results with min-

imal disruption of the surrounding blood supply and soft tissues. Jaberg *et al.*[15] reported on results of this method of treatment for unstable fractures of the proximal humerus. This treatment is based on the premise that an acceptable closed reduction of the fracture fragments can be obtained. Once this is achieved, the fragments are held in position with multiple percutaneous wires. This allows for limited internal fixation which ideally protects the vascular supply to the humeral head, and hence prevents the risk of avascular necrosis.

A review of the patients managed with this form of treatment demonstrated 70% satisfactory results. Unfortunately, this series of displaced proximal humeral fractures represented a disproportionate number (75%) of two-part fractures. These results, therefore, are skewed in favour of less severe fractures, which have a propensity for more favourable results. Thus, this study may not be indicative of the outcome which can be expected for displaced three-part fractures. The head and shaft can often be reduced and pinned, but reduction of the tuberosity segment is extremely difficult.

This technique has been noted by its authors to be technically demanding and technique dependent. Although described as minimally invasive, it is not without complications which include loss of fixation, malunion/non-unions, superficial and deep wound infections, as well as avascular necrosis.

Open reduction and internal fixation

T-Plate

This form of treatment was once very popular, but several recent studies have reported high rates of failure with inferior results when compared to tension-band wiring[14,16,17]. There are several disadvantages of this method of treatment. First, this technique involves extensive soft tissue dissection, which may potentially disrupt the remaining blood supply to the humeral head leading to osseous necrosis. Secondly, depending on age, there is a great variability in the quality of cancellous bone stock in the humeral head and shaft. This affects screw purchase and ultimate fixation of the fracture fragments. Patients who are older and are known to have osteoporosis may have too high a fracture rate for this form of treatment. Lastly, there can be a tendency to place the hardware too proximal which will result in secondary impingement. In these cases, a second surgical procedure is required for removal of hardware after the fracture has healed. It is for these reasons that this technique has fallen out of favour for the treatment of most displaced three-part proximal humeral fractures. However, in a young patient with good bone stock, it remains an option.

Tension-band wire technique

This form of treatment was popularized by Hawk-

ins and co-workers[18] who reported satisfactory results in a series of 14 patients with three-part proximal humeral fractures. The advantages of this method of management include adequate visualization of the fracture fragments, ensuring appropriate reduction with minimal soft tissue stripping, preservation of the vascular supply to the humeral head, and secure fixation of the fracture fragments relying on soft tissue and not bone. Complications with this treatment have been reported to be minimal. Avascular necrosis of the humeral head did develop in two patients, only one of whom was symptomatic enough to require revision to hemiarthroplasty. It is unknown if the avascular necrosis was secondary to the initial trauma or a result of surgery. But despite these two cases, the overall complication rate was low and functional results were good.

Tension-band wiring has become the accepted method of treatment for three-part proximal humeral fractures since it allows for reduction and secure enough fixation of the fracture fragments to allow early passive range of motion. It is important to let the reader know that tension-band wiring alone is not satisfactory for two-part shaft displacement fractures. For some reason, the fracture construct is too often unstable, hinging on the tension-band side. This has been our experience and has been recently reported by Koval *et al.*[19].

Immediate hemiarthroplasty

Infrequently, patients with displaced three-part humeral fractures may be candidates for immediate prosthetic replacement. In some rare cases, older patients may have soft tissue attachments which are poor and not capable of providing adequate blood supply to the head or serving as a means of rigid fixation. It is in these special cases that Tanner and Cofield[20] have suggested that shoulder function may be more predictable if immediate hemiarthroplasty is performed. It should be noted, however, that these cases are usually the exception and, in most cases, the quality of the rotator cuff tissue is adequate for blood supply as well as a means for fixation.

Operative procedure

The patient is positioned on the operating room table in a semi-sitting 'beach chair' position, intubated, and the head is rotated to the contralateral side. To prevent the patient from sliding down the operating room table, a pillow is placed behind the knees and a seat belt across the patient's thighs. A bladder of a blood pressure cuff may be positioned underneath the ipsilateral scapula and inflated to bring the shoulder into the most advantageous position for surgical approach. A sterile drape is placed across the neck to prevent hair and saliva from contaminating the wound. Intravenous antibiotics are administered to the patient 30 min prior to surgical incision and two doses postoperatively. Preoperatively, the patient is instructed to scrub the shoulder and axillary region for a total of 5 min with a Hibiclens solution. This allows for the use of a single step preparation, consisting of a Betadine solution in an alcohol base, to provide antimicrobial properties as well as enhancing the ability for the drapes to stick to the patient, maintaining a sterile field. A sterile stockinette allows for free manipulation of the arm. A large sterile drape may be applied anteriorly and then wrapped completely and circumferentially to seal off the axilla and to hold the drapes in the appropriate position.

Surgical approach

Bony landmarks are outlined with a surgical marker. An extended deltopectoral approach is employed, measuring 12–15 cm in length, originating at the anterolateral corner of the acromion, curving toward the coracoid and ending at the deltoid insertion (Figure 5.3). The cephalic vein in this case is taken medially so that it is not traumatized during the extensive dissection. If the vein is taken laterally, often excessive tension is placed on the vein, leading to rupture. The insertion of the pectoralis major is partially released for exposure. Abducting the humerus during the procedure aids in relaxing the deltoid. If excessive deltoid tension is present, a transverse division of the anterior 1 cm of the deltoid insertion distally improves exposure, and more importantly, lessens damage to the deltoid. Blunt dissection is then carried out in the subacromial space to free up any adhesions. A deltoid retractor is placed deep to the deltoid and acromion and superficial to the rotator cuff and humeral head. The coracoacromial ligament may be released superiorly for improved exposure.

The long head of the biceps tendon serves as the key landmark in separating the greater and lesser tuberosity segments, allowing for identification of the fracture fragments. Almost all of these fractures involve the greater tuberosity. The fracture pattern is visually confirmed by verifying that the

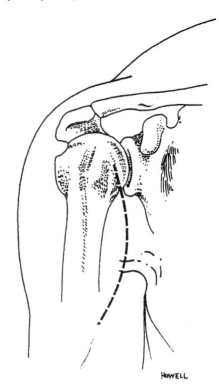

Figure 5.3 Extended deltopectoral approach.

lesser tuberosity remains attached to the humeral head, the displaced greater tuberosity with its attached supraspinatus tendon lies laterally and posteriorly and there is displacement between the humeral head and shaft. The articular surface of the humeral head is usually directed posteriorly, directed away from the glenoid fossa, often facing lateral (Figure 5.4a, b). It is necessary to free the humeral head by blunt dissection and confirm that the head does not have a rare impaction or head-splitting fracture.

Mobilization of the fracture fragments

A stay suture is placed into the supraspinatus tendon and greater tuberosity, allowing for mobilization of this fragment. This will aid in reduction of the fragment back to the bed from which it was avulsed. The humeral head can then be reduced with external rotation of the arm and pushing on the head fragment while rotating it into the glenoid fossa. Simultaneously, the greater tuberosity frag-

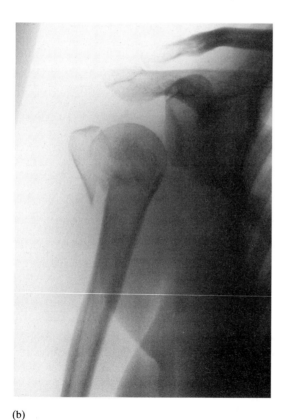

(a)

(b)

Figure 5.4 (a, b) A three-part fracture with a displaced greater tuberosity and an unimpacted, displaced segment of the head

ment is brought down to its anatomical position, which assists in holding the head reduced.

Reduction of fracture fragments

A 14-gauge large-bore colpotomy needle, with its stylet in place, is passed through the supraspinatus tendon and its attached greater tuberosity, through the head and out through the lesser tuberosity and subscapularis tendon. An 18-gauge wire is then passed into the bore of the colpotomy needle after the stylet is removed (Figure 5.5). The needle is then withdrawn to deliver the wire through the above segments. A second wire is then passed in a similar manner by placing the colpotomy needle 1 cm above and parallel to the first wire.

Two sets of drill holes are made perpendicular to the long axis of the shaft through the anterior aspect of the proximal portion of the distal shaft fragment, on each side of the bicipital groove, to accept the two previously passed wires (Figure 5.5). The head is then reduced onto the humeral shaft. The free end of the first wire, which lies lateral to the humerus, is then crossed over the fracture site to the medial aspect of the distal fragment segment and passed through the drill hole from medial to lateral. This forms a figure-of-eight pattern, and provides tension-band wiring of the fracture (Figure 5.6). The second wire is then passed in an identical fashion through the remaining holes. With the fracture reduced, the wires are secured using a wire tightener. Occasion-

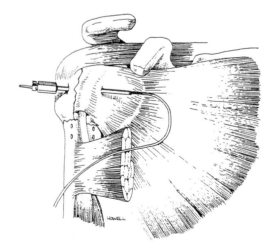

Figure 5.5 Reduction of fracture fragments and preparation for tension-band wiring

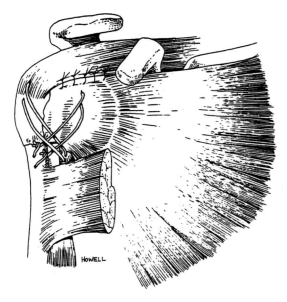

Figure 5.6   Figure-of-eight tension-band wiring technique

ally, in more stable constructs, one wire is sufficient.

Crossing the wires over the site of the fracture brings the segments of the head and shaft together and also compresses the segments of the head and greater tuberosity, thus converting the three-part pattern to a stable one-piece unit. Strong non-absorbable suture such as a no. 5 could be employed, but in our experience it does not cinch down as effectively and does not provide as much stability as wire. The rent between the supraspinatus and subscapularis tendon is then repaired, and the shoulder is carefully moved through a range of motion to confirm the stability of the fracture. Prior to closure, it is imperative to confirm that the humeral head is reduced within the glenoid.

Postoperative care

Usually, secure fixation of the fracture fragments is obtained and passive range of motion can begin immediately. If, as rarely occurs, the bone is found to be excessively osteoporotic or the rotator cuff is of poor quality, thereby making the fixation tenuous, the patient may be left relatively immobilized in a sling until secure, usually for 3 weeks.

Rehabilitation

Progression of the rehabilitation programme must be individualized to optimize the recovery of shoulder function. The surgeon and the physiotherapist must convey to the patient a clear understanding of what is expected for short- and long-term goals. The postoperative management programme has three well-defined phases: phase I consists of passive or assisted range of motion; phase II is active range of motion with terminal stretching; phase III is a resisted programme with ongoing active motion and terminal stretching.

Phase I begins on day 1, especially with the aid of an interscalene block for early pain control, and continues for 6 weeks. It is essential to confirm that the fracture fragments move in unison, signifying fracture stability. This phase may rarely need to be delayed for up to 4 weeks in some cases if the fixation is not rigid. This phase consists of passive forward elevation, and external and internal rotation of the involved shoulder with the assistance of the contralateral extremity. Assisted exercises begin in the supine position with early emphasis on elevation and external rotation. Pendulum exercises are used as a warm-up after a few days. Several days later, those exercises are performed sitting or standing. Towards the end of this initial 6-week phase, isometric strengthening may be added. These are performed by applying gentle resistance to inward and outward rotation when the arm is at the side and the elbow is flexed to 90°. Similar exercises are performed for flexion and extension. These activities need to be monitored carefully by the physician and the physiotherapist. They are taught to the patient and the patient's spouse so that they can be carried out at home.

Phase II, commencing at 6 weeks, consists of active range of motion exercises with terminal stretching, beginning once early union has been achieved, confirmed clinically and radiographically. When commencing phase II, resumption of the supine position permits concentration on forward elevation and is often advisable when starting the second phase of the programme, at least for a few days until the patient is strong enough to elevate in the upright position. Full active range of motion in all planes is sought during this phase.

Phase III, resisted strengthening, begins 10 weeks after surgery when union is assured and adequate range of motion has been obtained. The challenge to achieve normal shoulder function is met with greater resistance during the strengthening exercises and the ongoing terminal stretching programme. Maximal recovery is rarely achieved before the first postoperative year. All too frequently, the exercise programme is abandoned too early which does not allow the patient to reach full recovery potential.

Complications

There have been many reported complications following closed and open treatment of displaced three-part proximal humeral fractures. These can be thought of as non-specific or specific to the fracture pattern. Infection, neurovascular injury, malunion/non-union, hardware failure, joint stiffness and heterotopic ossification can result after the treatment of any proximal humeral fracture. Avascular necrosis, on the other hand, is more likely to occur in four-part displaced proximal humeral fractures and rarely with three-part fractures[1].

Infection is rare with open reduction and internal fixation of displaced three-part proximal humeral fractures. Fortunately, the proximal humerus has adequate soft tissue coverage with good vascular supply to the tissues, decreasing the risk of infection. However, infection is still possible and it is for this reason care should be taken to maintain sterility, administer prophylactic antibiotics and minimize excessive soft tissue dissection. Obtaining haemostasis at the time of closure and appropriately draining the wound is important to prevent haematoma formation which increases the potential risk for infection.

Neurovascular injuries have been well documented following displaced proximal humeral fractures. Stableforth[21] reported a 5% incidence of axillary artery compromise and a 6.2% incidence of brachial plexus injuries. Vascular injury most often is associated with penetrating or violent blunt trauma caused by the initial injury, but also occurs after open reduction and internal fixation[22]. If a vascular disruption occurs, the lesion is usually found at the junction of the anterior humeral circumflex and axillary artery. The diagnosis is often difficult to make, since peripheral pulses may be normal as a result of collateral circulation. Paraesthesiae may be a helpful clinical sign. Since early diagnosis and repair are crucial to the outcome, angiography and exploration should be performed without delay when a vascular injury is suspected.

The axillary nerve is the most susceptible to injury following fractures with and without dis-location of the proximal humerus. The axillary nerve provides motor supply to the deltoid and teres major with sensory distribution over the lateral aspect of the upper arm. Sensation over the lateral deltoid region is not a reliable means of determining if there is an axillary nerve injury. A more reliable means of testing the axillary nerve is palpating all three leaves of the deltoid muscle for contraction. Due to pain in an acute fracture, this is often difficult to accurately assess. Electromyelography should be obtained if a nerve injury is suspected. This study should be obtained no earlier than 3 weeks after the injury when the results are most accurate, both for documentation and as a baseline for subsequent comparisons of recovery. The majority of these injuries are secondary to a neuropraxia and improve with time. If a complete axillary nerve injury does not improve within a three- to six-month period, surgical exploration may be considered.

Malunion of the proximal humerus can cause significant functional limitations. In the case where the greater tuberosity heals in a superior or medial position, the space beneath the subacromial arch will be limited and impingement will occur when the arm is abducted. This problem can be corrected with a salvage surgical procedure which requires an osteotomy of the greater tuberosity and mobilization of the rotator cuff. This is often difficult because the anatomy is quite distorted and there is often extensive scarring.

Non-union at the surgical neck is not an infrequent complication, more common with two-part displaced shaft fractures but occasionally with three-part fractures. Interposition of soft tissue, excessive soft tissue dissection, inadequate immobilization, poor patient compliance or over-aggressive physical therapy may contribute to non-union. Treatment in these cases usually includes open reduction and internal fixation, autogenous bone grafting and spica cast immobilization. Intra-medullary (Rush) nails with tension-band wiring is a preferred method of internal fixation for these difficult cases. Rarely, arthroplasty is performed.

Joint stiffness can occur as a result of either closed or open treatment. Prolonged immobilization can result in bursal or capsular adhesions. Prominent hardware (i.e. rods/plates) can contribute to limited mobility. Persistence with daily terminal stretching programmes is the best management, but may require up to 18 months for full benefit. Forced manipulation risks refracture and is rarely indicated.

Heterotopic ossification appears to be related to

both repetitive forceful attempts at closed reduction and delay in open reduction beyond 1 week for fracture/dislocations. Inadequate irrigation to wash out bony fragments following open reduction and internal fixation may also increase the risk. Exercises to maintain range of motion should be the mainstay of treatment. After 1 year if a negative bone scan indicates quiescence, excision of the heterotopic bone with soft tissue releases may be considered.

Avascular necrosis of the head is one of the most severe complications following displaced three-part proximal humeral fractures. It results from disruption of the vascular supply to the humeral head. This is generally considered to be a complication of four-part fractures, but may occur after three-part fractures and can even occur in some two-part fractures. Avascular necrosis is reported to be as high as 90% in four-part fractures and anywhere from 3% to 25% in three-part fractures[1,22]. The incidence of avascular necrosis was noted to be slightly higher in those patients undergoing open reduction and internal fixation compared to closed treatment. Factors responsible for disruption of blood supply may include the initial trauma of the injury, the extensive soft tissue dissection for open reduction or damage by methods of internal fixation. It is uncertain how many individuals who develop avascular necrosis will become symptomatic enough to warrant further surgery. If resorption or collapse of the articular segment occurs, pain and loss of motion may result. In these cases, hemiarthroplasty can usually provide pain relief and functional improvement. Total shoulder arthroplasty may be necessary if joint incongruity involves the glenoid surface.

Conclusion

Operative treatment is indicated for the healthy, active individual who has a three-part displaced fracture of the proximal humerus. We believe the best results of these difficult fractures are obtained with the use of a figure-of-eight tension-band wiring technique. Adequate exposure provided by the extended deltopectoral approach helps to identify, reduce and stabilize the fracture. It is essential to incorporate the attachment of the subscapularis and supraspinatus tendons in the repair to provide the primary fixation to aid in stabilizing the fracture. A total reliance on bone for fixation with wire would likely lead to failure. Finally, a prolonged, closely monitored and well-defined programme of rehabilitation is necessary to obtain the best functional results. The ultimate outcome may be limited for many of these patients because of their age or concomitant medical problems, but in general a near full range of motion and normal function should be the goal.

References

1. Neer, C.S. II. Displaced proximal humeral fractures, part II: treatment of three-part and four-part displacement. *J. Bone Joint Surg.*, **52A**, 1090 (1970)
2. Gerber, C., Schneeberger, A.G. and Vinh, T. The arterial vascularization of the humeral head. *J. Bone Joint Surg.*, **10A**, 1486–1494 (1990)
3. Laing, P.G. The arterial supply of the adult humerus. *J. Bone Joint Surg.*, **38A**, 1105 (1956)
4. Moseley, H.F. and Goldie, I. The arterial pattern of the rotator cuff on the shoulder. *J. Bone Joint Surg.*, **45B**, 780 (1963)
5. Rathburn, J.B., and McNabb, I. The microvascular pattern of the rotator cuff. *J. Bone Joint Surg.*, **52B**, 540 (1970)
6. Rockwood, C.A. and Matsen, F.A. *The Shoulder*. W.B. Saunders, Philadelphia (1990)
7. Drapanas, T., MacDonald, J. and Hale, H.J. Jr. A rational approach to classification and treatment of fractures of the surgical neck of the humerus. *Am. J. Surg.*, **99**, 617 (1960)
8. Knight, R.A. and Mayne, J.A. Comminuted fractures and fracture/dislocations involving the articular surface of the humeral head. *J. Bone Joint Surg.*, **39A**, 1343 (1957)
9. Kocher, T. *Beitrage zur Kenntnis Einigen Praktisch Wichtigen Fracturenforman*. Carl Sallman Verlag, Basel (1896)
10. Watson-Jones, R. *Fractures and Joint Injuries*, 5th edn, Williams and Wilkins, Baltimore (1955)
11. Codman, E.A. *The Shoulder*. Thomas Todd, Boston (1934).
12. Neer, C.S. II. Displaced proximal humeral fractures, part I: classification and evaluation. *J. Bone Joint Surg.*, **52A**, 1077 (1970)
13. Horak, J. and Nilsson, B.E. Epidemiology of fracture of the upper end of the humerus. *Clin. Orthop.*, **112**, 250 (1975)
14. Kristiansen, B., Barfod, G., Bredesen, J. *et al*. Epidemiology of proximal humeral fractures. *Acta Orthop. Scand.*, **50**, 75 (1987)
15. Jaberg, H., Warner, J.P. and Jakob, R. Percutaneous stabilization of unstable fractures of the humerus. *J. Bone Joint Surg.*, **74A**, 508 (1992)
16. Paavolainen, P., Bjorkenheim, J.M., Slatis, P. *et al*. Operative treatment of severe proximal humeral fractures. *Acta Orthop. Scand.*, **54**, 374 (1983)
17. Sturzenegger, M. Fornaro, E. and Jakob, R.P. Results of surgical treatment of multi-fragmented fractures of the humeral head. *Arch. Orthop. Traumat. Surg.*, **100**, 249 (1982)
18. Hawkins, R.J., Bell, R.H. and Gurr, K. The three-part fracture of the proximal part of the humerus: operative treatment. *J. Bone Joint Surg.*, **68A**, 1410 (1986)

19. Koval, K.J., Sanders, R., Zuckerman, J.D. *et al.* Modified tension band wiring of displaced surgical neck fractures of the humerus. *J. Shoulder Elbow Surg.*, March/April (1993)

20. Tanner, M.W. and Cofield, R.H. Prosthetic arthroplasty for fracture and fracture-dislocations of the proximal humerus. *Clin. Orthop.*, **179**, 116 (1983)

21. Stableforth, P.G. Four-part fractures of the neck of the humerus. *J. Bone Joint Surg.*, **66B**, 104 (1954)

22. Hagg, O. and Lundberg, B. Aspects of prognostic factors of comminuted and dislocated proximal humeral fractures. In *Surgery of the Shoulder* (eds J.E. Bateman and R.P. Welsh), B.C. Decker, Philadelphia (1984)

6

Four-part and head-splitting fractures of the proximal humerus: treatment with prosthetic replacement

Edward B. Self and Louis U. Bigliani

Fractures of the proximal humerus are most commonly non-displaced or minimally displaced, and are best treated non-operatively[1–7]. Results of treatment of the most severely displaced fractures of the proximal humerus, however, have not been consistently satisfactory when treated with non-operative measures[3,6,8,11,12] or with open reduction and internal fixation (ORIF)[8,11–14]. The four-segment classification of proximal humeral fractures developed by Neer in 1970[8], which he later simplified[5,9], made the descriptive account of proximal humeral fractures by Codman[10] clinically relevant. This classification is now widely accepted, can guide in the treatment of these fractures[5,8] and has prognostic significance. Because of the poor results of non-operative treatment or ORIF for these severe fractures, Neer introduced prosthetic arthroplasty with tuberosity reconstruction[15]. Numerous reports in the literature have documented the results of this procedure[3,8,11,12,16–24].

This chapter reviews the indications for humeral head replacement for displaced four-part fractures of the proximal humerus, head-splitting fractures and head-impression fractures. The review includes initial evaluation, indications for prosthetic arthroplasty, surgical technique and postoperative rehabilitation. Complications of humeral head replacement for fracture are reviewed in a separate chapter.

Initial evaluation

Initial evaluation includes a thorough examination of the patient as well as of the fracture radio-graphically. Evaluation of the patient begins with a close examination of the injured shoulder, including neurovascular assessment of the extremity. Axillary and musculocutaneous nerve function, both motor and sensory, as well as the other peripheral nerves should be specifically examined. Injury to the axillary artery may occur, particularly in fracture dislocations, and can be limb threatening. Closed injury to the brachial plexus or peripheral nerves requires documentation and may be treated expectantly. Electromyography at 3–4 weeks following injury may help clarify the extent of involvement. Neurological injury should not delay the definitive management of the fracture, as most nerve injuries are neuropraxias and will resolve sufficiently to allow adequate function[19,25]. Nerve exploration and reconstruction can be done later, between 3 and 6 months, if necessary. The patient's general medical condition must also be carefully evaluated, and possible additional occult associated injuries must be ruled out or identified and treated. One must also evaluate the mental status of the patient to determine whether or not the patient will be able to understand and complete the rigorous and extensive postoperative rehabilitation programme necessitated by prosthetic replacement. This is the appropriate time to discuss the expected surgical outcome with the patient, and to educate the patient regarding the extensive postoperative rehabilitation that will be necessary to ensure a satisfactory outcome. What are the functional demands and activities of daily living performed by the patient, and what are the patient's expectations regarding surgical care?

Proper X-ray evaluation should include the trauma series of the shoulder, consisting of a true anteroposterior view of the glenohumeral joint perpendicular to the scapula and a true lateral or Y-view of the shoulder, parallel to the scapula[8]. These views may be supplemented with an axillary view performed by abducting the arm 20–30° and placing the tube in the axilla with the plate above the shoulder. There is no need to fully abduct the arm. Often the physician must personally position the patient for this X-ray, as the patient is apprehensive and the X-ray technician fearful to move the injured extremity. Alternatively, a Velpeau axillary view[26] can be obtained, with the patient remaining in the sling and leaning back over the plate with the tube directed downwards. A CT scan may also be helpful in selected cases to better evaluate the articular surface of the humeral head. With these views, the surgeon is able to identify the four fragments and classify the fracture. The location of the head fragment in relation to the tuberosities and shaft must be determined. A part must be displaced greater than 1 cm or angled greater than 45° to be considered 'displaced'. Loss of blood supply to the head fragment due to fracture displacement can lead to avascular necrosis[2,5,8,11,13,16,27–29]. The head can also be split (Figure 6.1) or have a significant impression defect (greater than 40% involvement) in it. This may often be only appreciated on the axillary projection radiograph or CT scan cuts (Figure 6.2).

In the so-called 'valgus impacted' four-part fracture, the articular segment is rotated laterally and impacted onto the shaft[30,31] (Figures 6.3a–c). The tuberosities overlie the joint surface and the articular surface of the head is out of contact with the glenoid. Often, the head fragment may not be impacted, but only displaced laterally. However, it is still not in contact with the glenoid. In true fracture dislocations, the head fragment is completely displaced from the glenoid – anteriorly, posteriorly or inferiorly. The other fragments or 'parts' are classified with reference to their position in relation to the head fragment. If the head fragment is displaced from the shaft, lesser tuberosity and greater tuberosity, it is classified a four-part fracture (Figures 6.4a, b). A not infrequent situation occurs when the head is displaced from the shaft and the tuberosities; however, the tuberosities remain attached to each other. Since the head has been totally displaced from all bone or soft tissue attachment, such a case is classified as a four-part fracture. Careful examination of the radiographs and understanding of the guidelines

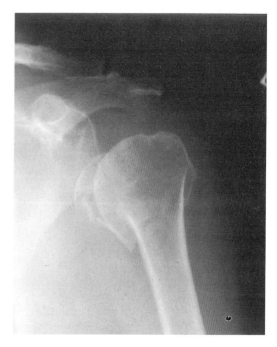

(a)

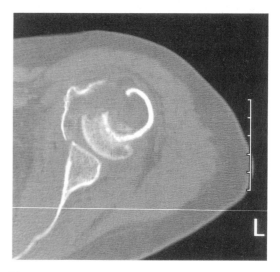

(b)

Figure 6.1 In a head-splitting fracture, the articular segment is split with displacement, causing a 'double crescent' sign. AP radiograph (a) and axial CT scan (b)

of Neer's classification will help the surgeon to classify the fracture correctly, assess the risk of avascular necrosis, and thus determine proper treatment.

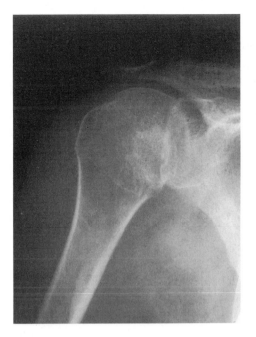

(a)

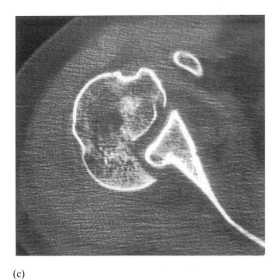

(c)

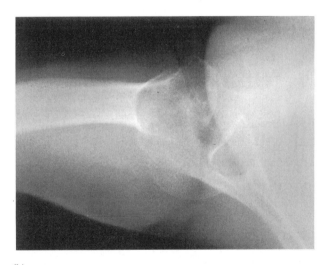

(b)

Figure 6.2 A head-impression or impaction fracture may not be easily identified on routine AP (a) radiographs. The axillary view (b) and CT scan (c) delineate this injury clearly. This is a posterior fracture-dislocation with significant impaction of the joint surface. This injury requires open reduction of the dislocation, and hemiarthroplasty. There may or may not be significantly displaced 'parts' associated with a head-impression fracture

Indications for prosthetic arthroplasty – acute cases

Prosthetic arthroplasty is indicated for certain severe acute fractures of the proximal humerus, including (a) four-part fractures and fracture dislocations, (b) selected three-part fractures in older patients with osteopenic bone, (c) head-splitting fractures, and (d) impression fractures involving greater than 40% of the articular surface. The great majority of severely displaced proximal humeral fractures occur in the older population with a female predominance[6,15,17–21,23,25]. In this population, bone stock is usually osteopenic and may not hold even minimal internal fixation of sutures or wires. Medical evaluation of these patients should be thorough but expeditious, and surgical treatment should be performed as soon as the patient

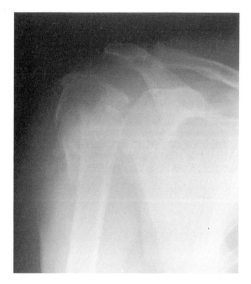

Figure 6.3(a)   This type of fracture has been termed a 'valgus impacted' four-part fracture[30,31]. The head segment is 'impacted' and laterally rotated at least 45°. The tuberosities are displaced and overlie the head. Although this injury initially can appear less displaced than classic four-part fracture dislocations, it may behave biologically as a four-part fracture as the head is significantly displaced from its blood supply

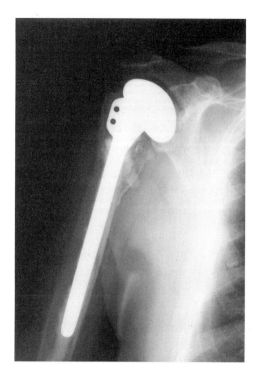

Figure 6.3(c)   Radiograph after tuberosities have united

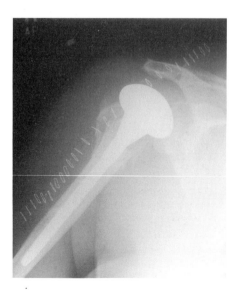

Figure 6.3(b)   Humeral head replacement was performed, with tuberosity reconstruction below the prosthetic head

is medically cleared. Expeditious surgery may decrease the problems of excessive scarring, contracture and bone deformity, and may decrease development of heterotopic ossification. The sur-

gery is technically easier in the acute setting and pain relief is more predictable[6,18]. The patient must be mentally and physically able to understand and follow through with a vigorous postoperative rehabilitation programme that is necessary to ensure a satisfactory outcome.

Four-part fractures

Prosthetic arthroplasty with tuberosity reconstruction and rotator cuff repair is well supported in a critical review of the literature as the best treatment option for four-part fractures and fracture dislocations in patients of all ages. When only true four-part fractures (both tuberosities displaced greater than 1 cm and the head out of contact with the tuberosities and shaft) are evaluated using a consistent grading scale[32], and less severe fractures have been excluded, management with prosthetic replacement is clearly the treatment of choice. Non-operative treatment of 97 four-part fractures from 5 series resulted in only 5 (5%) satisfactory outcomes[3,6,11,12,15]. Operative treatment with ORIF of 56 four-part fractures in 5 series resulted in only 17 (30%) satisfactory outcomes[11–15]. However,

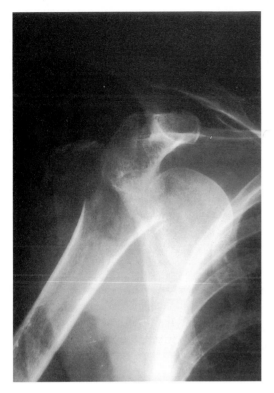

Figure 6.4(a) In a classic four-part fracture dislocation, the head segment is dislocated from the glenoid and separated from all soft-tissue attachments

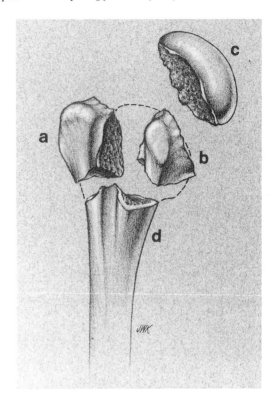

Figure 6.4(b) The four major anatomical segments are the (a) greater tuberosity, (b) lesser tuberosity, (c) articular head, and (d) humeral shaft

prosthetic replacement with tuberosity reconstruction in 171 cases in 9 series were similarly evaluated, and satisfactory results were obtained in 136 cases (80%)[4,6,11,12,18,20,22–25].

ORIF of 'valgus impacted' four-part fractures with disimpaction and elevation of the articular segment and fixation of the tuberosities below the head has been advocated by some authors[30,31]. In selected young patients, an attempt at ORIF may be reasonable to consider. However, risk for avascular necrosis is high and postoperative results have not been comparable to those of humeral head replacement[4,11,12,24,27,33]. Patients who mentally or physically cannot participate properly with the rigorous postoperative rehabilitation may be better treated conservatively, as the result of a technically well-performed operation followed by improper or inadequate physical therapy is often worse than the result of no surgery at all[19,21].

Head-splitting fractures

Head-splitting fractures, in which the articular surface is split and the fragments are displaced, is the result of violent compression of the head against the glenoid, and is more common than previously thought[19]. Head-splitting fractures may or may not have additional displaced 'parts' as components to the injury; however, 'part analysis' is difficult. For example, when half the head is with the greater tuberosity and half is with the lesser tuberosity and both are displaced from the shaft and each other, there are three fragments. However, this would not be classified a three-part fracture, but as a head-splitting fracture. Reduction of this fracture anatomically with internal fixation may be quite difficult, and the final outcome unsatisfactory. We prefer prosthetic replacement in most of these severe injuries.

Head-impression fractures

Fractures that result from large impression defects in the articular surface of the humeral head are usually secondary to posterior fracture dislocations. Treatment is determined by the size of the head defect. A head-impression defect of greater than 40% of the head surface area is best treated by prosthetic replacement. A smaller (but also significant) defect of 20–40% is best treated by transfer of the lesser tuberosity (and attached subscapularis tendon) into the head defect[2,4,16]. A CT scan may be helpful to evaluate the degree of head-impression defect, and can aid in preoperative planning.

Three-part fractures

Some three-part fractures and fracture dislocations of the proximal humerus may be considered for prosthetic replacement of the proximal humerus. This fracture pattern indication is discussed in another chapter.

Surgical technique

Prosthetic replacement for fractures of the proximal humerus is technically demanding. The anatomy is distorted due to soft tissue swelling, fracture haematoma and displaced bone fragments. The bone of the proximal humerus and tuberosities is often comminuted and osteoporotic. The rotator cuff may be torn. The physician must restore both soft tissue and bony fragments as anatomically as possible.

Preoperatively, the shoulder and axilla must be prepared and shaved as cleanly as possible. We prefer scalene block anaesthesia, which is safe and effective and results in excellent muscle relaxation. General anaesthesia may also be used. The patient is placed in a beach chair position. The head is supported by a well-padded headrest and the operative limb is supported by a short arm board that can be moved to provide both maximum support and mobility for the limb. All bony prominences, including the heels, must be protected. The opposite extremity may be elevated across the abdomen to decrease dependent oedema of the hand. A small roll is placed under the medial border of the scapula to stabilize it laterally. The patient is positioned at the edge of the table to allow shoulder extension and adduction,

which allows easier passage of the prosthetic stem into the medullary canal of the humerus (extension allows the prosthetic head to clear the anterior acromion, and adduction allows the head to clear the coracoid process). Prophylactic broad-spectrum antibiotics are administered preoperatively, and continued for 24 hours after drain removal.

The preparation includes the shoulder, lateral neck, axilla, chest wall, front and back toward the midline, and ipsilateral arm to the wrist. The shoulder is draped with the arm free to allow repositioning during surgery.

A deltopectoral approach is made, with the incision extending from the inferior aspect of the clavicle across the coracoid process toward the deltoid insertion. The deltopectoral interval is utilized with preservation of the cephalic vein. The deltoid origin is preserved. The pectoralis major insertion may be partially released to allow increased exposure as necessary. The arm is abducted to relax the deltoid and provide adequate exposure, thus maintaining the deltoid origin and insertion intact.

Utilizing the coracoid process as a guide, the clavipectoral fascia is now incised lateral to the coracoid muscles, exposing the haemorrhagic bursa and fracture haematoma. The coracoid muscles are gently retracted medially and the deltoid muscle is retracted laterally. The subacromial space is now developed, irrigating the haematoma away and excising the haemorrhagic bursal tissue. With great care to avoid glove puncture from sharp bone fragments, the displaced tuberosities are identified. The musculocutaneous nerve and the axillary nerve may be identified by palpation and are protected. The leading edge of the coracoacromial ligament may be partially excised to facilitate exposure. The surgeon must expect some difficulty initially identifying the tuberosities, rotator cuff and head. However, patience and care will be rewarded. The long head of the biceps tendon as well as the bicipital groove (palpable along the upper aspect of the humeral shaft) will guide the surgeon to the rotator cuff interval. The lesser tuberosity is usually displaced medially in four-part fractures, and the greater tuberosity may be displaced superiorly (beneath the acromion) or posteriorly. The biceps tendon is carefully preserved and the tuberosities with their rotator cuff attachments are identified. Small skin hooks carefully placed through the rotator cuff attachment at the tuberosities may be of assistance in gently mobilizing the tuberosities and rotator cuff. Stay sutures may then be placed through the tendon bone attachment for control and mobilization of the fragments. The rotator cuff tendon may be stronger and hold these sutures better than small comminuted or osteoporotic fracture fragments. Great care must be taken both to prevent further comminution of the osteoporotic tuberosity fragments and proximal humeral shaft, and to prevent further weakening or tearing of the rotator cuff attachment to the tuberosity fragments. It is critical to maintain the rotator cuff attachments to the tuberosities during the tuberosity mobilization.

The fracture site is entered by retracting the subscapularis with the attached lesser tuberosity medially. The head fragment is then removed. When the head fragment is located deep to the greater and lesser tuberosities, these tuberosities are first gently retracted, developing the rotator interval as necessary, to allow head extraction. When the tuberosities remain attached to each other with an intact rotator interval, but cover the displaced head fragment like a hood, one attempts to extract the head without incising the rotator interval and without dividing the tuberosities if possible. If this cannot be done, the head is extracted after opening the interval and separating the tuberosities. When the head has been dislocated anteriorly (and is located wedged beneath the coracoid process against the brachial plexus and neurovascular structures), great care must be taken to identify the position of the neurovascular structures prior to a very gentle extraction of the head fragment. Adhesions may be present, especially in the chronic setting, and one must be prepared for bleeding. Patience and careful dissection, however, will allow the head fragment to become free and be removed. This head fragment is saved as a source for possible cancellous bone graft. When the head fragment has been dislocated posteriorly, the shaft and greater tuberosity are gently retracted laterally, allowing exposure of the head. A blunt retractor is often necessary to carefully lever the head fragment free from the posterior glenoid rim, reducing it into the joint, from which location removal is possible.

Once the tuberosities have been identified with the rotator cuff attachment and the head has been removed, attention is directed to the proximal humeral shaft. The arm board is now moved to allow the limb to be extended and externally rotated. This manoeuvre brings the shaft into the wound and the medullary canal is prepared with sequential rasps and reamers. Great care must be exercised during reaming in the presence of osteo-porotic bone to prevent fracture or extension of a non-displaced fracture line of the proximal humeral shaft. The prosthetic trials are now used to determine the proper stem size and head size, and to determine the proper degree of retroversion and length. Proper stem size is determined by pre-operative review of X-rays as well as by the humeral trials, determining which stem best fills the medullary canal. Proper head size is determined by evaluating the removed head fragment, as well as by evaluating the rotator cuff tension and tuberosity placement after insertion of the trial prosthesis and reapproximating the tuberosities and cuff. By achieving proper height and retroversion, satisfactory length and tension will be restored to the myofascial sleeve and allow placement of the tuberosities beneath the prosthetic head against the shaft of the proximal humerus. If the prosthesis is placed deep into the remaining shaft and not left appropriately 'proud', especially in fractures with marked comminution and loss of bone substance, the myofascial sleeve will be too lax. However, the joint should not be 'overstuffed' by placing the prosthesis too proud or by utilizing too large a head size, as postoperative stiffness may result. Proper soft tissue tension will allow about 50% translation of the prosthetic head both anteroposteriorly and superoinferiorly. The prosthesis should be positioned at approximately 30–40° of retroversion in routine acute cases for stability (Figure 6.5). This position can be identified by comparing the head position with the distal epicondylar axis of the humerus, and usually involves placing the fin just posterior to the bicipital groove.

The proper head diameter will achieve stability and also allow closure of the rotator cuff around the prosthesis without undue tension. The previously placed stay sutures in the greater and lesser tuberosities and cuff which aided in the mobilization of the tuberosities now assist with the reduction of the tuberosities to the humeral shaft beneath the prosthetic head. When proximal shaft comminution exists, these shaft fragments must be reduced and held with sutures or wires to reconstruct the proximal bony envelope. Cancellous bone graft from the humeral head may be utilized as necessary.

Secure fixation of the prosthesis within the medullary canal of the proximal humerus routinely requires cement fixation. Prior to cementing, drill holes are made in the proximal shaft and non-absorbable no. 2 or no. 5 sutures are placed. These are the tuberosity 'pull-down' sutures, and 3–4

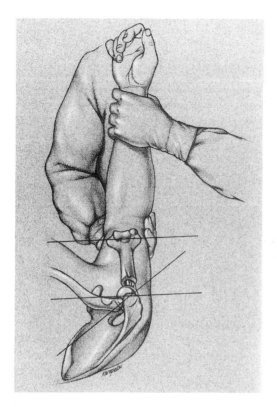

Figure 6.5 The prosthesis should be placed in 30–40 degrees of retroversion for acute fractures. This position can be determined by palpating the distal epicondylar axis of the humerus and positioning the prosthesis accordingly

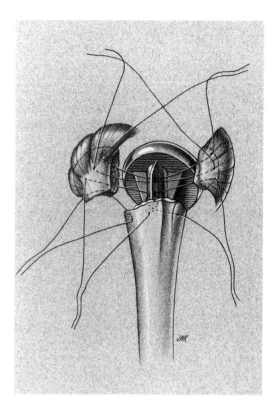

Figure 6.6 With the prosthesis placed in proper height and retroversion, the tuberosities must fit below the head. The previously placed 'pull-down' sutures are now used to secure the tuberosity segments to the shaft. The tuberosities are also secured to the prosthetic fin and to each other

sutures are used for the greater tuberosity and 2–3 are used for the lesser tuberosity. The prosthesis is now cemented in place with proper retroversion and height maintained. Excess cement is carefully removed at the site of tuberosity–shaft fixation, to allow bone-to-bone contact necessary to achieve tuberosity union. Secure prosthetic fixation to the shaft with cement is necessary for rotational stability, and will prevent possible subsequent prosthetic rotation within the osteoporotic shaft of the proximal humerus with resulting loss of proper version and possible postoperative prosthetic instability or dislocation.

Once the prosthesis has been properly cemented within the proximal humeral shaft, attention is focused to tuberosity reconstruction and rotator cuff repair. The previously placed large non-absorbable sutures are now utilized to reduce the tuberosities and secure them to the fin of the prosthesis and the proximal humeral shaft (Figure 6.6). One must be careful not to excise the tuberosities, as they are necessary to achieve bony union to the

shaft (and thus rotator cuff fixation). The tuberosities must be secured below the prosthetic head or impingement in the subacromial space will occur with attempted overhead limb motion. The greater tuberosity is repaired first, followed by repair of the lesser tuberosity. The tuberosity 'pull-down' sutures prevent the muscle forces of the rotator cuff from displacing the tuberosity segments off the shaft, with resulting superior or posterior displacement and subsequent non-union or malunion. Displacement superiorly within the subacromial space will result in impingement symptoms, and displacement posteriorly will result in loss of external rotation due to bony block against the glenoid.

Secure tuberosity reconstruction and cuff repair must be accomplished in order to allow the early passive motion essential to achieve satisfactory function postoperatively. Portions of the humeral head may be used as bone graft beneath the tuberosity fragments. Proper tuberosity reconstruction will include fixation through the holes in the fin of the prosthesis as well as to each other and to the proximal shaft. The biceps tendon is placed back in its groove and the rotator cuff interval between the supraspinatus and subscapularis tendon is closed (Figure 6.7). The arm is now placed through a careful range of motion and the reconstruction is observed. This evaluation aids the surgeon in planning the limits of the postoperative early passive motion programme. Suction drains are placed in the subacromial space adjacent to the tuberosities and rotator cuff repair. The deltopectoral interval is reapproximated. Skin closure is obtained and the limb is immobilized in a carefully padded sling and swathe.

The critical technical points of this procedure have been discussed by Neer and McIlveen, and by Bigliani and McCluskey[16,21,22]: the origin of the deltoid is preserved and not elevated. Minimal bone removal is utilized and any bone graft required is obtained from the head segment that has been excised. The proper height and retrover-

sion of the implant restores the mechanical advantage of the shoulder joint, allowing proper tension in the myofascial sleeve and stability of the construct. The tuberosities repaired must be secured with non-absorbable suture fixation to the prosthesis, to each other, and most importantly to the humeral shaft. Last, but equally important, early passive motion as planned at surgery is begun under close physician supervision.

Postoperative rehabilitation

Proper postoperative rehabilitation is essential to ensure the achievement and maintenance of satisfactory range of motion, strength and function of the shoulder[34,35,41]. This goal is achieved by a carefully planned and extensive rehabilitation programme directed by the operating surgeon. The programme is determined by the quality of the tissues, strength of repair and range of motion achieved at surgery. It is then modified in the postoperative period, as indicated by X-ray evidence of healing, patient compliance and successful progress. Each patient's rehabilitation programme is individualized to their specific needs. The successful execution of the therapy programme is equally as important in achieving a satisfactory outcome as the technical aspects of the surgical procedure performed[19].

The three-phase system of postoperative rehabilitation devised by Hughes and Neer[36] is widely accepted. Phase I, passive glenohumeral motion, is initiated in the first postoperative day, including passive and active motion exercises for the ipsilateral hand, wrist and elbow. A sling is worn during the initial 6-week period of time postoperatively, except when performing the phase I exercises. The limits of early motion have been determined by the surgeon at the time of surgery. It is helpful for the surgeon to include an outline of the planned postoperative rehabilitation programme in the operative dictation. At that time, the details of the operative procedure are clear in the surgeon's mind. These details include bone quality, strength of rotator cuff and deltoid repair, range of motion, and strength of tuberosity repair to the proximal humeral shaft and prosthesis[19,23]. Restoration of range of motion of the glenohumeral joint is the initial goal of therapy. It is critical that the patient be able to understand the goal as well as the restrictions of activity necessary in the early postoperative period to achieve it successfully. The patient must clearly understand the difference

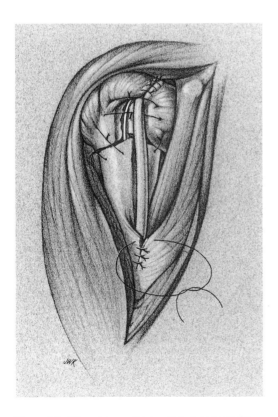

Figure 6.7 The rotator cuff interval is closed and the biceps tendon, which has been preserved, is placed back in the groove. If the pectoralis major tendon was partially released, it is also repaired

between early *passive* motion (performed in the immediate postoperative period), and later active motion and strengthening (to be performed after tuberosity union). The patient must understand that too vigorous early exercise may result in tuberosity pull-off – a devastating complication[39]. Regaining strength of the shoulder girdle must be delayed until healing of the tuberosities is complete. This is usually evident radiographically after approximately 6–8 weeks.

Initial exercises are performed 3 times daily for approximately 5–7 min each time, and may be assisted by prior application of a heat pack to the shoulder. Gravity-assisted pendulum exercises are performed initially to warm up, and give the patient confidence. Passive elevation in the scapular plane by the surgeon, a physical therapist, or a a trained family member within defined limitations is begun. Passive supine external rotation with a stick within limits may also be allowed depending on the stability of the tuberosity reconstruction. These passive exercises are continued for approximately 6 weeks. Assisted forward elevation against gravity with a pulley system and internal rotation exercises are not initiated for a 6-week period of time postoperatively, to allow adequate tuberosity union and to decrease the risk of tuberosity pull-off. At the time of discharge from the hospital, the patient should have a good understanding of how to perform the exercise programme properly, and should have achieved 140° of forward elevation and 20–30° of external rotation. The wound should be healing well, the patient should be afebrile, and the postoperative pain should be well controlled with oral analgesia. Whether or not the patient should continue to work with a physiotherapist immediately after hospital discharge, or whether the patient is able to perform the early passive motion exercise programme independently at home with the assistance of a family member, is a decision the surgeon must make at the time of discharge and is based upon observation of the patient's progress while in the hospital.

Phase II exercises, including active assisted elevation with a pulley and isometric strengthening for the rotator cuff and deltoid, are initiated when there is evidence of tuberosity healing at approximately 6 weeks. The patient is taught to assist the elevation of the involved shoulder with the opposite extremity through the pulley system or the use of a stick. Gradually the patient is taught to use the involved extremity muscles more actively and the contralateral extremity muscles less assistively. Shoulder extension and

internal rotation stretching are now initiated. Activities of daily living, including personal hygiene, eating and washing, are advanced and build muscle strength and endurance. The patient is instructed to utilize the arm initially at waist level close to the body, and then gradually (in the ensuing weeks) begin to reach outwards and upwards, utilizing the other arm for support as necessary and as dictated by comfort and lack of pain. Gentle stretching is encouraged during this phase to ensure motion is maintained and improved upon. These stretches are gentle and emphasize full glenohumeral and scapulothoracic elevation. Supine forward elevation while lying on the floor and holding a stick in both hands for assistance is an excellent exercise to be performed after a hot shower to gain further elevation.

Phase III resistive strengthening and more aggressive stretching exercises are initiated at approximately 12 weeks postoperatively. Theraband progressive resistance and light weights of 1–3 lb (0.5–1.4 kg) are utilized when the patient has achieved almost complete motion and experiences no pain. The patient requires encouragement at each of the three phases and should be congratulated upon successful progress. The patient must also understand that maximum benefits are often not achieved until 12–18 months postoperatively.

Indications for prosthetic arthroplasty – chronic cases

Prosthetic replacement may also be utilized for the reconstruction of old fractures where previous treatment has failed. This includes cases of failed previous non-operative treatment or of previous ORIF, with resulting malunion, non-union, avascular necrosis or post-traumatic arthritis. Prosthetic arthroplasty for 'old trauma' may be among the most technically demanding and difficult reconstructions. The surgeon must address not only the distorted bony and soft tissue anatomy but also the extensive adhesions of the subacromial space, rotator cuff contraction and capsular tightness. Adhesions must be released and the soft tissues must be rebalanced. The blood loss may be greater and the complication rates are higher with less predictable function postoperatively[6,18,40]. However, pain relief is often satisfactory. It is therefore important that the patient understand that pain relief is the primary goal of this surgery and that functional improvement is secondary.

Malunion of the greater tuberosity may result

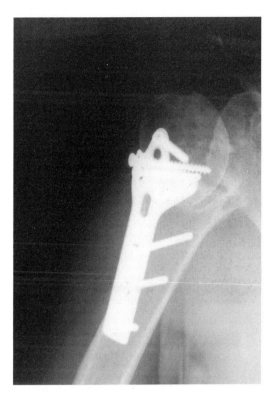

Figure 6.8(a) A malunion of a proximal humerus fracture after open reduction and internal fixation. The medial shaft is articulating with the inferior aspect of the glenoid, the greater tuberosity is prominent, and the head has cystic changes and softening

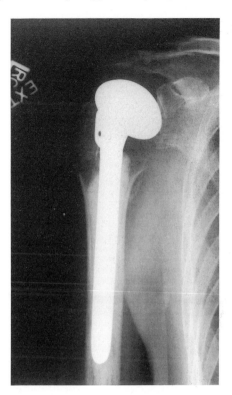

Figure 6.8(b) A humeral head replacement was performed with minimal bone removal. The prosthesis was placed so that it was medial to the proximal shaft. The greater tuberosity was 'excavated' so that the prosthesis could fit into it and above it to prevent 'lateralization' of the tuberosity, and to avoid impingement. An acromioplasty was also performed

in impingement symptoms when the tuberosity is displaced superiorly into the subacromial space. When displaced and malunited posteriorly, however, the greater tuberosity fragment may abut against the glenoid with progressive external rotation, resulting in a bony block and limitation to external rotation. When performing humeral head replacement for post-traumatic arthritis in this situation, tuberosity osteotomy may be necessary to obtain proper prosthetic replacement and motion. However, it is usually best to avoid osteotomy if possible (Figures 6.8a, b). Anterior acromioplasty may be utilized to open the subacromial space as necessary. Soft tissue adhesions must be lysed and the rotator cuff mobilized and repaired as necessary. Release of the coracohumeral ligament may be necessary to allow adequate rotator cuff mobilization and repair.

Non-unions of the surgical neck may occur with two-part fractures or as a component of a more severe fracture pattern. Cases documented in the literature have been treated primarily with ORIF and iliac bone grafting[25,37,38]. In a recent review of 20 surgical neck non-unions treated on the Shoulder Service of the New York Orthopedic Hospital, humeral head replacement with bone grafting was found to be comparable in treatment outcome to ORIF and bone grafting, but without the subsequent hardware problems and reoperations that follow ORIF[40]. In those cases that had a failed early open attempt at fracture fixation, results were not as satisfactory when compared to cases that had been treated initially non-operatively[40]. Currently, we perform prosthetic replacement for a surgical neck malunion when the head is eroded or of poor bone quality (and unable to hold internal fixation hardware adequately) or when advanced post-traumatic glenohumeral arthritis is present (Figures 6.9a–c). ORIF with bone grafting is reserved for patients with preserved glenohumeral articular surfaces and good bone stock. The principles discussed earlier when

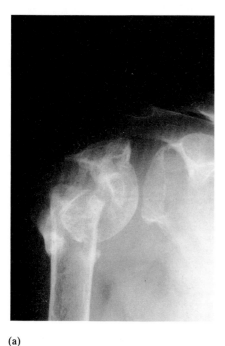

(a)

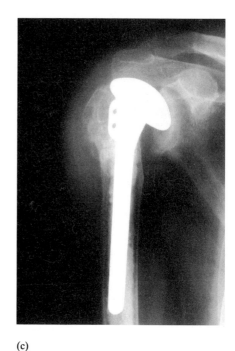

(c)

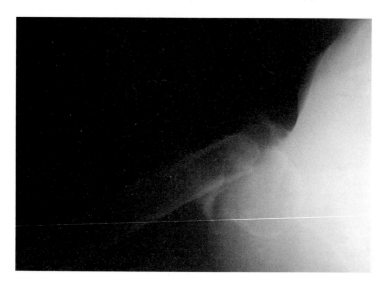

(b)

Figure 6.9 (a,b) Non-union of the surgical neck of the humerus with malposition and osteopenia of the proximal (head) fragment. (c) The osteopenic, malpositioned scarred head has been removed, but large tuberosity bone–rotator cuff segments have been maintained. The non-union has been eliminated with the placement of a cemented prosthetic replacement. The tuberosities are reconstructed below the head and heal to the shaft. The need for immobilization, to allow an internally fixed non-union time to heal, is eliminated. Early passive motion can begin

dealing with acute fractures are also applicable to the chronic case: attention to soft tissue release and reconstruction, cement fixation of the prosthesis and meticulous tuberosity fixation. With prosthetic replacement and tuberosity reconstruction for chronic fracture problems, prolonged immobilization of the shoulder girdle is not required, and early passive motion may be instituted. The need for hardware removal is not required, and the need for fracture fixation in an osteopenic head fragment is eliminated.

Results

Results of prosthetic replacement for treatment for fractures of the proximal humerus are reported extensively in the literature. Neer reported 91%

satisfactory results in a series of 43 patients in 1970[8]. He and McIlveen subsequently reported improved results of 98% excellent or satisfactory in 61 patients. They credited technical improvements for the improved results, especially preservation of the deltoid origin, emphasis on maintenance of normal humeral length, and early passive motion postoperatively[22]. Tanner and Cofield noted pain relief in 93% of cases in a series of 43 patients in 1983[23]. However, some other early reports documented a 60–82% failure rate due to persisting pain, stiffness and disability[20,24]. Our recent experience confirms the results of Neer, and document that good results may be consistently obtained by careful patient selection, meticulous operative technique and closely monitored postoperative care. Patients must be motivated, and document ability to follow instructions. Principles of the operative technique, as outlined above, are critical to ensure this successful result, and include: maintenance of deltoid origin and length, gentle tissue handling with maintenance of tuberosity bone stock and humeral length, proper prosthetic replacement, and secure fixation of the prosthesis and tuberosities. Proper postoperative rehabilitation, as discussed above, is also critical to ensure a good result, with emphasis placed on early passive motion, protection of the repair and close communication between the patient, therapist and physician. Recent review of 70 cases of prosthetic replacement for severely displaced proximal humeral fractures on our service, following the above principles, has documented a satisfactory or excellent outcome in 83% of the cases, and an unsatisfactory outcome in 17%[19]. The unsatisfactory results were associated with lack of patient compliance in 50% of the cases.

Conclusion

Prosthetic replacement with tuberosity reconstruction is indicated for certain displaced fractures of the proximal humerus in the patient who is medically stable and able to follow the difficult postoperative physical therapy programme. These fractures include four-part and certain three-part fractures and fracture-dislocations, head-splitting fractures, and head-impression fractures where greater than 40% of the articular surface is involved.

Surgical treatment is demanding and requires meticulous attention to many details. The postoperative programme of physical therapy is very important, and must be specific, requiring close communication between the orthopaedist, physiotherapist and patient. When the above principles are adhered to, prosthetic replacement for these fractures appears the most satisfactory method of restoring range of motion, strength and function.

References

1. Bigliani, L.U. Fractures of the proximal humerus. In *The Shoulder*, Vol. 1 (eds C.A. Rockwood Jr and F.A. Matsen II), Saunders, Philadelphia (1990), pp. 278–334
2. Bigliani, L.U. Fractures of the proximal humerus. In *Fractures in Adults*, Vol. 1, 3rd edn (eds C.A. Rockwood Jr D.P. Green and R.W. Bucholz), J.B. Lippincott, Philadelphia (1990), pp. 871–927
3. Leyshon, R.L. Closed treatment of fractures of the proximal humerus. *Acta Orthop. Scand.*, **55**, 48–51 (1984)
4. Neer, C.S. II. Displaced proximal humeral fractures, part II. Treatment of three-part and four-part displacement. *J. Bone Joint Surg.*, **52A**, 1090–1103 (1970)
5. Neer, C.S. II. Fractures about the shoulder. In *Fractures*, Vol. 1, 1st edn (eds C.A. Rockwood Jr and D.P. Green), J.B. Lippincott, Philadelphia (1984), pp. 585–623
6. Svend-Hansen, H. Displaced proximal humeral fractures. A review of 49 patients. *Acta Orthop. Scand.*, **45**, 359–364 (1974)
7. Young, T.B. and Wallace, W.A. Conservative treatment of fractures and fracture-dislocations of the upper end of the humerus. *J. Bone Joint Surg.*, **67B**, 373–377 (1985)
8. Neer, C.S. II. Displaced proximal humeral fractures, part I. Classification and evaluation. *J. Bone Joint Surg.*, **52A**, 1077–1089 (1970)
9. Neer, C.S. II. Four-segment classification of displaced proximal humeral fractures. *Instruct. Course Lect.*, **XXIV**, 160–168 (1975), American Academy of Orthopaedic Surgeons/C.V. Mosby, St Louis
10. Codman, E.A. *The Shoulder*, Thomas Todd, Boston, MA (1934)
11. Kristiansen, B. and Christiansen, S.W. Proximal humeral fractures. Late results in relation to classification and treatment. *Acta Orthop Scand.*, **58**, 124–127 (1987)
12. Stabletorth, P.G. Four-part fractures of the neck of the humerus. *J. Bone Joint Surg.*, **66B**, 104–108 (1984)
13. Paavolainen, P. Bjorkenheim, J.M., Slatis, P. and Paukka, P. Operative treatment of severe proximal humeral fractures. *Acta Orthop. Scand.*, **54**, 374–379 (1983)
14. Yamano, Y. Comminuted fractures of the proximal humerus treated with hook plate. *Arch. Orthop. Trauma Surg.*, **105**, 359–363 (1986)
15. Neer, C.S. II. Articular replacement for the humeral head. *J. Bone Joint Surg.*, **37A**, 215–228 (1955)
16. Bigliani, L.U. and McCluskey, G.M. Prosthetic replacement in acute fractures of the proximal humerus. *Sem. Arthroplasty*, **1**, 129–137 (1990)
17. Cofield, R.H. Comminuted fractures of the proximal humerus. *Clin. Orthop.*, **230**, 49–57 (1988)
18. Frich, L.H., Sojbjerg, J.O. and Sneppen, O. Shoulder

arthroplasty in complex acute and chronic proximal humeral fractures. *Orthopaedics*, **14**, 949–954 (1991)

19. Fischer, R.A, Nicholson, G.P., McIlveen, S.J. *et al.* Primary humeral head replacement for severely displaced proximal humerus fractures. Presented at American Academy of Orthopaedic Surgeons, 59th Annual Meeting, Washington, D. C. (February 1992)

20. Kraulis, J. and Hunter, G. The results of prosthetic replacement in fracture-dislocations of the upper end of the humerus. *Injury*, **8**, 129–131 (1976)

21. Neer, C.S. II and McIlveen, S.J. Recent results and techniques of prosthetic replacement for 4-part proximal humeral fractures. *Orthop. Trans.*, **10**, 475 (1986)

22. Neer, C.S. and McIlveen, S.J. Replacement de la tête humérale avec réconstruction des tubérosités et de la coiffe dans les fractures déplacées à 4 fragments. Resultats actuels et techniques. *Rev. Chir. Orthop.*, **74** (Suppl. II), 31–40 (1988)

23. Tanner, M.W. and Cofield, R.H. Prosthetic arthroplasty for fractures and fracture-dislocations of the proximal humerus. *Clin. Orthop.*, **179**, 116–128 (1983)

24. Willems, W.J. and Lim, T.E. Neer arthroplasty for humeral fractures. *Acta Orthop. Scand.*, **56**, 394–395 (1985)

25. Sorensen, K. Pseudarthrosis of the surgical neck of the humerus. Two cases. One bilateral. *Acta Orthop Scand.*, **34**, 132–138 (1964)

26. Bloom, M.H. and Obata, W.G. Diagnosis of posterior dislocation of the shoulder with use of Velpeau axillary and angle-up roentgenographic views. *J. Bone Joint Surg.*, **49A** 943–949 (1967)

27. Fourrier, P. and Martini, M. Post-traumatic avascular necrosis of the humeral head. *Int. Orthop.*, **1**, 187–190 (1977)

28. Gerber, C., Schneeberger, A.G., and Vinh, T.S. The arterial vascularization of the humeral head. An anatomic study. *J. Bone Joint Surg.*, **72A**, 1486–1494 (1990)

29. Sturzenegger, M., Fornaro, E. and Jakob, R.P. Results of surgical treatment of multifragmented fractures of the humeral head. *Arch. Orthop. Trauma Surg.*, **100**, 249–259 (1982)

30. Jakob, R.P., Kristiansen, T., Mayo, K. *et al.* Classification and aspects of treatment of fractures of the proximal humerus. In *Surgery of the Shoulder* (eds J.E. Bateman and R.P. Welsh), B.C. Decker, Philadelphia, PA (1984), pp. 330–343

31. Jakob, R.P., Miniaci, A., Anson, P.S. *et al.* Four-part valgus impacted fractures of the proximal humerus. *J. Bone Joint Surg.*, **73B**, 295–298 (1991)

32. Neer, C.S., II, Watson, K.C. and Stanton, F.J. Recent experience in total shoulder replacement. *J. Bone Joint Surg.*, **64A**, 319–337 (1982)

33. Marotte, J.H., Lord, G. and Bancel, P. L'arthroplastie de Neer dans les fractures et fractures-luxations complexes de l'épaule: Apropos de 12 cas. *Chirurgie*, **104**, 816–821 (1978)

34. Cuomo, F., Flatow, E.L., Miller, S.R. *et al.* Open reduction and internal fixation of 2- and 3-part proximal humerus fractures. *Orthop. Trans.*, **14**, 588 (1990)

35. Hawkins, R.J., Bell, R.H. and Gurr, K. The three-part fracture of the proximal part of the humerus. Operative treatment. *J. Bone Joint Surg.*, **68A**, 1410–1414 (1986)

36. Hughes, M. and Neer, C.S. II. Glenohumeral joint replacement and postoperative rehabilitation. *Phys. Ther.*, **55**, 850–858 (1975)

37. Coventry, M.B. and Laurnen, E.L. Ununited fractures of the middle and upper humerus. Special problems in treatment. *Clin. Orthop.*, **69**, 192–198 (1970)

38. Scheck, M. Surgical treatment of nonunions of the surgical neck of the humerus. *Clin. Orthop.*, **167**, 255–259 (1982)

39. Bigliani, L.U., Flatow, E.L., McCluskey, G.M. *et al.* Failed prosthetic replacement for displaced proximal humerus fractures. *Orthop. Trans.*, **15**, 747–748 (1991)

40. Bigliani, L.U., Nicholson, G.P., Pollock, R.G. *et al.* Operative treatment of nonunions of the surgical neck of the humerus. *Ortho. Trans.*, **17**, 937 (1993)

41. Bigliani, L.U., Nicholson, G.P. and Flatow, E.L. The management of fractures of the proximal humerus. In *Arthroplasty of the Shoulder* (ed. R.J. Friedman), Thieme, New York (1994).

7

Complications of prostheses for proximal humeral fractures

Richard J. Friedman and Stephen Ridgeway

Fractures of the proximal humerus are usually responsive to simple non-operative treatment modalities. However, when severe fragment displacement with or without dislocation is present, conservative treatment often does not provide satisfactory results. In an effort to develop a classification system that had some prognostic predictive value for treatment, Neer developed his anatomical classification scheme for displaced proximal humeral fractures[1,2]. This classification has been used extensively in developing guidelines for treatment, and evaluating treatment outcomes and complications of proximal humeral fractures[3]. Less confusion now exists in the literature, and analyses of treatment results have helped in our understanding of the various therapeutic modalities towards improving patient care.

The indications for a humeral hemiarthroplasty in the treatment of proximal humeral fractures are not universally agreed upon. However, a review of the current literature reveals some consensus[4]. Generally, four-part fractures and fracture-dislocations, anatomical neck fractures, three-part fractures and fracture-dislocations in osteoporotic patients, head-splitting fractures, and impression fractures in which more than 45% of the articular surface is involved, are considered indications for a hemiarthroplasty.

Historically, four-part fractures and fracture-dislocations have been treated by various methods. Closed reduction has resulted in a high incidence of osteonecrosis, ranging between 13% and 34%[2,5–10]. Malunions and degenerative post-traumatic osteoarthritis also occur with a high frequency, both with closed reduction as well as open

reduction and internal fixation (ORIF). The results of ORIF are generally unsatisfactory, with osteonecrosis and malunion common complications. While two-part and some three-part fracture-dislocations have been treated by more conservative methods such as ORIF, four-part fracture-dislocations have had much less satisfactory results from these methods, and therefore a proximal humeral hemiarthroplasty is indicated[4].

Two-part anatomical neck fractures are rare and therefore there have been few series on which to base any clinical decisions. Some believe that ORIF should be attempted in a young patient[11–14]. However, survival of the humeral head is poor since the blood supply has been completely disrupted. If the humeral head cannot be securely reattached to the proximal humerus to allow for early range of motion, or this injury occurs in an elderly patient with osteoporotic bone, then a prosthesis is indicated.

Three-part fractures and fracture-dislocations are often satisfactorily treated with ORIF. In certain patients, when the bone quality is poor, such as with osteoporosis, stable internal fixation to allow early range of motion is not possible, and a primary humeral hemiarthroplasty is the treatment of choice. Head-splitting fractures usually are associated with fractures of the surgical neck or either of the tuberosities. ORIF may be attempted in a young patient with otherwise healthy bone, but this will often fail, and a hemiarthroplasty is usually indicated. Fractures associated with a large humeral head defect involving greater than 45% of the articular surface are also best treated with a hemiarthroplasty. Proximal humeral hemiarthro-

Table 7.1   Potential complications of hemiarthroplasty for proximal humerus fractures. (From Norris[20], by permission)

Problem	Potential result	Solution
Prosthesis too low	Functionally weakens deltoid; inferior subluxation	Place tuberosities between shaft and head or bone graft to full humeral height
Prosthesis stem too narrow	Pistoning or spinning	Larger stem or methylmethacrylate fixation
Uncemented prosthesis without metaphyseal bone support	Loosening prior to tuberosity healing; subsidence	Larger stem or methylmethacrylate fixation
Prosthesis in varus	Greater tuberosity prominent; impingement; shaft penetration	Redirect prosthesis at proper height and version
Subsidence	Greater tuberosity prominent; impingement; shaft penetration	Cement at proper height; bone graft as necessary
Too much retroversion	Difficult greater tuberosity attachment; posterior instability	Correct version; cement as necessary
Too much anteversion	Anterior instability	Correct version; cement as necessary
Tuberosity avulsion	Cuff retear; weakness; loss of elevation	Delay rehabilitation; trim tuberosity for fit; vertical and horizontal repair; bone graft
Intraoperative shaft fracture below prosthesis stem	Unstable fracture	Long-stem prosthesis with or without cement
Cerclage wiring of upper shaft fracture	Bone necrosis or wire breakage	Wire removal, bone graft

plasty has also been used to treat the complications of either non-operative treatment or ORIF, such as osteonecrosis, post-traumatic arthritis, non-unions and malunions[15–17].

Generally, satisfactory results have been reported for proximal humeral hemiarthroplasty following various displaced fractures and fracture-dislocations about the shoulder. Following his initial description of an articular replacement for fractures of the humeral head[18], Neer reported on the results of 43 shoulders with displaced proximal humeral fractures. Ninety-one per cent had good or excellent results after prosthetic humeral head replacement[2]. Subsequent follow-up studies with a newer version of the prosthesis demonstrated excellent results, with no unsatisfactory outcomes[19]. It was concluded that the results of a technically well-done proximal humeral hemiarthroplasty with reattachment of the tuberosities and rotator cuff reconstruction are better than previously reported. Other recent studies have supported this conclusion, demonstrating 93% satisfactory pain relief following proximal humeral hemiarthroplasty for fractures and fracture-dislocations[17].

As the use of hemiarthroplasty for the treatment of displaced proximal humerus fractures increased, it became obvious that patients had a better outcome and fewer complications than with non-operative treatment. However, studies have given only brief descriptions of the complications occurring while concentrating on the clinical results. Also, no standardized methods exist for reporting complications, and not all authors agree on what is and is not a complication. Few long-term studies exist, and therefore the incidence of certain time-dependent complications such as component loosening are not well documented. This chapter presents the documented complications following proximal humeral hemiarthroplasty for displaced fractures and fracture-dislocations, and includes a discussion of their prevention and/or treatment[20] (Table 7.1). A complication is defined as any adverse outcome affecting the clinical result, but not necessarily leading to revision surgery. With this knowledge, the physician will be able to discuss the indications, risks and benefits of the procedure with the patient, and individualize treatment accordingly.

Incidence of complications

Despite the satisfactory improvements in pain relief and shoulder function that have been reported following hemiarthroplasty for displaced proximal humeral fractures, several studies include a significant number of patients with an unsatisfactory result secondary to pain, limited range of motion and disability[17,21,22]. There are numerous potential postoperative complications that can affect the outcome of a hemiarthroplasty and lead to an unsatisfactory result. Complications following hemiarthroplasty for proximal humeral fractures are related to many factors, including choice of prosthesis, surgical technique, type of fracture, time period between the acute fracture and surgery, and patient factors such as age, bone quality and their ability to participate in the demanding postoperative physical therapy programme.

Complications following humeral hemiarthroplasty for displaced fractures of the proximal humerus can be classified as early or late. Early complications include infection, neurovascular injury, subluxation and/or dislocation, wound haematoma, reflex sympathetic dystrophy, prosthesis malposition, intraoperative or postoperative humerus fracture and poor compliance with the postoperative rehabilitation protocol. Late complications include heterotopic bone formation, myositis ossificans, rotator cuff tears, prosthetic loosening, greater and/or lesser tuberosity detachment, non-union or malunion of the greater and/or lesser tuberosities, glenoid erosion, broken wires, acromioclavicular joint problems and subacromial impingement[2,4,9,15–17,19,21–29].

A review of the English literature found 13 studies reporting results of hemiarthroplasty for the treatment of acute and chronic proximal humeral fractures and fracture-dislocations (Table 7.2). There were a total of 349 hemiarthroplasties, with 239 being acute and 110 chronic. However, the mean follow-up period was only 38 months, with the range being 26–73 months. Since the follow-up periods were relatively short, the incidence of late complications was low. In fact, only one of the 13 series reported an episode of component loosening, yet it has been clearly documented elsewhere that this does occur, particularly with uncemented prostheses implanted for four-part fractures and fracture-dislocations[24]. Overall, the percentage of satisfactory results (or satisfactory pain relief if this was not stated) was 80%. In the acute group, the mean follow-up was 41 months, and there were 82% satisfactory results. For the chronic group, 77% had satisfactory results at a mean follow-up of 30 months.

It is difficult to calculate the incidence of various complications, as there was no standardization to reporting and complications were often not reported. What is clear is that these complications do occur, but their true incidence cannot be determined based on a review of the literature. A recent study reviewed 29 shoulders with failed hemiarthroplasties originally implanted for displaced fractures and fracture-dislocations of the proximal humerus, and while this does not allow one to calculate the true incidence of these complications, it does show that they occur more often than has been reported in the literature[24]. The causes of failure were identified, and multiple causes were found in 24 of the 29 shoulders. The exact causes of failure could be determined more accurately in 18 shoulders that underwent revision surgery. All of these were found to have multiple causes, with the mean number being 3.4 (range 2–6). In the shoulders that were not revised, the mean number of identifiable causes was 1.8 (range 1–3).

In the 29 failed hemiarthroplasties, the frequency of complications was as follows: greater tuberosity detachment (15); humeral prosthetic loosening (12) – aseptic (11, of which all were uncemented) and septic (1, cemented); inadequate or non-compliant rehabilitation (9); nerve injury (9); glenoid erosion (7); malposition of humeral prosthesis (8) – 3 inferior (1 uncemented, 2 cemented), 3 excess retroversion (2 uncemented, 1 cemented), 1 superior (uncemented), 1 excess anteversion (cemented); lesser tuberosity detachment (7); dislocation (5); ectopic bone (4); infection (4); greater tuberosity prominence (2); arterial injury (1); acromial non-union (1); postoperative humeral shaft fracture (1); acromioclavicular joint tenderness (1); broken wires (1); rotator cuff incompetence (1).

Tanner and Cofield[17] examined the causes of failure and results of hemiarthroplasty in patients with complex acute fractures and fracture-dislocations compared to those with chronic fractures and fracture-dislocations of the proximal humerus. Of the 16 patients in the acute group, tuberosity non-union accounted for 4 complications, rotator cuff stretching for another 4, and wound haematoma for one. Of the 28 in the chronic group, there were the following complications: rotator cuff stretching (4); malunion following tuberosity osteotomy (2); rotator cuff tear (3); instability (2); wound haematoma and ectopic ossification (1); reflex sympathetic dystrophy (1); and intraoperative radial nerve injury (1).

Another series treated 14 shoulders with chronic post-traumatic changes following proximal humeral fractures with a hemiarthroplasty[15]. While satisfactory results were obtained in 90% of cases,

Table 7.2 Complications following hemiarthroplasty for proximal humerus fractures

Author	Type	No.	Follow-up (months)	Satisfactory results (%)	Loosening	Instability	Tuberosity non/malunion	N-V injury	Infection	Rotator cuff stretch/tear	Fracture	RSD	Haematoma	Calcification	Wire breakage	Contracture
DesMarche	Acute	18	36	66												
Dines	Chronic	14	33	90		1	1	1						4		
Frich	Acute	15	23	87		4										
	Chronic	27	26	67					2							
Green	Acute	24	37	83			3								1	
Kraulis	Acute	11	36	18					2		1	2		4		
Moeckel	Acute	22	36	91		1	1							1		
Neer 1970	Acute	43	58	91			2		1							
Neer 1982	Chronic	41	31	71			1	1	1							
Neer 1986	Acute	44	73	100										5	9	
Stableforth	Acute	16		70	1								2			
Switlyk	Acute	20	40	70				1								1
Tanner	Acute	16	36	100			4			4			1			
	Chronic	28	30	90		2	2	1		7		1	1	1		
Willems	Acute	10	30	40												
Totals		349	38	80	1	8	14	4	6	11	1	3	4	15	10	1

N-V, neurovascular; RSD, reflex sympathetic dystrophy.

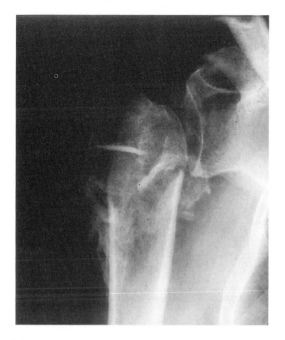

(a)

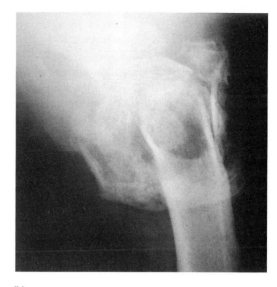

(b)

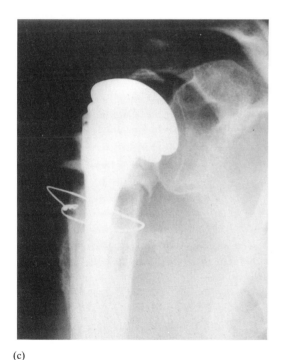

(c)

Figure 7.1 Anteroposterior and axillary lateral roentgenograms of the right shoulder in a 61-year-old male: (a,b) a 4-month-old four-part fracture of the proximal humerus demonstrating malunion of the tuberosities; (c) following hemiarthroplasty of the proximal humerus with osteotomy and reattachment of the tuberosities, the greater tuberosity fragment has displaced superiorly, with weakness and limitation of elevation

several complications were noted. These included myositis ossificans, non-union of the tuberosity osteotomy, superior subluxation and impingement, postoperative axillary neuropathy, and posterior glenohumeral subluxation with glenoid sclerosis. Several of these complications occurred in two patients.

Complications

Tuberosity detachment/non-union/malunion

Greater tuberosity detachment or non-union was the most common complication reported following hemiarthroplasty for complex fractures of the proximal humerus in two series[17,24]. In another series of 43 hemiarthroplasties, 2 of the 4 complications were greater tuberosity malunions, which accounted for 2 of the 4 failures[2]. These types of complications are the greatest cause of failure in the majority of reported cases of prosthetic failure in the treatment of complex proximal humeral fractures.

While some studies separate detachment and malunion into two groups, it is not clear whether the malunited tuberosities were originally attached in a prominent, malunited position or became detached following surgery and either went on to a non-union or subsequently healed in a malunited position[27]. Malunion in a prominent position results in impingement and rotator cuff insufficiency[15,24,30]. Greater tuberosity detachment also results in inadequate rotator cuff function with weakness in active elevation and external rotation (Figure 7.1).

Based on the high number of these complications resulting in failure, it appears that proper reconstruction of the rotator cuff and attachment of the tuberosities following trauma are crucial in achieving good results following hemiarthroplasty. However, fixation of the tuberosities in the acute situation can be very difficult secondary to fragmentation and osteoporosis. It is recommended that in order to secure the tuberosities, a heavy non-absorbable suture with adequate tensile strength be used to attach the tuberosities to the shaft of the humerus as well as to each other and the prosthesis[17] (Figures 7.2 and 7.3).

While heavy gauge wire has been recommended in the past, it tends to break and has caused problems requiring reoperation to relieve symptoms, and may be related to tuberosity non-union[19]. With the strict use of heavy, braided, non-absorbable sutures instead of wire suture since 1982, there have been only two documented cases of tuberosity detachment due to breakage in one series[24]. In addition, those cases were in patients known to be non-compliant with the postoperative physical therapy protocol in the early postoperative period. Others recommend the use of a modular humeral prosthesis which is thought to allow easier reduction of the tuberosities in a more anatomical position with appropriate soft tissue tension around the shoulder[30].

In chronic cases following complex displaced proximal humeral fracture that require hemiarthroplasty for relief of symptoms, it is often necessary to osteotomize the tuberosities (Figure 7.4). This is indicated when the greater tuberosity is posteriorly displaced blocking external rotation, or is superiorly displaced blocking elevation[15]. However, the functional results are improved if the tuberosities are left attached to the shaft with an intact rotator cuff in these chronic cases undergoing hemiarthroplasty. When this is not possible, great care must be taken to leave enough bone attached to the rotator cuff tendons to facilitate secure attachment to the humeral shaft and decrease the incidence of detachment, non-union or malunion.

Humeral prosthesis loosening

Humeral prosthesis loosening accounted for 12 of 29 complications in a series of failed hemiarthroplasties for displaced fractures, placing it second to tuberosity problems in incidence[24]. Eleven cases of component loosening were aseptic and 1 case was due to septic loosening. All of the aseptic loosenings were in press-fit components, one being porous coated. When both tuberosities are displaced, there is little remaining in the proximal humerus to provide any rotational stability for the prosthesis if it is press-fit and not secured with methylmethacrylate. The lateral fin of the prosthesis is frequently used for tuberosity reattachment, which places excessive torque on the pros-

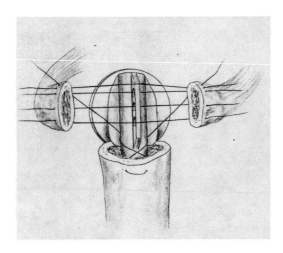

Figure 7.2 Fixation of the tuberosities should be to each other and the humeral shaft using the holes in the lateral fin of the prosthesis (From Dines *et al.*[15], by permission)

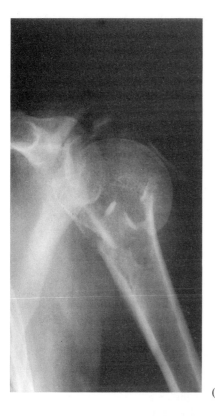

(a)

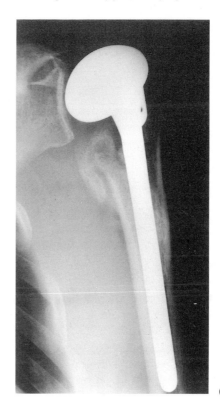

(b)

Figure 7.3 Anteroposterior and axillary lateral roentgenograms of the left shoulder in a 42-year-old male: (a) an acute four-part fracture of the proximal humerus; (b,c) secure reattachment of the tuberosities has resulted in healing to the proximal humerus, with good elevation and external rotation

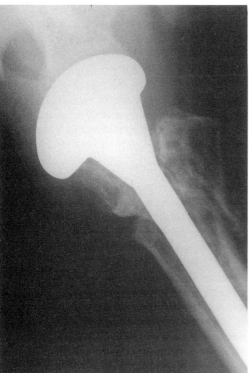

(c)

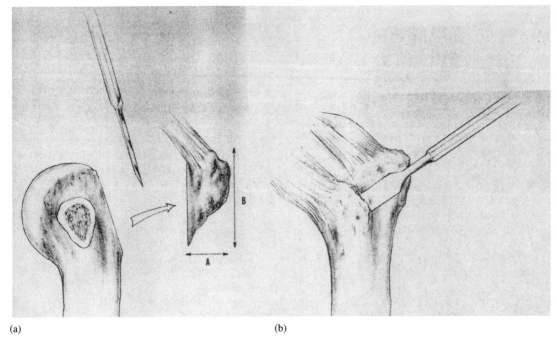

(a)   (b)

Figure 7.4 (a) Osteotomy of the tuberosities should leave enough bone attached to the rotator cuff for a strong repair (A) and should be long enough to allow contact with the humeral shaft for healing to occur (B). (b) The bicipital groove is an important landmark for placing the tuberosity osteotomy following malunion. (From Dines *et al.*[15], by permission)

thesis once active rotator cuff function is restored. This is a problem in the typical patient who sustains a complex displaced fracture of the proximal humerus and who is older with osteopenic bone and widened medullary canals that provide limited support and stability for the humeral component in a severely comminuted fracture. This can be significant enough for loosening to result.

As a result, many recommend against a press-fit technique for humeral component fixation in the treatment of proximal humerus fractures except in the rare, young patient with good bone stock that provides sufficient rotational stability[24]. The reliability of humeral component fixation is increased with methylmethacrylate. In several series, loosening was not noted to be a problem, but in the majority of cases the prosthesis was cemented[2,16,17,21,22,26]. In the 13 series reviewed, there was only 1 case of early loosening reported and no cases of late loosening[29]. While the rate of early loosening was probably low due to the use of methylmethacrylate, the follow-up was short and therefore the rate of late component loosening could not be determined.

In order to increase the long-term survival of the humeral component and decrease late loosening,

modern cementing techniques should be used. These include using a cement restrictor 1–2 cm distal to the tip of the prosthesis to help pressurize the methylmethacrylate, a cement gun to inject the methylmethacrylate down the humeral canal, preparation of the methylmethacrylate in some environment to decrease porosity such as vacuum mixing or centrifuging, preparation of the humeral canal with removal of all cancellous bone, pulsatile lavage to remove any debris, and thorough drying of the humeral canal prior to injection of the methylmethacrylate.

Inadequate or non-compliant rehabilitation

While many rehabilitation programmes for prosthetic replacement following complex proximal humeral fractures have been described, it is of paramount importance to individualize the programme for each patient based on the status of the tuberosities and condition of the rotator cuff[15,26,31]. In one series of 11 hemiarthroplasties, 3 of the failures were in chronic alcoholics who refused to participate in the rehabilitation programme[22]. Tanner and Cofield had 2 poor results secondary to patient refusal to participate in a physical therapy programme[17]. In a review of 29 failed hemiarthroplasties, 9 shoulders were affected by an inadequate physical therapy protocol or non-compliance[24]. Some of these patients did not attend physiotherapy, while others actively used their shoulders immediately postoperatively. Noncompliance may have resulted in later detachment of the greater tuberosity.

Most studies reviewed report difficulties with compliance in the rehabilitation programme[15,17,22,24,30]. Rehabilitation following this procedure is long, and patients should be told that it can take up to 1 year for them to achieve their final functional result. Good communication with the patient prior to and after surgery about the demands and expectations of the rehabilitation programme is necessary for patient compliance and obtaining a satisfactory result. Constant reinforcement of this message is also important. However, some patients are simply not going to comply with any physical therapy programme and their functional result from this procedure will be compromised. Consequently, any patient who is identified as one likely to be non-compliant should be considered a poor surgical candidate.

Neurovascular injury

Neurovascular injury is a recognized complication following displaced complex fractures and fracture-dislocations of the proximal humerus, and a careful neurovascular examination must be performed and documented when the patient is first seen. These injuries have also been reported following proximal humeral hemiarthroplasty, and can contribute to failure of the procedure. Neurovascular injuries can involve the axillary nerve, musculocutaneous nerve, suprascapular nerve, brachial plexus and radial nerve, and should be documented and followed with electromyography and nerve conduction studies[17,24].

Neer[2] reported 10 patients with neurological deficits following complex fractures of the proximal humerus, and only 4 of these did not recover with conservative treatment. These involved the axillary and median nerves in 4 patients, axillary and radial nerves in 2 ulnar nerve in 2 and three nerves in 2 patients. Only 1 patient treated with a hemiarthroplasty developed a postoperative neurological lesion, and received an unsatisfactory rating because of poor function. There are several other instances of similar injuries in the literature[15,22,26]. There is also a report of spontaneous relocation of a dis-located hemiarthroplasty following recovery of a brachial plexus lesion[32].

Nerve lesions should be considered as possible aetiologies for unexplained weakness following proximal humeral hemiarthroplasty. Even with a careful preoperative evaluation, it can sometimes be difficult to determine whether a neurological lesion is present because the patients are in pain and cannot move their extremity. Stableforth[9] noted that 6.1% of four-part anterior fracture dislocations of the shoulder resulted in a nerve injury, but it is likely that some of these injuries were the result of treatment, whether a closed reduction, open reduction or hemiarthroplasty was performed[2]. Many of these lesions recover spontaneously, but it can take a long period of time before it is known if the end result will be affected.

Reflex sympathetic dystrophy has also been reported as a postoperative complication following proximal humeral hemiarthroplasty[17,22]. In most cases, this is treated non-operatively with physiotherapy and sympathetic ganglion blocks as needed. It is important to try to maintain as much motion as possible during this time, and patients should be counselled that the treatment period can be prolonged but that in most cases their symptoms will eventually resolve.

Humeral component malposition

Malposition of the humeral component can include being too superior or inferior in the intramedullary canal of the humerus, excessive anteversion and excessive retroversion[24]. The incidence of malposition following the treatment of fractures and fracture-dislocations is increased with press-fit prostheses, but it is not clear if they were originally malpositioned or migrated into another position. The humeral component should generally be placed in 30° to 40° of retroversion, but this will vary depending on the fracture pattern, length of time between the fracture and treatment, and intraoperative stability of the prosthesis as it articulates with the glenoid.

Precise positioning can be difficult because the anatomical landmarks used are disturbed due to the displaced fracture fragments. With poor anatomical positioning of the humeral component, erosion of the glenoid fossa can result, and was present in 24% of 29 failed hemiarthroplasties[24]. One of 2 failures in a series of 20 patients treated with a hemiarthroplasty for complex fractures of the proximal humerus involved glenoid erosion, which occurred secondary to a postoperative axillary neuropathy and posterior subluxation leading to posterior erosion[15].

Restoration of the anatomical length of the humerus is crucial to restoring normal musculoskeletal tension of the deltoid and rotator cuff muscles, as this is key for regaining shoulder function[16]. Improper articulation of the humeral head against either the inferior or superior portion of the glenoid can result in uneven wear leading to a poor result, with decreased glenohumeral motion and pain. When this occurs, revision to total shoulder arthroplasty is often indicated[24].

Instability

Instability of the humeral component can result from many factors related to both the patient as well as the surgical technique. If the instability results from displacement of the tuberosities, this must be recognized early and surgically corrected. A similar approach must be taken if the rotator cuff tears and leads to instability. Provided these aetiologies have been excluded, a closed reduction will often be successful, followed by patient re-education and physical therapy. Patient factors such as non-compliance and pre-existing medical problems such as seizure and movement disorders will also influence the incidence of instability.

In a series of 27 patients with chronic complex fractures of the proximal humerus treated with a hemiarthroplasty, 2 dislocations occurred[17]. One of these was in a patient suffering from alcohol withdrawal with confusion and agitation, and the other was an elderly patient who had a dislocation in the early postoperative period. Both of these were treated with closed reduction and immobilization. There was good pain relief but limited function in the alcoholic, while the other patient reported extensive pain and poor function but refused further evaluation. In another series, there were 5 instances of instability, 3 anterior and 2 posterior[24]. Four of the unstable hemiarthroplasties were in patients who experienced postoperative seizures, and 1 occurred in a patient with Parkinson's disease. All of these shoulders initially had a four-part posterior fracture-dislocation.

In these patients, all but one had a pre-existing movement disorder, seizure disorder or predisposition to agitation. It seems prudent, then, to use aggressive prophylaxis against or to treat any pre-existing condition that may impact negatively on the procedure postoperatively. It must be remembered that in all likelihood, these pre-existing medical conditions that predispose to postoperative complications were predisposing factors for the fracture. With this connection in mind, a high index of suspicion should exist for these disorders in patients with complex fractures and especially fracture-dislocations of the proximal humerus, and they should be aggressively sought after and treated.

Infection

Infection is a constant concern following joint arthroplasty. Predisposing factors include previous shoulder surgery such as open reduction and internal fixation, malnourishment, immunocompromised patients, and those with debilitating medical conditions. Many reports of hemiarthroplasty for complex proximal humerus fractures report infection leading to prosthetic failure[9,16,22,24]. Kraulis and Hunter[22] reported 2 cases of deep infection in their group of 11 patients. Frich *et al.*[16] had two instances of infection in their group of 42 hemiarthroplasties, resulting in persistent instability and failure. Both of these were in the chronic fracture group who had open reduction and internal fixation initially for their injury, and had an average delay between injury and hemiarthroplasty of 14 months.

The treatment of a prosthetic joint infection often requires removal of the components, irrigation and debridement and subsequent reimplantation, either immediate or delayed. A review of the literature does not allow one to determine if immediate reimplantation is a more successful approach for an infected shoulder hemiarthroplasty than for an infected hip or knee arthroplasty. At the first sign of infection, however, irrigation and debridement followed by antibiotic therapy sensitive to the organism cultured at the time of surgery may be sufficient to eradicate the infection if performed very early in the course of infection.

In a series of failed hemiarthroplasties, there were 4 prosthetic infections found postoperatively, and they were all treated with removal of the component, irrigation and debridement and immediate reimplantation, followed by 4–6 weeks of intravenous antibiotics appropriate for the organism cultured at the time of revision surgery[24]. The diagnosis was often very difficult to make preoperatively, despite a high index of suspicion and attempts to culture an organism with repeated aspirations. Intraoperative cultures were the most reliable when it came to establishing a diagnosis of infection. At follow-up periods ranging from 3 to 55 months, all four patients have remained free of infection.

It has been suggested that the increased incidence of instability and infection leading to failure in a series of chronic reconstructions argues for less reluctance on the part of surgeons to perform primary hemiarthroplasties for complex proximal humeral fractures[16]. It is felt that the practice of treating these types of fractures conservatively, with the thought that they could be revised to a hemiarthroplasty, leads to poorer results, including the complication of infection. Others have observed that since preoperative pain reduces the efficiency of skin preparation, it should be thoroughly cleansed under anaesthesia[22]. They felt that prophylactic antibiotics would have been of help in lowering the incidence of infection in their patients, and this is something that is routinely practised today.

Miscellaneous complications

In most series, heterotopic bone formation, myositis ossificans and wound haematoma have been reported as complications[15,17,19,24]. In one series reporting 5 cases of heterotopic bone formation in 44 hemiarthroplasties, all had delayed treatment[19]. However, these patients achieved excellent range of motion and did not require further surgery. Tanner and Cofield[17] had 1 case of wound haematoma and heterotopic ossification in their group of 28 hemiarthroplasties with chronic fractures and fracture-dislocations of the proximal humerus. In another series, 20% of patients with chronic complex fractures developed myositis ossificans, but only one of these was considered clinically significant and resulted in a poor result[15]. Bigliani *et al.*[24] found that heterotopic bone contributed to failure in 4 hemiarthroplasties, but the average time from injury to treatment was only 14 days (range 2–42 days). All of these patients developed sufficient bone to limit motion of the hemiarthroplasty.

In the majority of the cases where heterotopic bone formation is clinically significant, patients have had a significant delay between injury and treatment. None of the patients in an acutely treated group suffered from this complication[17]. However, Kraulis and Hunter[22] had 4 instances of what they termed pericapsular calcification in their 11 patients, and 10 were treated acutely. They felt that the calcification was perhaps due to retention of bony fragments from the tuberosities, thus explaining the high incidence of this complication

in their group of acutely treated patients. Therefore, it has been recommended by various authors that a shoulder hemiarthroplasty should not be delayed greater than 2 weeks after injury and that loose bone fragments should not be left in the fracture site[16,17,19,28,33]. Surgical delays over 2 weeks can compromise the results of a shoulder hemiarthroplasty for various reasons[28].

Conclusion

Hemiarthroplasty for repair of complex proximal humeral fractures provides results superior to those of more conservative therapies in properly chosen patients[2,9,15–17,21,24]. The complications described above, however, show that there are many potential pitfalls to this type of treatment. Some general recommendations have been made, aimed at reducing the number of complications and therefore improving the results of this procedure[30]. Patients must have the proper physical and mental capability to undergo surgery and a long period of postoperative rehabilitation. Surgical technique must be meticulous and precise, with strict maintenance of appropriate humeral height, proper humeral retroversion (30–40°), and secure fixation and healing of both tuberosities with rotator cuff repair. Rehabilitation requires properly monitored physical therapy with the knowledge that improvement is slow and may continue for as long as 1 year. To obtain the best results with this procedure, it should be performed within 2 weeks of injury. Chronic fractures undergo changes that make anatomical reconstruction more difficult and result in a higher complication rate and greater incidence of poor results and failure.

Finally, in the case of unsatisfactory results that require revision surgery, the primary indication should be severe pain and not restoration of function. In a study of 18 failed shoulder hemiarthroplasties that underwent revision surgery, pain relief was good, as 10 of the 18 had only slight or occasional pain[24]. Range of motion and functional improvements, though, were not very significant. Overall, there was 1 excellent, 2 good, 13 fair and 2 poor results. The results of revision surgery emphasize the importance of the primary hemiarthroplasty, and that it be done as expertly and precisely as possible since the best results are obtained with the initial procedure.

References

1. Neer, C.S. Displaced proximal humerus fractures, part I. Classification and evaluation. *J. Bone Joint Surg.*, **52A**, 1077–1089 (1970)

2. Neer, C.S. Displaced proximal humerus fractures, part II. Treatment of three-part and four-part displacement. *J. Bone Joint Surg.*, **52A**, 1090–1103 (1970)

3. Kristiansen, B. and Christensen, S.W. Proximal humerus fractures. Late results in relation to classification and treatment. *Acta Orthop. Scand.*, **58**, 124–127 (1987)

4. Bigliani, L.U. Fractures of the proximal humerus. In *The Shoulder* (eds C.A. Rockwood and F.A. Matsen), W.B. Saunders, Philadelphia (1990), pp. 278–334

5. Geneste, R., Durandeau, A., Gauzere, J.M. *et al.* Closed treatment of fracture-dislocations of the shoulder joint. *Rev. Chir. Orthop.*, **66**, 383–386 (1980)

6. Hagg, O. and Lundberg, B. Aspects of prognostic factors in comminuted and dislocated proximal humerus fractures. In *Surgery of the Shoulder* (eds J.E. Bateman and R.P. Welsh), B.C. Decker, Philadelphia (1984), pp. 51–59

7. Knight, R.A. and Mayne, J.A. Comminuted fractures and fracture-dislocations involving the articular surface of the humeral head. *J. Bone Joint Surg.*, **39A**, 1347–1355 (1957)

8. Pilgaard, S. and Oster, A. Four part segment fractures of the humeral neck. *Acta Orthop. Scand.*, **44**, 124 (1973)

9. Stableforth, P.G. Four-part fractures of the neck of the humerus. *J. Bone Joint Surg.*, **66B**, 104–108 (1984)

10. Svend-Hansen, H. Displaced proximal humeral fractures. A review of 49 patients. *Acta Orthop. Scand.*, **45**, 359–364 (1974)

11. DePalma, A.F. and Cautilli, R.A. Fractures of the upper end of the humerus. *Clin. Orthop.*, **20**, 73–93 (1961)

12. Jakob, R.P., Kristiansen, T., Mayo, K. *et al.* Classification and aspects of treatment of fractures of the proximal humerus. In *Surgery of the Shoulder* (eds J.E. Bateman and R.P. Welsh), B.C. Decker, Philadelphia (1984) pp. 330–343

13. Kofoed, H. Revascularization of the humeral head. A report of two cases of fracture-dislocation of the shoulder. *Clin. Orthop.*, **179**, 175–178 (1983)

14. Neer, C.S. and Rockwood, C.A. Fractures and dislocations of the shoulder. In *Fractures* (eds C.A. Rockwood and D.P. Green), J.B. Lippincott, Philadelphia (1984), pp. 675–707

15. Dines, D.M., Warren, R.F., Altchek, D.W. *et al.* Post-traumatic changes of the proximal humerus: malunion, nonunion, and osteonecrosis. Treatment with modular hemiarthroplasty or total shoulder arthroplasty. *J. Shoulder Elbow Surg.*, **2**, 11–21 (1993)

16. Frich, L.H., Sojbjerg, J.O. and Sneppen, O. Shoulder arthroplasty in complex acute and chronic proximal humeral fractures. *Orthopedics*, **14**, 949–954 (1991)

17. Tanner, M.W. and Cofield, R.H. Prosthetic arthroplasty for fractures and fracture-dislocations of the proximal humerus. *Clin. Orthop.*, **179**, 116–128 (1983)

18. Neer, C.S. Articular replacement for the humeral head. *J. Bone Joint Surg.*, **37A**, 215–228 (1955)

19. Neer, C.S. and McIlveen, S.J. Recent results and technique of prosthetic replacement for 4-part proximal humerus fractures. *Orthop. Trans.*, **10**, 476 (1986)

20. Norris, T. Fractures of the proximal humerus and dislocations of the shoulder. In *Skeletal Trauma* (eds B.D. Browner, J.B. Jupiter and A.M. Levine), W.B. Saunders, Philadelphia (1992), pp. 1201–1290

21. Willems, W.J. and Lim, T.E. Neer arthroplasty for humeral fractures. *Acta Orthop. Scand.*, **56**, 394–395 (1985)

22. Kraulis, J. and Hunter, G. The results of prosthetic replacement in fracture-dislocation of the upper end of the humerus. *J. Trauma*, **21**, 788–791 (1976)

23. Bigliani, L.U. and McCluskey, G.M. Prosthetic replacement in acute fractures of the proximal humerus. *Sem. Arthroplasty*, **1**, 129–137 (1990)

24. Bigliani, L.U., Flatow, E.L., McCluskey, G.M. *et al.* Failed prosthetic replacement for displaced proximal humerus fractures. *Orthop. Trans.*, **15**, 747–748 (1991)

25. Des Marchais, J.E. and Benazet, J.P. Evaluation of Neer's hemiarthroplasty in the treatment of humeral fractures. *Can. J. Surg.*, **26**, 469–471 (1983)

26. Neer, C.S., Watson, K.C. and Stanton, F.J. Recent experience in total shoulder replacement. *J. Bone Joint Surg.*, **64A**, 319–337 (1982)

27. Green, A., Barnard, W.L. and Limbird, R.S. Humeral head replacement for acute, four-part proximal humerus fractures. *J. Shoulder Elbow Surg.*, **2**, 249–254 (1993)

28. Moeckel, B.H., Dines, D.M., Warren, R.F. *et al.* Modular hemiarthroplasty for fractures of the proximal part of the humerus. *J. Bone Joint Surg.* **74A**, 884–889 (1992)

29. Switlyk, P. and Hawkins, R.J. Hemiarthroplasty for treatment of severe proximal humerus fracture. *Orthop. Trans.*, **13**, 235 (1989)

30. Dines, D.M. and Altchek, D.W. Hemiarthroplasty techniques for for proximal humerus fractures. *Complications Orthop.*, **3**, 25–31 (1991)

31. Hughes, M. and Neer, C. Glenohumeral joint replacement and postoperative rehabilitation. *Phys. Ther.*, **55**, 850–858 (1975)

32. Rao, J.P., Berkman, A.R. and LaPilusa, S.J. A spontaneous relocation of a dislocated Neer prosthesis. Occurs with recovery of brachial plexus lesion. *Orthop. Rev.*, **15**, 453–456 (1986)

33. Mills, H.J. and Horne, G. Fractures of the proximal humerus in adults. *J. Trauma*, **25**, 801–805 (1985)

8

Alternatives to hemiarthroplasty in the treatment of complex proximal humeral fractures

Jon J.P. Warner and Christian Gerber

Only about 20% of proximal humeral fractures represent a therapeutic challenge for orthopaedic surgical management. These often occur in active, middle-aged individuals and may result in significant functional deficiencies[1-3]. These injuries are usually the result of high-energy trauma and are comminuted and displaced, sometimes with an associated glenohumeral dislocation. Conservative treatment gives poor results[4-9]. Standard techniques of open reduction and rigid internal fixation may be technically possible only in select cases due to difficulties resulting from osteoporotic, comminuted bone[2,4,6,10-22]. In three- and four-part fractures in particular, the additional surgical devascularization through exposure and implant positioning places the articular segment at increased risk for avascular necrosis, thereby compromising the final outcome[23-25]. While hemiarthroplasty is considered to be the procedure of choice in older individuals with three- and four-part fractures, the documented clinical short and mid-term results, and the concerns about prosthesis longevity, suggest the need to develop and study optimal joint preserving reconstructive techniques.[26-34]

Rational treatment decisions for these fractures requires insight into the mechanical and biological problem in each case, as well as an appreciation of the displacement types and natural history of individual fractures[6,35-38]. It is the experience of the senior author (C.G.) that *certain* complex proximal humerus fractures can be treated successfully using reduction and fixation techniques which minimize trauma the residual vascular supply to the articular segment. These techniques, which

minimally traumatize the periarticular soft tissues, may yield not only long-term excellent clinical results, but also allow successful secondary prosthetic reconstruction in cases complicated by avascular necrosis[38-42]. This chapter considers these issues and presents the authors' concepts for joint-preserving surgery for complex proximal humeral fractures.

The problem of classification/ prediction of outcome

A rational decision concerning treatment of a fracture is based on an appreciation of the prognosis of this particular fracture type. Two detailed classification systems are currently employed by most practising orthopaedic surgeons and are used as a guide for selecting treatment, namely the Neer[8,9] and the AO/ASIF classification[43].

The Neer[8,9] classification depends on a standard radiographic evaluation, if necessary aided by special imaging techniques[44-47]; it distinguishes four groups of displaced fractures and a group of fracture-dislocations. Subgroups are included for displaced segments in the three- and four-part fractures and articular surface impression fractures. Displacement is arbitrarily defined based on Neer's extensive clinical experience, and is considered to be present if segments are displaced linearly more than 10 mm or rotated more than 45°. The decision not to consider impacted fragments with a displacement of more than 1 cm or a tilt of more than 45° has thereby created considerable confusion[47]. The justification for these particular values remains unsubstantiated by experimental or clinical data; however, it has never been the concept to apply these values in an unreflected way, but as guidelines for discriminating displaced from undisplaced fractures in the recognized continuum of segment displacement. Indeed, it is often difficult to determine, on X-rays, if a segment is 'displaced', but this decision has relevant implications for treatment. Due to individual interpretation, there may be an unjustified impression that all 'four-part' fractures do poorly after joint-preserving surgery and should be treated with hemiarthroplasty due to development of avascular necrosis.

The AO alphanumeric system of A, B, C describes fractures of increasing severity, with each alpha group subgrouped numerically – higher numbers reflecting greater severity of injury[43]. For each group, subgroup 1 corresponds to undisplaced or minimally displaced fractures, subgroup 2 to displaced fractures, and subgroup 3 to displaced fractures with comminution or dislocation. The purpose of this classification system was to provide a more detailed method for fracture documentation and offer a more specific algorithmic approach to treatment.

Several recent studies have documented that even excellent preoperative routine X- ray analysis does not allow reproducible classification of these fractures according to these two systems[6,35–38]. Fractures classified similarly on the basis of preoperative X-rays may therefore be different fractures, and comparing series from different institutions must be considered to be invalid. The problems associated with classification may indeed largely account for the variability of the treatment results of allegedly similar fractures[3,8,9,33,47–49].

In addition, it is also likely that the wide variation in reported treatment outcome also reflects the variability of surgical techniques used to reconstruct these fractures. These observations suggest that our knowledge of classification, natural history and results of various treatments is insufficient to form the basis of conclusive guidelines for treatment of these fractures.

Consideration of outcome of treatment

Quality of maintained ('anatomical') reduction

In general, it is preferable to anatomically reconstruct complex proximal humeral fractures with an 'alive' rather than a 'dead' (prosthetic) articular segment. In active, middle-aged individuals the functional outcome of the latter approach is often not satisfactory[26–28,30,31,33,34,50,51]. Open reduction and rigid fixation using traditional AO concepts with plates[9,18,52–55] is also often unsatisfactory for many cases. Both open reduction and internal fixation (ORIF) and prosthetic replacement approaches require anatomical reconstruction of tuberosities and rotator cuff while maintaining soft tissue integrity and mobility in order to restore good function[56].

All methods of reduction and fixation must consider the following inherent problems in operating in this region:

- *the bone of the proximal humerus is osteoporotic*, which makes it difficult to obtain and particularly to maintain anatomical reduction and may render rigid internal fixation almost impossible[2,5,11,14,15,18–22,25,57,58].
- residual vascularity of the articular segment may be tenuous, and soft tissue stripping for fixation may increase *chances of avascular necrosis* (AVN)[6,20,42].
- the anatomy somewhat limits the use of protruding fixation devices due to *potential impingement* and therefore interference with an early active rehabilitation programme[6,18].

For these reasons a variety of fixation techniques have been proposed as alternatives to rigid internal fixation with plate and screws. These include external fixation[4,52,59,60], intramedullary nails[6,9,61–64], tension-band fixation[1,49,53,65,66], tension-band fixation combined with intramedullary nails[67–71], and closed reduction and percutaneous pinning[44,72–76].

It has been our experience that, provided that the anatomical relationship between head segment and the tuberosities are restored, rotational and angular deformities between the head and the shaft are well tolerated in healed proximal humeral fractures[73]; and if these are functionally relevant, they are amenable to surgical management with a good to excellent prognosis[39]. Furthermore, anatomical restoration of the tuberosities is as important a factor in overall functional outcome as is vascular integrity of the articular segment.

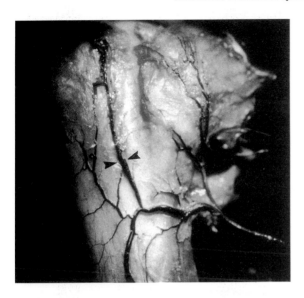

Figure 8.1 The ascending branch (arrows) of the anterior humeral circumflex artery forms the major blood supply to the articular segment of the humeral head in this right shoulder. (From Gerber *et al.*[23], by permission)

Consequences of avascular necrosis

The reported rate of avascular necrosis following operative treatment of three- and four-part fractures is 12–25% and 41–59%, respectively[1,6,7,9,15,33,48,57,60,74–80]. In general, ORIF with plate and screws has been associated with a higher rate of AVN than ORIF with minimal dissection and fixation or closed reduction and internal fixation (CRIF)[42,48,73,75,76,81]. The major blood supply to the articular segment comes from the anterolateral ascending branch of the anterior humeral circumflex artery running in the bicipital groove lateral to the long head of the biceps tendon. This vessel enters the humeral head at the proximal end of the bicipital groove at its junction with the greater tuberosity (Figure 8.1)[23,24]. This is precisely the region where dissection is necessary for application of a plate.

It has been reported that certain fractures which were classified as a four-part in the Neer system have a lower incidence of AVN[78]. Therefore, in these particular incidences, careful ORIF with minimal disruption of soft tissue can give good results. Jakob *et al.*[78] reported on what they called the 'valgus-impacted' four-part fracture and suggested that valgus angulation of the articular segment >45° may not disrupt its vascular supply (Figure 8.2(a-c). In these fractures, repair by a lim-ited open reduction and fixation technique yielded good and excellent results in the majority of patients, and resulted in an AVN rate of only 26%. Furthermore, Jaberg and colleagues[73] and others[48,82] have observed that some individuals with three- or four-part fractures may develop a form of subtotal AVN which is manifest as reversible sclerocystic changes in the humeral head. In these cases, they feel that careful limited dissection and fixation were responsible for preserving some residual vascularity and avoiding collapse due to AVN.

The natural history of AVN following proximal humeral fracture has remained controversial. The consensus has been that this is a catastrophic complication attended by advancing humeral head collapse and pain and dysfunction[57,77,83,84]. Recently, the senior author (C.G.) has examined this opinion by comparing 25 patients with AVN after ORIF for three- or four-part fractures with a group of 15 undergoing immediate hemiarthroplasty for similar fractures[40]. Postoperative follow-up was 6.5 years and 3.5 years, respectively, for each group. These groups were found to be statistically similar with regard to overall clinical function (age and sex-adjusted Constant Score)[85], active range of motion and complaints of pain. If the avascular necrosis cases were divided into one group in which AVN had ensued after anatomical reduction and into a second group with AVN after non-anatomical reduction, it was shown that the clinical results after anatomical reduction were at least as good as after hemiarthroplasty; however, the results of AVN in the setting of an additional malunion were poor. It is therefore our impression that a shoulder can function satisfactorily over many years despite post-traumatic AVN, provided that the fracture had initially been reduced anatomically and that this reduction had been maintained until healing of the fracture (Figure 8.3a-g).

Other factors

Miscellaneous other factors must be considered when selecting treatment and/or predicting outcome. These include the presence of other local (rotator cuff tear, nerve injury, dislocation) and systemic (brain injury, compliance in postoperative care) injuries. Patient factors such as alcoholism, metabolic bone disease (osteopenia, renal osteodystrophy, etc.), old age, and dependence on crutches, are not favourable factors for internal fixation of proximal humeral fractures and these factors should be taken into account when alterna-

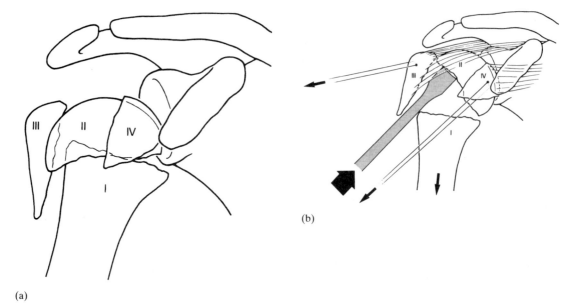

(a)

(b)

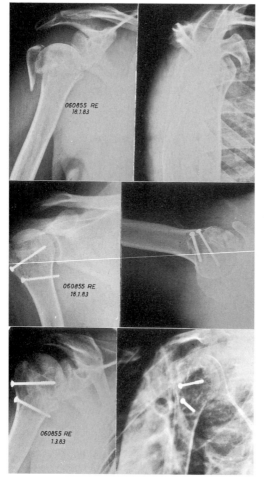

(c)

Figure 8.2   (a,b) Valgus-impacted four-part fracture anatomy and technique of open reduction and repair (see text for additional explanation). (From Jakob *et al.*[78], by permission). (c) Four-part valgus, impacted fracture fixed with two screws

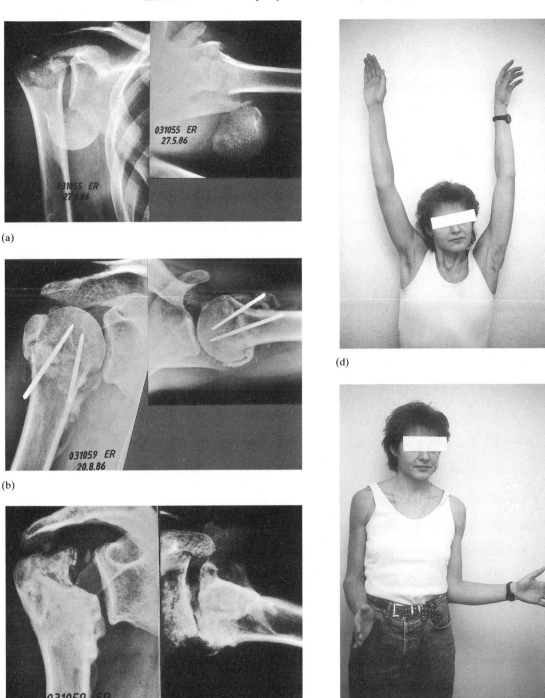

Figure 8.3 (a) Anatomical neck fracture in a 31-year-old woman. (b) Open reduction and minimal dissection with fixation using two pins; (c) Four years following surgery there is global collapse of the humeral head secondary to avascular necrosis, but the tuberosities are anatomical. (d–g) Clinical function at 4 years is good, though this patient has some limitation of rotation. There is only occasional mild pain

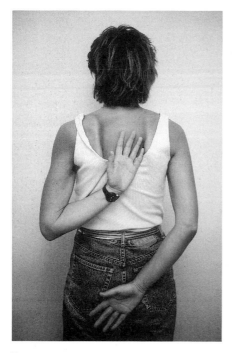

(f)

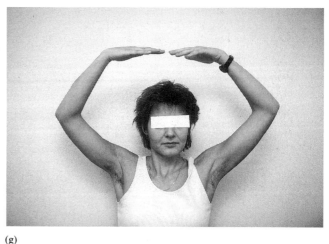

(g)

Figure 8.3 *cont.*

tives to hemiarthroplasty are considered. It is our experience that severe osteoporosis is associated with a high rate of complications of closed reduction and internal fixation, and the methods to be presented are mainly considered in the young patient with good bone quality and a reasonable potential for compliance with a postoperative regimen.

Authors' preferred methods of treatment

Closed reduction and percutaneous pinning

This technique is mainly used to treat two- and three-part fractures of patients with good bone quality which can be reduced closed but cannot be maintained in a close to anatomical position without stabilization[44,73]. The main advantage of this technique is that it limits soft tissue trauma with its additional morbidity (postoperative shoulder stiffness), and that it does not constitute a significant risk to the vascular supply of the articular segment. The technique is technically demanding and requires a co-ordinated team effort by anaesthesia, radiology, and the operating surgeon and his assistants.

Reduction manoeuvre

The patient is positioned supine on the operating table with the arm abducted to about 70–80°. The patient must be positioned and supported with the shoulder over the edge of the operating table so that the C-arm image intensifier can visualize the joint in both anteroposterior and axillary planes. A vacuum mattress is helpful for maintaining this position and preventing the patient from slipping. Image intensification *must* allow true anteroposterior and true axillary lateral imaging of the fracture. *Failure to test whether these two projections are easily possible on the table before draping is considered to be a formal technical error* (Figure 8.4 a–e). The reduction manoeuvre consists of progressive longitudinal traction applied to the abducted arm, while posterior pressure is applied to the humeral shaft to reduce it underneath the humeral head. In most cases the humeral shaft is displaced anteriorly or angulated anteriorly by the pull of the pectoralis major, and posterior pressure on the shaft will correct this deformity (Figure 8.4). Failure of reduction is usually the result of soft tissue interposition (periosteum or long head of biceps) or irreducible displacement of tuberosity fragments. If this technique does not allow reduction, a 2.5 mm pin with a threaded tip is brought through the greater tuberosity into the humeral head and used as a 'joystick' for reducing the humeral head–tuberosity part to the shaft.

Pinning technique

An attempt is made to reduce the humeral head slightly medial to the shaft allowing for placement of one pin centrally in the head segment (Figure 8.4). Terminally threaded AO pins (2.5 mm) are used for fixation, since the terminal threads reduce the risk of migration. To determine proper pin placement, a pin is held over the anterior shoulder and visualized with the image intensifier. In varus displacements, a first pin is introduced through the greater tuberosity coming from a position immedi-

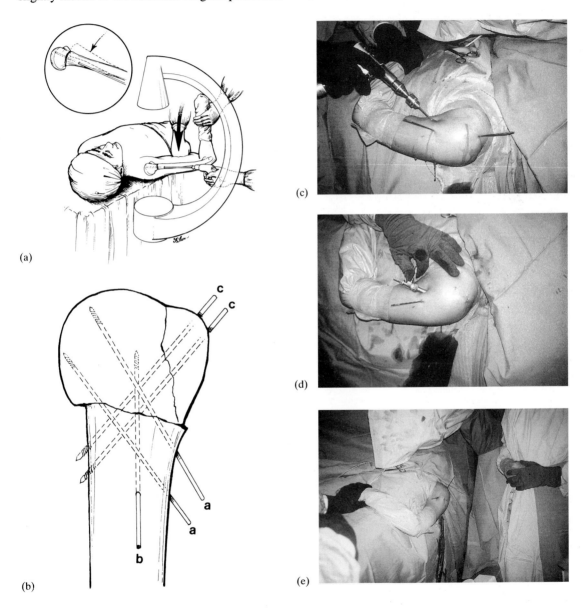

(a)

(b)

(c)

(d)

(e)

Figure 8.4 (a) Patient positioning and reduction manoeuvre for closed reduction and percutaneous pinning (see text for further explanation). (From Jaberg *et al.*[73], by permission). (b) Three terminally threaded AO pins, 2.5 mm in diameter, are inserted. Two are passed through the lateral aspect of the humeral shaft just above the deltoid insertion (**a**), and a third is placed through the anterior cortex (**b**). If the greater tuberosity is displaced, two more pins are inserted retrograde for reduction and fixation (**c**). (From Jaberg *et al.*[73], by permission). (c–e) Clinical example of pinning technique (see text for explanation)

ately adjacent to the lateral acromion into the humeral head. After the malalignment is corrected, it becomes obvious that this pin would exit above the shaft segment if driven further. A second pin is then introduced again from a new skin incision immediately adjacent to the lateral acromion and

introduced from above downwards with the reduction being maintained using the first pin as a 'joy-stick'. This second pin can then usually be driven further into the shaft segment which has been reduced manually. A small incision is then made along the lateral shaft of the humerus, being care-

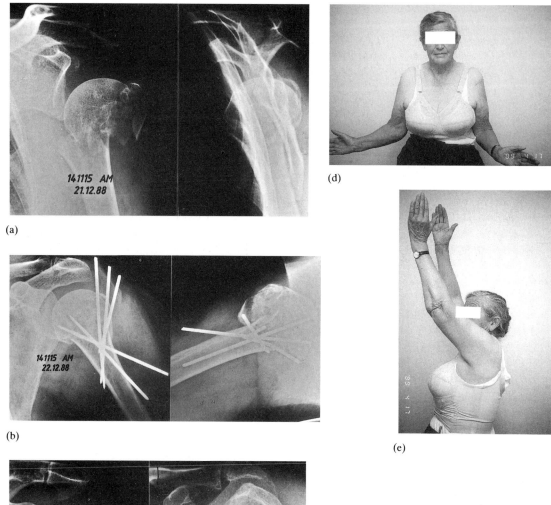

(a)

(b)

(c)

(d)

(e)

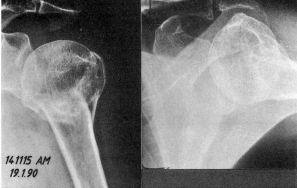

Figure 8.5 Displaced two-part fracture which could be reduced closed but was unstable. (b) Closed reduction and percutaneous pinning was performed. (c) Two years after surgery there is radiographic union with satisfactory alignment. (d, e) Clinical function at 2 years is excellent

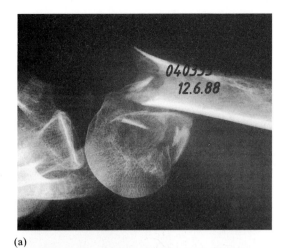

(a)

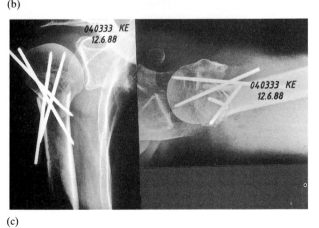

(b)

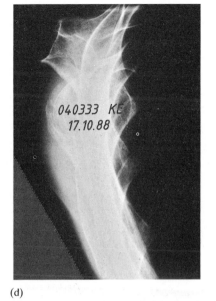

(d)

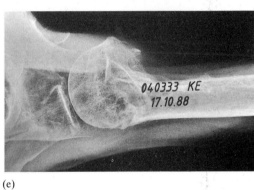

(e)

(c)

Figure 8.6   (a, b) Displaced, unstable two-part fracture. (c) Closed reduction and percutaneous fixation. (d, e) Four months after surgery there is radiographic union and satisfactory alignment. (f–i) This patient is wheel-chair dependent and has excellent function with independent transfer ability

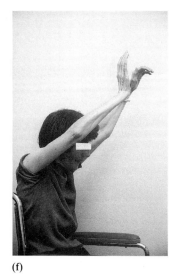

(f)

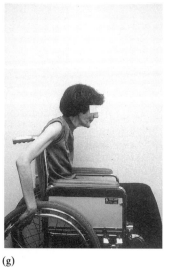

(g)

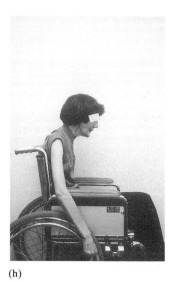

(h)

Figure 8.6 *cont.*

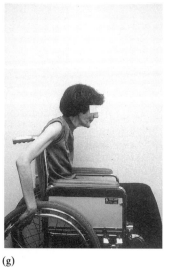

(i)

ful to remain above the deltoid insertion so as not to risk injury to the radial nerve. A straight clamp is then placed into the incision and the soft tissue is spread down to the lateral cortex of the humeral shaft. The angle of insertion of each pin relative to the lateral cortex is about 45°, and usually three pins are placed from the shaft into the head segment in as wide a spread as possible. The normal 30° retroversion of the humeral head is considered when inserting the pins. Two to three pins coming from distal to proximal are used to stabilize the shaft-head segment reduction. If the arm is held in internal rotation, it should be realized that a pin introduced in the frontal plane is placed too anteriorly in the head segment. The pin should be directed from anterior and lateral to posterior and medial. After each pin is inserted, an axillary image is made to ensure proper placement. A displaced greater tuberosity fragment is stabilized with two pins (to the shaft, not only to the head) (Figure 8.5 a–c). The pins are then trimmed to a subcutaneous position and the arm is placed in a Velpeau dressing.

Postoperative care

The arm remains immobilized for 3 weeks. Any physiotherapy within the first 2–3 weeks is considered to be an error. Serial X-rays are taken at 10-day intervals to check for pin loosening and migration. If pins have been placed in a greater tuberosity fragment these are removed at 3 weeks and then gentle pendulum exercises are begun. The remaining pins are removed after 1–3 additional weeks, at which time active-assisted range of motion is instituted.

Clinical examples of this technique are illustrated in Figures 8.5 (a–e) and 8.6 (a–i).

Complications and contraindications

Loss of fixation due to pin loosening or migration is rare[73] (Figure 8.7 a, b) in young patients with adequate bone. When this occurs it is usually due to inappropriate selection of a patient, and less frequently to technically inadequate pinning or to early mobilization after surgery. The most

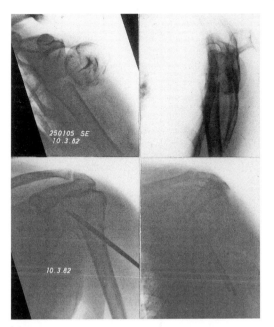

(a)

Figure 8.7 (a) Two-part displaced fracture closed, reduced and fixed with too few pins, too close together, and placed too medially. (b) Displacement of the fracture occurred with loss of fixation and, with the exception of breakage of one pin intramedullary, the fracture was successfully managed with a revision closed reduction and pinning using a correct technique

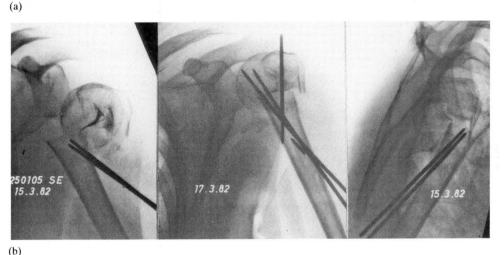

(b)

common technical error is to place too few pins or pins too close together (Figure 8.7). Malunion of the shaft–articular segment in the coronal, sagittal or rotational planes is usually not problematic, though displacement of a greater tuberosity fragment may sometimes lead to impingement and loss of motion (Figure 8.8 a–e). The presence of metaphyseal comminution is a contraindication to this technique, as loss of fixation and failure of union are likely to occur (Figure 8.9 a–d). Even though pin migration is a concern, we have not had a problem with this since serial X-rays allow us to identify and remove any loose pins. Pin-track infection has not been observed since we cut the

pins underneath the skin. We have not had a problem with permanent loss of motion due to scarring with this form of postoperative care; and in our experience immobilization after this technique of transcutaneous fixation is not detrimental to ultimate function. Fracture through pin holes after removal is a rare but a potential complication which has recently been reported[86].

Open reduction and minimal fixation

This type of surgical approach might be more appropriately described as open reduction with minimal soft tissue dissection followed by surgical

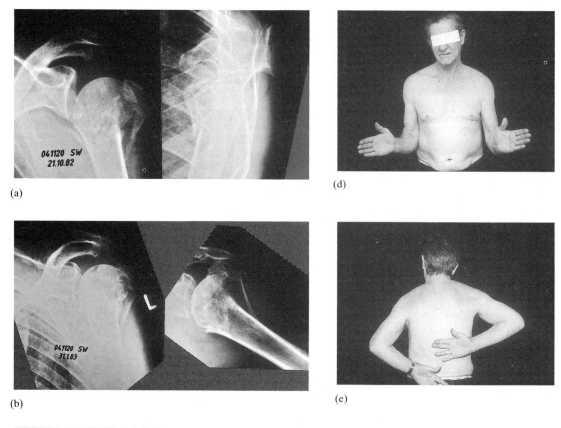

(a)

(b)

(d)

(e)

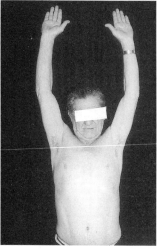

(c)

Figure 8.8 (a) Two-part fracture with cephalad displacement of the greater tuberosity. (b) Malunion of the greater tuberosity in a proximal, displaced position occurred. (c–e) This patient, however, had no symptoms of impingement

stabilization. As we have previously suggested, there are many three- and four-part fractures which may have sufficient vascularity to the articular segment through retained soft tissue attachments that AVN is not a certainty. However, we feel strongly that aggressive surgical dissection and reduction with soft tissue stripping required to apply a plate to the lateral cortex or even detachment of the subscapularis and opening the joint may destroy this residual soft tissue and its vascularity, thus pro-

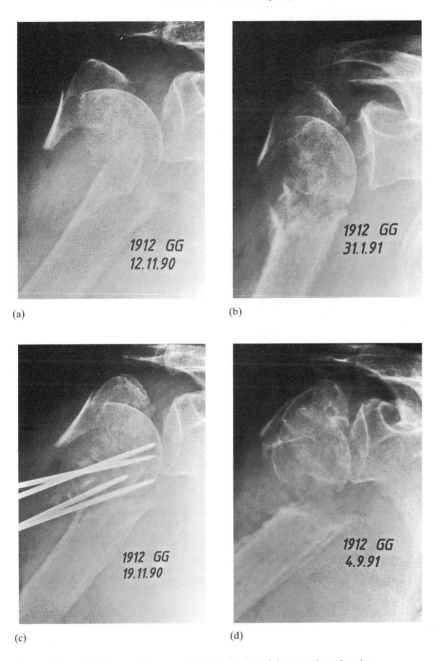

(a)

(b)

(c)

(d)

Figure 8.9   (a, b) Three-part fracture with comminution of the metaphyseal region.
(c) Inadequate reduction and pinning with failure to stabilize any of the three segments.
(d) Progression to non-union

moting AVN (Figure 8.10 a–d). One type of fracture which we believe may be treated by a limited open approach is the 'valgus-impacted four-part' fracture[78] (see Figure 8.2). By the AO classification this would be called a C2.1 or C2.2 fracture,

and Jakob observed an AVN rate of only 5 of 19 (26%) when such fractures were treated with limited dissection and fixation. Reduction is achieved through a deltopectoral approach with use of a bone punch or laminar spreader to reposition the

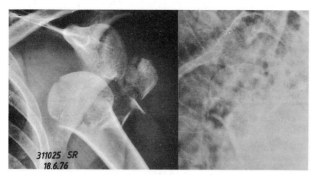

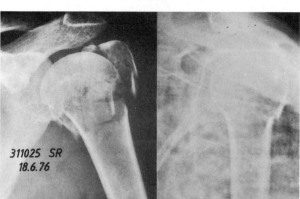

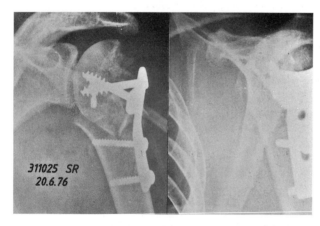

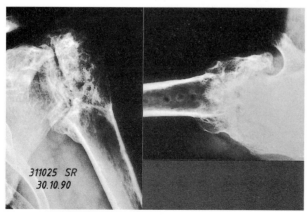

Figure 8.10 (a) Three-part anterior fracture-dislocation. (b) Closed reduction of the dislocation. (c) Open reduction and internal fixation with an AO plate and screws. (d) Progressive avascular necrosis and humeral head articular segment collapse over 14 years.

(a)

(b)

(c)

(d)

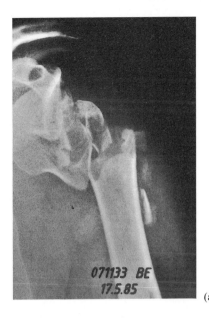

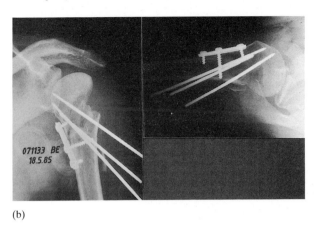

(b)

(a)

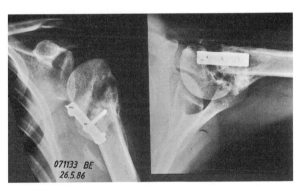

(c)

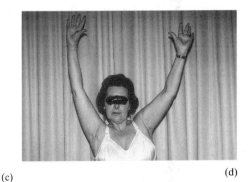

(d)

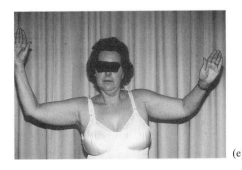

(e)

Figure 8.11 (a) Three-part fracture dislocation with extensive metaphyseal comminution. (b) This was reduced and fixed using combined medial plate with bone graft and percutaneously placed pins in order to preserve residual soft tissue connections and articular segment vascularity. (c) After removal of the pins the fracture healed with some medially bridging callus. The articular segment remained viable. (d, e) The patient has excellent function 3 years after surgery

articular segment out of its valgus attitude (see Figure 8.2). In cases where valgus correction leaves a significant bony defect underneath the humeral head, a bone graft from the iliac crest is used to buttress the reduced articular segment. Large non-absorbable sutures are placed in the tuberosity fragments to reposition them and the

fixation is achieved using sutures alone, or occasionally screws or (wire) suture cerclages, carefully avoiding injury to the ascending branch of the anterior humeral circumflex artery (see Figure 8.1).

For some three-part fractures we apply a modified tension-band technique similar to that described by Hawkins[1,13], but we always perform only minimal soft tissue dissection around the bicipital groove area.

Management of extensive comminution

Some proximal humeral fractures may be very difficult to treat due to extension of comminution into the metaphysis or even the diaphysis. In certain cases these will be three- or four-part fractures. Surgical treatment by either hemiarthroplasty or ORIF can be problematic due to poor bone stock (Figure 8.11a–e). We have found it useful to individualize treatment by combining techniques of closed reduction and open reduction with internal fixation (Figure 8.11). In cases where we think we can preserve the articular segment viability, we still apply the standard AO techniques[54] of rigid internal fixation (Figure 8.12a, b).

Management of head-splitting fractures and articular impression fractures

In complex head-splitting fractures, the only alternative is hemiarthroplasty replacement. In most cases these fractures occur in older individuals with osteoporotic bone that comminutes when subjected to a forceful central impaction injury[87] (Figure 8.13). However, this injury may also occur in a young individual. In the case of extensive articular comminution in a young labourer, we would recommend arthrodesis. In some cases where there is a single fracture line through the articular surface, we would treat this with open reduction just as we might apply to an intra-articular fracture in the knee or ankle. Fortunately, younger patients usually have bone with a density sufficient to permit fixation by screws (Figure 8.14a–c).

Traditional teaching is that an impression fracture involving more than 40% of the articular sur-

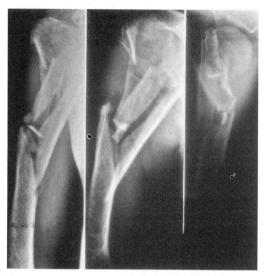

(a)

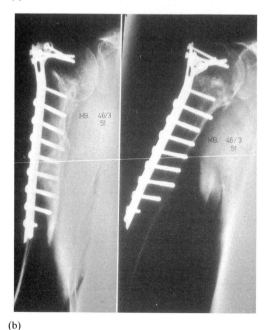

(b)

Figure 8.12 Comminuted metaphyseal–diaphyseal fracture in a young patient. (b) Open reduction and internal fixation with an AO plate and screw

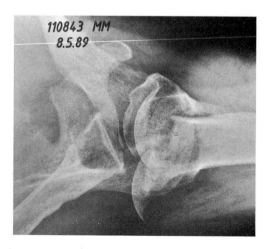

Figure 8.13 Articular head-splitting fracture in an elderly patient. This required a hemiarthroplasty

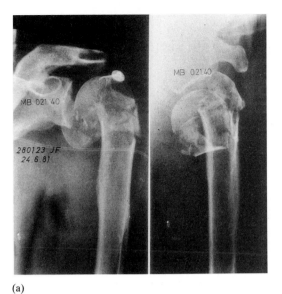

(a)

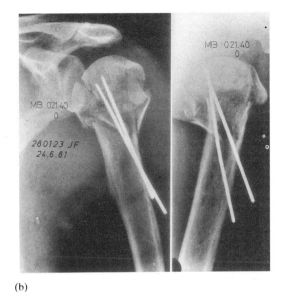

(b)

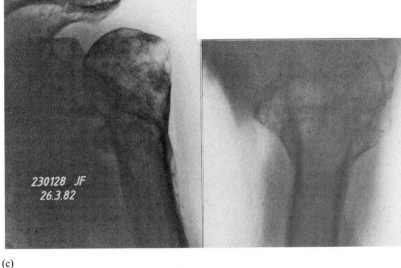

(c)

Figure 8.14 (a) Proximal humerus fracture with intra-articular displaced fracture component. (b) This fracture was reduced through a limited open approach and stabilized with two percutaneous pins. (c) The fracture has healed with acceptable joint congruity

face of the humerus, as might occur with a locked posterior dislocation, requires hemiarthroplasty. This is considered as undesirable in a young patient and has led the senior author (C.G.) to attempt reconstruction of the humeral head with a matched osteochondral allograft. This has been found to be a valuable alternative to hemiarthroplasty in selected cases.[88] (Figure 8.15a–c).

Management of anatomical neck fractures

Isolated anatomical neck fractures are rare. In the AO series both non-displaced and displaced isolated anatomical neck fractures accounted for only 0.3% (2/730) of all proximal humeral fractures treated surgically. Non-displaced anatomical neck fractures may not progress to AVN; however, we have seen cases where an unrecognized anatomical

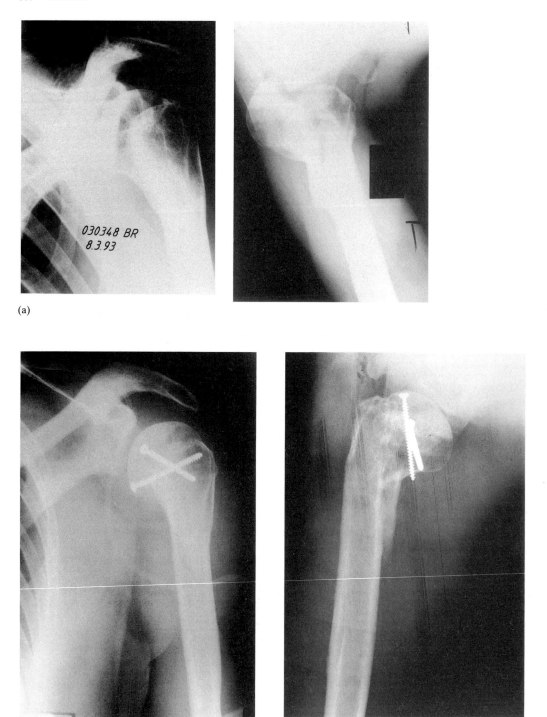

(a)

(b)   (c)

Figure 8.15   (a) Chronic, locked, posterior dislocation with a large reverse Hill–Sachs lesion. (b, c) This was reduced through an anterior approach and the articular segment was reconstructed with a matched humeral head osteochondral allograft

neck fracture displaced during closed reduction of a dislocated shoulder (Figure 8.16a–d) and documented the results of this condition[89]. In older individuals with an anatomical neck fracture we recommend hemiarthroplasty, while in younger individuals we will conservatively treat non-displaced anatomical neck fractures, and occasionally attempt open reduction and fixation in the hopes that articular collapse may be minimal (Figure 8.16). The anatomical neck fracture should, however, usually be treated with hemiarthroplasty, and joint preservation surgery must be looked at as experimental.

Conclusion

The classification of fractures remains an important problem which hinders critical review of results of fracture treatment. While the four-segment concept appears to be an excellent one, allowing meaningful description and communication, we do not yet have reliable methods of imaging to reproducibly describe the position of each segment and thereby assign the fracture a specific place in a classification system. In our experience, the quality of the bone is a factor that has to be taken into account if optimal treatment

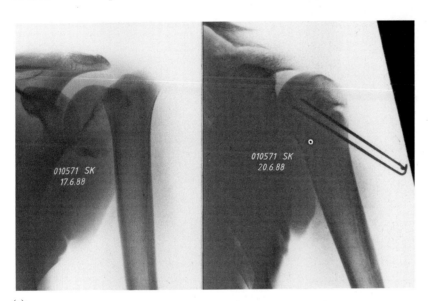

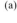

(a)

Figure 8.16 (a) Anatomical neck fracture which displaced with reduction of an anterior dislocation. This was fixed using open reduction and percutaneous pin fixation. (b) The fracture united. (c) MRI demonstrates avascular necrosis after surgical stabilization. (d) At 1 year there was no humeral head collapse, but with subsequent follow-up the humeral head has demonstrated progressive collapse

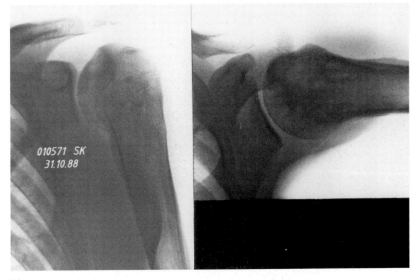

(b)

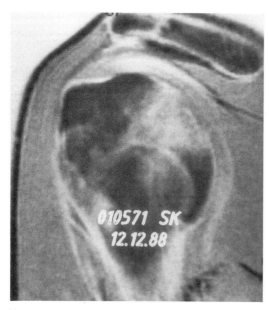

(c)

Figure 8.16 *cont.*

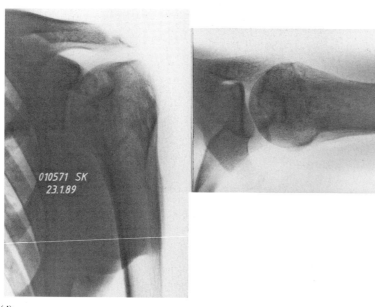

(d)

is to be selected, and it may well be that the same fracture accurately classified in two different patients requires different treatment.

Neither hemiarthroplasty nor open reduction and internal fixation yields consistently satisfactory results in the treatment of complex ('three- and four-part') fractures of the humerus. Assessment, operative technique and postoperative care are continuously evolving, and thus lead to stepwise improvements of the results of these fractures treated with hemiarthroplasty as well as with open or closed reduction and internal fixation. We feel that reduction and internal fixation techniques have radically evolved and possibly made more progress than the techniques of hemiarthroplasty. These conceptual changes must be implemented if

ORIF or CRIF are applied to the treatment of these fractures; and it should be understood that the results of modern reduction and internal fixation techniques are not comparable to those currently quoted in the literature. The main advances are the understanding that any reduction and internal fixation must respect the biology of the anatomical region and the fracture, and that surgical approach, reduction techniques and implants have to be selected accordingly[41]. We now know that non-anatomical reductions of complex fractures must not be accepted, and that anatomical reduction is absolutely critical if good function of the shoulder is to be maintained. This factor even takes precedence over the development of AVN[49]. It is our opinion that if such a reduction is obtained without soft tissue trauma, revision to hemiarthroplasty or total shoulder is possible with a good functional result[39,40]. This is, however, not the case if the anatomy of the proximal humerus is distorted, and the soft tissues have been compromised. Furthermore, we have observed that when fixation is extra-articular without soft tissue stripping, it is not necessary to move the shoulder immediately. Rather, the maintenance of the obtained reduction is of much higher priority than obtaining very early motion. Many complex fractures of the proximal humerus, however, especially in alchoholics and elderly patients with relevant osteopenia, should *not* be treated with ORIF or CRIF, even if they are to be classified similarly to a comparable fracture of a young individual which can be treated with joint-preserving surgery. There is no doubt that for such patients hemiarthoplasty is superior; and we need to continue to improve our technique of surgery and rehabilitation. It is the authors' feeling that the current controversy whether hemiarthroplasty or ORIF/CRIF are better for the treatment of complex proximal humeral fractures is artificial. These two methods are complementary and it is our mission to improve both methods and to define which method is best for which fracture in which patient.

References

1. Hawkins, R.J., Bell, R.H. and Gurr, K. The three-part fracture of the proximal humerus: operative treatment. *J. Bone Joint Surg.*, **68A**, 1410–1414 (1986)
2. Horak, J. and Nilsson, B.E. Epidemiology of fractures o the upper end of the humerus: an experimental and clinica study. *J. Bone Joint Surg.*, **32**, 1–29 (1934)
3. Jakob, R.P. and Ganz, R. Proximale humerusfrakturer *Helv. Chir. Acta.*, **48**, 595–610 (1981)
4. Kristiansen, B. External fixation of proximal humerus fractures: clinical and cadaver study of pinning technique. *Acta Orthop. Scand.*, **58**, 645–648 (1987)
5. Kristiansen, B., Angermann, P. and Larsen, T.K. Functional results following fractures of the proximal humerus. A controlled clinical study comparing two periods of immobilization. *Arch. Orthop. Trauma Surg.*, **108**, 339–341 (1989)
6. Kristiansen, B. and Christiansen, S.W. Proximal humerus fractures. Late results in relation to classification and treatment. *Acta Orthop. Scand.*, **58**, 124–127 (1987)
7. Mouradian, W.H. Displaced proximal humerus fractures: seven years' experience with a modified Zickel supracondylar device. *Clin. Orthop.*, **212**, 209–218 (1986)
8. Neer, C.S. II. Displaced proximal humerus fractures. Part I: Classification and evaluation. *J. Bone Joint Surg.*, **52A**, 1077–1089 (1970)
9. Neer, C.S. II. Displaced proximal humerus fractures. Part II: Treatment of three-part and four-part displacement. *J. Bone Joint Surg.* **52A**, 1090–1103 (1970)
10. DuParc, J. and Largier, A. Les luxations-fractures de l'extrémité supérieure de l'humérus. *Rev. Chir. Orthop.*, **62**, 91–110 (1976)
11. Hall, M.C. and Rosser, M. The structure of the upper end of the humerus with reference to osteoporotic changes in senescence leading to fractures. *Can. Med. Ass. J.*, **88**, 290–294 (1963)
12. Hawkins, R.J. and Angelino, R.L. Displaced proximal humeral fractures: selecting treatment, avoiding pitfalls. *Orthop. Clin. N. Am.*, **18**, 421–431 (1987)
13. Hawkins, R.J. and Kiefer, G.N. Internal fixation techniques for proximal humeral fractures. *Clin. Orthop.*, **223**, 77–85 (1987)
14. Keene, J.S., Huizenga, R.E., Engber, W.B. and Rogers, S.C. Proximal humerus fractures: a correlation of residual deformity with long-term function. *Orthopaedics*, **6**, 173–178 (1983)
15. Kristiansen, B. and Christiansen, S.W. Plate fixation of proximal humerus fractures. *Acta Orthop. Scand.*, **57**, 320–323 (1986)
16. Lyons, F.A. and Rockwood, C.A. Jr. Migration of pins used in operations on the shoulder. *J. Bone Joint Surg.*, **72A**, 1262–1267 (1990)
17. Paavolainen, P., Bjorkenheim, J.M., Slatis, P. and Pavkku, P. Operative treatment of severe proximal humerus fractures. *Acta Orthop. Scand.*, **54**, 374–379 (1983)
18. Poilleux, F. and Courtois-Suffit, M. Des fractures du Col Chirurgical de L'Humérus. *Rev. Chir.*, **75**, 133–158 (1954)
19. Savoie, F.H., Geissler, W.B. and Vander Greind, R.A. Open reduction and internal fixation of three-part fractures of the proximal humerus. *Orthopaedics*, **12**, 65–70 (1989)
20. Svend-Hansen, H. Displaced proximal humerus fractures: a review of 49 patients. *Acta Orthop. Scand.*, **45**, 359–364 (1974)
21. Watson, K.C. Complications of internal fixation of proximal humerus fractures. In *Complications of Shoulder Surgery* (ed. L.U. Bigliani), Williams and Wilkins, Baltimore, (1993) pp. 190–201
22. Watson, K.C. Modification of rush pin fixation for frac-

tures of the proximal humerus. Presented at A.S.E.S. Meeting, Santa Fe, New Mexico (November 1988)

23. Gerber, C., Schneeberger, A.G. and Vinh, T-S. The arterial vascularization of the humeral head. *J. Bone Joint Surg.* **72A**, 1486–1493 (1990)

24. Laing, P.G. The arterial supply of the adult humerus. *J. Bone Joint Surg.*, **38A**, 1105–1116 (1956)

25. Saitoh, S. and Nakatsuchi, Y. Osteoporosis of the proximal humerus: comparison of bone-mineral density and mechanical strength with the proximal femur. *J. Shoulder Elbow Surg.*, **2**, 78–84 (1993)

26. Desmarchais, J.E. and Morais, G. Treatment of complex fractures of the proximal humerus by Neer hemiarthroplasty. In *Surgery of the Shoulder* (eds J.E. Bateman and R.P. Welsh), C.V. Mosby, Toronto (1984), pp. 60–62

27. Fischer, R.A., Nicholson, G.P., McIlveen, S.J., McCann, D., Flatow, E.L. and Bigliani, L.U. Primary humeral head replacement for severely displaced proximal humerus fractures. Presented at the 8th Open Meeting of the A.S.E.S. Washington, D.C. (23 February 1992)

28. Green, A., Bernard, W.L. and Limbird, R.S. Humeral head replacement for acute, four-part proximal humerus fractures. *J. Shoulder Elbow Surg.*, **2**, 249–254 (1993)

29. Hawkins, R.J. and Switlyk, P. Acute prosthetic replacement for severe fractures of the proximal humerus. *Clin. Orthop.*, **289**, 156–160 (1993)

30. Kraulis, J. and Hunter, G. The results of prosthetic-replacement in fracture-dislocations of the upper end of the humerus. *Injury*, **8**, 129–131 (1976)

31. Moekel, B.H., Dines, D.M., Warren, R.F. and Altchek, D.W. Modular hemiarthroplasty for fractures of the proximal humerus. *J. Bone Joint Surg.*, **74**, 884–889 (1992)

32. Neer, C.S. II and McIlveen, S.J. Recent results and techniques of prosthetic replacement for four-part proximal humerus fractures. *Orthop. Trans.*, **10**, 475 (1986)

33. Stableforth, P.G. Four-part fractures of the neck of the humerus. *J. Bone Joint Surg.* **66B**, 104–108 (1984)

34. Tanner, M.W. and Cofield, R.H. Prosthetic arthroplasty for fractures and fracture-dislocations of the proximal humerus. *Clin. Orthop.*, **179**, 116–128 (1983)

35. Ackerman, C., Lam, Q., Linder, P., Kull, C. and Regazzoni, P. Problematik der Frakturklassifikation am proximalen humerus. *Z. Unfallchir. Vers. Med. Berufskr.*, **79**, 209–215 (1986)

36. Sidor, M.L., Zuckerman, J.D., Lyon, T., Koval, K. and Schoenberg, N. Neer classification of proximal humerus fractures and assessment of inter-observer and intra-observer reliability. Presented at the 8th Annual Open Meeting of the A.S.E.S. Washington, D.C. (23 February 1992)

37. Siebenrock, K.A. and Gerber, C. The reproducibility of classification of fractures of the proximal humerus. *J. Bone Joint Surg.* **75A** 1751–1755 (1993)

38. Siebenrock, K.A. and Gerber, C. Frakturklassification und Problematik bei proximalen Humerusfrakturen. *Orthopäde*, **21**, 98–105 (1992)

39. Gerber, C. Rekonstruktive Chirurgie nach fehlverheilten Frakturen des proximalen Humerus bei Erwachsensen. *Orthopäde*, **19**, 316–323 (1990)

40. Gerber, C. and Berberat, C. The clinical relevance of post-traumatic avascular necrosis of the humeral head. *J. Shoulder Elbow Surg.*, **2** (Supply. 1), 30 (1993)

41. Gerber, C., Mast, J.W. and Ganz, R. Biological fixation of fractures. *Arch Orthop. Trauma Surg.* **109**, 295–303 (1990)

42. Sturzenegger, M., Fornaro, E. and Jakob, R.P. Results of surgical treatment of multifragmented fractures of the humeral head. *Arch. Orthop. Traumat. Surg.*, **100**, 249–259 (1982)

43. Muller, M.E., Nazarian, S., Koch, P. and Schatzker, J. *The Comprehensive Classification of Fractures of Long Bones*, Springer-Verlag, Berlin (1990), p. 54

44. Benirschke, S.K., Urst, G.G., Healey, M.B. and Mago, K.A. Percutaneous pin fixation of surgical neck fractures of the humerus. Presented at the Annual Meeting of the Orthopaedic Trauma Association, Seattle, WA. (October 1991)

45. Kilcoyne, R.F., Shuman, W.P., Matsen, F.A. III, Morris, M. and Rockwood, C.A. Jr. The Neer classification of displaced proximal humerus fractures: spectrum of findings on plain radiographs and C.T. scans. *Am. J. Roentgenol.*, **154**, 1029–1033 (1990)

46. Kuhlman, J.E., Fishman, E.K., Ney, D.R. and Magial, D. Complex shoulder trauma: three-dimensional CT imaging. *Orthopaedics*, **11**, 1561–1563 (1988)

47. Neer, C.S. II. Fractures. In *Shoulder Reconstruction* (ed. C.S. Neer II), W.B. Saunders, Toronto (1990), p. 363.

48. Lee, C.H. and Hansen, H.R. Post-traumatic avascular necrosis of the humeral head in displaced proximal humerus fractures. *J. Trauma*, **21**, 788–791 (1981)

49. Mills, H.J. and Horne, J.G. Fractures of the proximal humerus in adults. *J. Trauma.* **25**(8), 801–805 (1985)

50. Cofield, R.H. Comminuted fractures of the proximal humerus. *Clin. Orthop.* **230**, 49 (1988)

51. deAnquin, C.L. and deAnquin, A. Prosthetic replacement in the treatment of serious fractures of the proximal humerus. In *Shoulder Injury* (eds I. Baley and L. Kessel), Springer-Verlag, Berlin (1965), pp. 206–217

52. Lentz, W. and Meuser, P. The treatment of fractures of the proximal humerus. *Arch. Orthop. Trauma Surg.*, **96**, 283–285 (1980)

53. Moda, S.K., Chadha, N.S., Sangwan, S.S., Khurana, D.K., Dahiya, A.S. and Siwaah, R.C. Open reduction and fixation of proximal humerus fractures and fracture-dislocations. *J. Bone Joint Surg.*, **72B**, 1050–1052 (1990)

54. Muller, M.E., Allgower, M., Schneider, R. and Willenegger, H. *Manual of Internal Fixation. Techniques Recommended by the A.O. Group*, Springer, New York (1979)

55. Sehr, J.R. and Szabo, R.M. Semitubular blade plate for fixation in the proximal humerus. *J. Orthop. Trauma*, **2**, 327–323 (1989)

56. Iannotti, J.P., Gabriel, J.P., Schneck, S.L., Evans, B.G. and Misra, S. The normal glenohumeral relationships. An anatomical study of one hundred and forty shoulders. *J. Bone Joint Surg.*, **74A**, 491–500 (1992)

57. Haag, O. and Lundberg, B. Aspects of prognostic factors in comminuted and dislocated proximal humerus fractures.

In *Surgery of the Shoulder* (eds J.E. Bateman and R.P. Welsh), Toronto, Decker (1984), pp. 57–59

58. Lind, T., Kroner, K. and Jensen, J. The epidemiology of fractures of the proximal humerus. *Arch. Orthop. Trauma Surg.*, **108**, 285–287 (1989)

59. Kristainsen, B. and Kofoed, H. Transcutaneous reduction and external fixation of displaced fractures of the proximal humerus: a controlled clinical trial. *J. Bone Joint Surg.*, **70B**, 821–824 (1988)

60. Lim, T.E., Ochsner, P.E., Marti, R.K. and Holscher, A.A. The results of treatment of comminuted fractures and fracture dislocations of the proximal humerus. *Neth. J. Surg.*, **35**, 139–143 (1983).

61. Grimes, D.W. The use of Rush pin fixation in unstable upper humeral fractures: a matched blind insertion. *Orthop. Rev.*, **9**, 75–79 (1980)

62. Haas, K. Displaced proximal humerus fractures operated by Rush pin technique. *Opuscula Medica*, **23**, 100–102 (1978)

63. Seidel, H. Humeral locking nail: a preliminary report. *Orthopaedics*, **12**, 219–226 (1989)

64. Weseley, M.S., Barenfeld, P.A. and Eisenstein, A.L. Rush pin intramedullary fixation for fractures of the proximal humerus. *J. Trauma*, **17**, 29–37 (1977)

65. Drapunas, T., McDonald, J. and Hale, H.W. Jr. A rationale approach to classification and treatment of fractures of the surgical neck of the humerus. *Am. J. Surg.*, **99**, 617–624 (1970)

66. Koval, K.J., Sanders, R., Zuckerman, J.D., Helfet, D.L., Kummer, F. and DiPasquale, T. Modified-tension band wiring of displaced surgical neck fractures of the humerus. *J. Shoulder Elbow Surg.*, **2**, 85–92 (1993)

67. Bigliani, L.U. Fractures of the proximal humerus. In *The Shoulder* (eds C.A. Rockwood and F.A. Matsen III), W.B. Saunders, Philadelphia (1990), pp 278–334

68. Bigliani, L.U. Treatment of two- and three-part fractures of the proximal humerus. *Instruct. Course Lect.* **38**, 231–244 (1989), American Academy of Orthopaedic Surgeons, Park Ridge, Ill

69. Contreras, D., Day, L., Bovill, D. and Appleton, A. Combined enders rods and tension banding for humeral neck fractures. Presented at 57th Annual Meeting, American Academy of Orthopaedic Surgeons, New Orleans, LA (9 February 1990)

70. Cuomo, F., Flatow, E.L., Maday, M.G., Miller, S.R., McIllveen, S.J. and Bigliani, L.U. Open reduction and internal fixation of two- and three-part proximal humerus fractures. *J. Shoulder Elbow Surg.* **1**, 287–295 (1992)

71. Norris, T.R. Fractures of the proximal humerus and dislocations of the shoulder. In *Skeletal Trauma* (eds B.D. Browner, J.B. Jupiter, A.M. Levine and P.G. Trafton), W.B. Saunders, Philadelphia (1992), pp. 1201–1290

72. Bohler, J. Les fractures récentes de l'épaule. *Acta Orthop. Belg.* **30**, 235–242 (1964)

73. Jaberg, H., Warner, J.J.P. and Jakob, R.P. Percutaneous stabilization of unstable fractures of the humerus. *J. Bone Joint Surg.*, **74A**, 508–515 (1992)

74. Jakob, R.P. Kristiansen, T., Mago, K., Ganz, R. and Muller, M.E. Classification and aspects of treatment of fractures of the proximal humerus. In *Surgery of the Shoulder* (eds J.E. Bateman and R.P. Welsh), B.C. Decker, Philadelphia (1984), pp. 330–343

75. Siebler, G., Walz, H. and Kuner, E.H. Minimal osteosynthese von oberarmkopffrakturen. Indikation, Technik, Ergebnisse. *Unfallchirurgie*, **92**, 162–184 (1989)

76. Siebler, G., and Kuner, E.H. Spatergebnisse nach operativer behandlung proximaler humerusfrakturen bei erwachsensen. *Unfallchirurgie*, **11**, 119–127 (1985)

77. Casey, K., Lee, H. and Hansen, H.A. Post-traumatic avascular necrosis of the humeral head in proximal humerus fractures. *J. Trauma*, **21**, 788–791 (1981)

78. Jakob, R.P., Miniaci, A., Anson, P.S., Jaberg, H., Osterwalder, A. and Ganz, R. Four-part-valgus impacted fractures of the proximal humerus. *J. Bone Joint Surg.*, **73B**, 295–298 (1991)

79. Lyshon, R.C. Closed treatment of fractures of the proximal humerus. *Acta Orthop. Scand.*, **55**, 48–51 (1984)

80. Seeman, W.R., Siebler, G. and Rupp, H.G. A new classification of proximal humerus fractures. *Eur. J. Radiol.*, **6**, 163–167 (1986)

81. Watson-Jones, R. *Fractures and Joint Injuries*, Vol. 2, 7th edn. Williams and Wilkins, Baltimore (1955), pp. 473–476

82. Kofoed, H. Revascularization of the humeral head. A report of two cases of fracture-dislocation of the shoulder. *Clin. Orthop.*, **179**, 175–178 (1983)

83. Cruess, R.L. Osteonecrosis of bone. Current concepts as to etiology and pathogenesis. *Clin. Orthop.* **208**, 30–39 (1986)

84. Cruess, R.L. Steroid induced avascular necrosis of the head of the humerus. *J. Bone Joint Surg.*, **58B**, 313–317 (1976)

85. Gerber, C. Integrated scoring systems for the functional assessment of the shoulder. In *The Shoulder: A Balance of Mobility and Stability* (eds F.A. Matsen III, F.H. Fu and R.J. Hawkins), American Academy of Orthopaedic Surgeons Rosemont, Ill. (1993), pp. 531–550

86. Stoller, C. and Gerber, C. Pathological fracture of the humerus after closed reduction and stabilization of subcapital fracture of the proximal humerus (in press)

87. Dehne, E. Fractures of the upper end of the humerus. A classification based on the etiology of the bone. *Surg. Clin. N. Am.*, **25**, 28–47 (1945)

88. Gerber, C. Locked inveterated posterior dislocations of the shoulder. Presented at the 7th Congress of the European Society of Surgery of the Shoulder and Elbow, Aarhus, Denmark (11 May 1993)

89. Hersche, O. and Gerber, C. Iatrogenic displacement of fracture-dislocations of the shoulder. *J. Bone Joint Surg.*, **76B**, 30–33 (1994)

9

Complications of non-operative management and internal fixation of proximal humeral fractures

Andrew Green and Tom R. Norris

Fractures of the proximal humerus are common and account for about 4% of all fractures[1]. Age- and sex-related osteopenic changes in the proximal humerus account for the predominance of fractures in elderly females[2–4]. Among young adults these fractures are more often the result of severe trauma. Fortunately, 60–80% are non- or minimally displaced and do not require operative treatment[1]. Non-operative treatment, including appropriate immobilization and rehabilitation, has been the usual treatment for most of these injuries.

Nevertheless, complications can occur after all types of fractures and methods of treatment. Although discussed in texts, complications of proximal humeral fractures have been less frequently emphasized in comprehensive studies that specifically address the aetiology and treatment[1,5]. The subject has been further confused by deficiencies in the earlier orthopaedic literature, especially failure to classify fractures or objectively assess outcome. Unfortunately, complications are not uncommon and lead to poor results.

Proximal humeral fractures can involve significant injury to the shoulder girdle. Neurological and vascular injury, rotator cuff tearing, instability, malunion, non-union, avascular necrosis and stiffness can occur after any form of treatment. However, each treatment modality is associated with specific complications (e.g. infection after operative treatment), and a greater proportion of complications occur among the relatively small number of displaced fractures. This chapter reviews the assessment and management of complications of the non-operative treatment and internal fixation of proximal humeral fractures.

Errors of diagnosis

The importance of accurate classification and diagnosis of proximal humeral fractures has been emphasized[1,6–8]. Inadequate evaluation often leads to error in diagnosis and inappropriate treatment. A detailed history, physical examination and plain radiographs form the basis of any shoulder evaluation[9,10]. Of all the classes of shoulder disorders, fractures are perhaps the most dependent upon accurate radiographic imaging techniques. The three views of the shoulder trauma series (glenohumeral anteroposterior (AP), axillary lateral and scapular lateral) should be obtained in all cases of shoulder injury[1,10]. If only two views can be obtained, then the true AP and axillary lateral are the most informative.

Posterior fracture dislocations and displaced greater tuberosity fractures are the most commonly missed fractures of the proximal humerus (Figures 9.1a,b). This usually occurs because an axillary lateral projection is not obtained. Although it can be difficult to position the shoulder due to pain or body habitus, there are many positions and projection techniques that can be used to obtain a good axillary lateral image. If there is any question about the anterior-posterior position of the humeral head or the position of the greater tuberosity, a computed tomography (CT) scan should be obtained. CT scans can be especially useful in evaluating complex fractures or malunion[11]. We have found three-dimensional imaging to be useful in occasional cases with especially complex fractures.

Patients with a locked posterior dislocation classically have limited forward elevation and external rotation (Figures 9.1c,d)[12]. A large anterior impression fracture ('reverse Hill–Sachs' lesion) in the humeral head prevents spontaneous or easy reduction of the dislocation. Occasionally, if the missed dislocation is recognized soon after the injury, a closed reduction can be successful. With longer delays, soft tissue contracture occurs and prevents closed reduction. Open reduction then becomes necessary. Eventually, with prolonged missed dislocation, degenerative changes affect the hyaline articular cartilage of the glenohumeral joint and prosthetic arthroplasty is required for treatment. Similarly, it is not uncommon for a posterior dis-

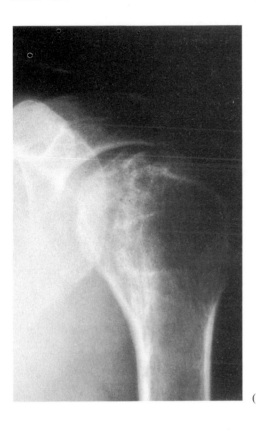

(a)

(b)

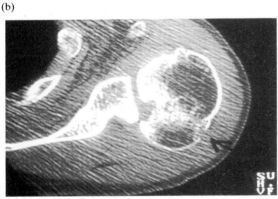

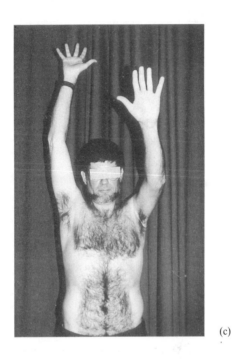

(c)

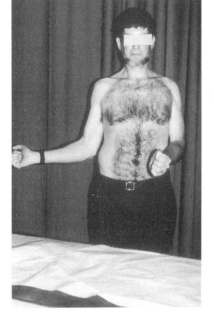

(d)

Figure 9.1 (a) AP radiograph and (b) CT scan of a shoulder with a locked posterior fracture-dislocation. The patient with a locked posterior fracture-dislocation classically has limitation of (c) elevation and (d) external rotation

location of the humeral head or articular segment that is associated with a displaced proximal humeral fracture to be missed.

Superior displacement of a greater tuberosity fracture can usually be demonstrated on an AP radiograph. In contrast, a medially displaced greater tuberosity can be missed on an AP projection if the humeral head overlies the fracture fragment. The infraspinatus and teres minor muscles pull the fragment medially and there is weakness of external rotation. Axillary radiographs or CT scans will best demonstrate the displacement.

Misinterpretation of radiographs can also be a problem. Although Neer[13] defined significant displacement as either 1 cm or 45°, a certain amount of judgment is involved in the evaluation of radiographs. There can be significant inter- and intra-observer variation in the interpretation of the radiographs of displaced proximal humeral fractures which may affect the choice of treatment and eventual outcome[14,15]. Thus, the decision of whether or not to perform surgery to obtain restoration of the normal anatomy is crucial.

Careful and systematic evaluation of the injured shoulder should reduce the incidence of misdiagnosis. In most cases, this may be accomplished with a complete history, a thorough physical examination and adequate plain radiographs. Less often, CT scanning is helpful. MRI scanning is rarely indicated in the setting of acute proximal humeral fractures.

Neurovascular complications

The intimate association of the glenohumeral joint and proximal humerus to the brachial plexus and peripheral nerves of the upper extremity place these important structures at considerable risk for injury. Neurological injury can occur at the time of initial trauma or secondary to closed or open treatment. Nerve injury is a not infrequent cause of delayed recovery after an otherwise less severe injury and can be the cause of permanent disability. In the setting of acute injury, nerve injuries are often overlooked because the physical examination is either cursory or limited by the clinical situation. All muscle groups should be examined for at least isometric contraction which can be elicited in most cases without significant discomfort. This is especially important for the axillary nerve, because the presence of intact superficial sensation over the proximal lateral arm does not always correlate with normal motor innervation.

Blom and Dahlback[16] have published the best information about the incidence and types of nerve injuries that occur with proximal humeral fractures. The axillary nerve is the most commonly injured. It passes inferior to the subscapularis muscle and then wraps around the surgical neck to travel on the deep surface of the middle and anterior deltoid muscle (Figure 9.2). Loss of deltoid function deprives the shoulder of 50% of the power for arm elevation and can have a devastating effect[17,18]. Nerve injuries are more frequent in individuals older than 50 years and with fracture dislocations. Infraclavicular brachial plexus lesions are not uncommon with shoulder girdle injuries, and have a relatively favourable prognosis[19].

The incidence of nerve injury after closed reduction or operative treatment of proximal humeral fractures has not been well documented. However, it is clear that there are circumstances that involve greater risk. Forceful closed reductions, especially with variations of Hippocrates' (foot-in-axilla) technique, endanger the peripheral nerves[20]. A change in the neurological status after the reduction manoeuvre may require operative exploration, but the indications for this remain unclear.

Operative treatment of proximal humeral fractures can be complicated by nerve injury. Percutaneous pin fixation can skewer the axillary nerve.

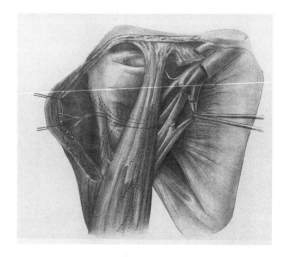

Figure 9.2 Drawing of the anatomy of the anterior aspect of the shoulder girdle. The axillary nerve is depicted branching from the posterior cord of the brachial plexus, passing posteriorly around the surgical neck of the humerus, and lying on the deep surface of the deltoid muscle. (From Bigliani[76], by permission).

This is best avoided by choosing the deltoid tubercle as the point of entry into the humerus. Deltoid-splitting approaches may also endanger the axillary nerve. Burkhead *et al.*[21] have demonstrated that the axillary nerve is an average of 5.4 cm in females and 6.2 cm in males from the midportion of the acromion. Glousman *et al.*[22] found similar distances and noted that the standard recommendation to split the deltoid fibres 5 cm distally would cross 44% of the axillary nerves in females. The axillary nerve is also exposed to danger anteriorly as it leaves the posterior cord of the brachial plexus and passes inferior to the subscapularis. Great care must be taken when operating in this region, especially when retrieving the humeral head in an anterior fracture-dislocation.

Occasionally, it is difficult to obtain adequate exposure of the proximal humerus through a deltopectoral approach. Several variations and additional surgical steps have been recommended to improve exposure. Some of these are associated with specific complications. Coracoid osteotomy has been recommended to improve access to the anterior glenoid. However, dissection on the medial side of the conjoint tendon or coracoid process can injure the musculocutaneous nerve. Flatow and colleagues demonstrated that the musculocutaneous nerve enters the coracoid muscles 3.1–8.2 cm (mean 6.6 cm) distal to the coracoid process[23]. Bach and co-workers found the mean distance in 61 specimens to be 4.9 cm with three nerves only 2.0–2.5 cm from the coracoid[24]. The coracoid process has been called 'the lighthouse of the shoulder' (F.A. Matsen III, personal communication). A helpful mnemonic for students and residents with respect to the coracoid is: 'the lateral side is the safe side and the medial is the suicide'. Conjoined tendon release and/or coracoid osteotomy sacrifice an important barrier for protecting the brachial plexus. Experience with the Bristow procedure exemplifies this problem[25].

Another step recommended to improve exposure is release of the anterior deltoid from the clavicle[26]. Unfortunately, this can lead not only to axillary nerve injury, but to complete dehiscence of the deltoid origin. This is best treated by prevention, as no surgical reconstruction can reliably restore the function of a missing anterior deltoid. Adequate operative exposure of the proximal humerus can usually be achieved by appropriately positioning the arm in abduction to relax the deltoid muscle. Release of the insertion of the anterior portion of the deltoid muscle and the cephalad portion of the pectoralis major muscle from the humerus can also improve exposure if necessary.

The treatment options for nerve injuries depend on the type of injury. In any case, careful and accurate documentation and follow-up of peripheral nerve function are essential. Electromyography and nerve conduction velocity testing aid in the diagnosis and can help to determine the prognosis. Electromyography is usually positive at 3 weeks after injury, once Wallerian degeneration occurs. Infraclavicular brachial plexus injuries usually have good recovery with non-operative management[19]. Nerve repair is indicated when there is actual disruption of the peripheral nerve, rather than just an injury in continuity. The results of early repair or nerve grafting are superior to those of late grafting[27]. Numerous muscle transfers have been described for paralysis about the shoulder girdle. Paralysis in combination with proximal humeral fracture is a difficult situation that cannot be easily treated.

Vascular injuries are less frequently associated with proximal humeral fractures. Axillary artery

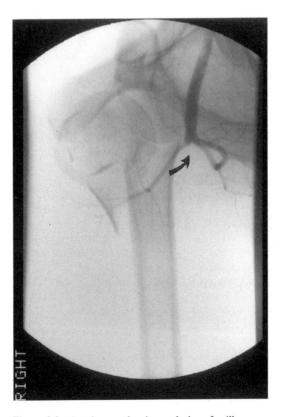

Figure 9.3 Arteriogram showing occlusion of axillary artery in association with a displaced surgical neck fracture

injury is more prevalent in older patients with fragile atherosclerotic vessels[28–30]. Acute thrombosis appears to be more common than laceration. The collateral circulation around the shoulder girdle may be sufficient to reconstitute the radial pulse. Diminished pulse or other sign of vascular insufficiency should be investigated with Doppler pressure measurements and arteriography (Figure 9.3). Restoration of arterial flow is generally indicated and failure to address vascular injury can lead to amputation.

Non-union

Non-unions of proximal humeral fractures are relatively uncommon. Most pertinent studies have reviewed the treatment of non-unions rather than the epidemiology. Several early studies of non-operative treatment of proximal humeral fractures, including hanging casts, abduction splints, slings and functional treatment, do not note a significant incidence of non-union[31–33]. However, when a surgical neck non-union does occur, it is generally after closed treatment[34]. Non-union usually involves the surgical neck or greater tuberosity.

Scheck considered a surgical neck fracture ununited if 'the fragments did not move as a unit after a minimum of eight weeks'[35]. Most surgical neck non-unions result from displaced two-part fractures (Figure 9.4a). A significant number also occur in association with more comminuted fractures. One-third of the surgical neck non-unions reported by Norris and co-workers were originally three- and four-part fractures[36]. Fracture displacement, osteopenia, motion at the fracture site, soft tissue interposition, and failed open reduction and internal fixation are contributing factors in the development of non-union. Closed reduction of displaced surgical neck fractures is commonly employed. However, the reduction is often unstable and redisplacement occurs due to the pull of the pectoralis major and deltoid muscles on the humeral shaft. If this is not recognized in a timely fashion, a non-union may result. Although hanging casts were advocated by many early orthopaedists, others have noted that excessive distraction at the fracture can lead to non-union[34].

Inadequate open reduction and internal fixation can lead to loss of fixation. The holding strength of screws and plates is compromised by comminuted and osteopenic bone in the proximal humerus. Similarly, Rush rods do not provide good rotational control in the proximal humerus. Neer[34] reported on 22 surgical neck non-unions after three- and four-part fractures. Sixteen had been treated closed and 6 with open reduction and internal fixation. In contrast, Hawkins *et al.*[37] reported far more predictable results with wire or heavy suture tension band fixation of three-part fractures by placing the fixation at the rotator cuff insertion rather than through the bone of the tuberosity.

Osteopenia of the proximal humerus renders the metaphyseal region of the surgical neck devoid of bone[2]. This is the probable aetiology of the apparent resorption of the proximal humerus and cavitation of the humeral head that occurs with non-union. Communication with the synovial fluid of the glenohumeral joint can further prevent bone healing. These factors, combined with excessive motion, create a poor healing environment. Lastly, interposition of soft tissue such as the deltoid and biceps muscles, rotator cuff tendons and periosteum can occur. The tendon of the long head of the biceps is the most commonly reported specific soft tissue interposed in the proximal humerus fracture site[38].

Surgical neck non-union causes marked functional disability and pain. The goals of treatment are the relief of pain and restoration of active motion which improves extremity function. Operative treatment is very difficult. The distorted anatomy and extensive scar tissue complicate the surgical exposure. The rotator cuff and capsular tissue become inelastic and unyielding as a result of inactivity and prevent normal glenohumeral motion even if reconstruction is performed. Open reduction and internal fixation and bone grafting of the non-union can be attempted if there is good bone stock. Our preferred technique is to combine intramedullary fixation with modified Ender rods and tension-band fixation with heavy sutures, with autogenous bone grafting[1] (Figure 9.4b). Other authors have reported on techniques using plate and screw fixation. Either technique can be very difficult, especially if the proximal fragment is small and osteopenic. Humeral head replacement is used for surgical neck non-unions when the bone is too osteopenic or the proximal fragment is too small to hold fixation. Pain relief is usually dramatic but the functional gains are modest[36,39].

Greater tuberosity non-union is less common but can be equally disabling. Displaced greater tuberosity fractures are often associated with a rotator cuff tear[13,40,41]. Failure of internal fixation of greater tuberosity fractures treated with screw

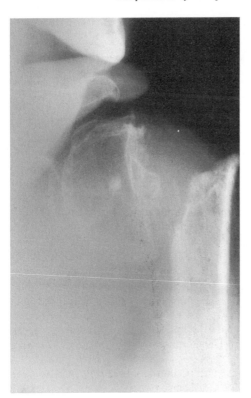

Figure 9.4 (a) Radiograph of a two-part surgical neck non-union that occurred with non-operative treatment. (b) Radiographs of a surgical neck non-union treated with intramedullary Ender rods and tension-band fixation

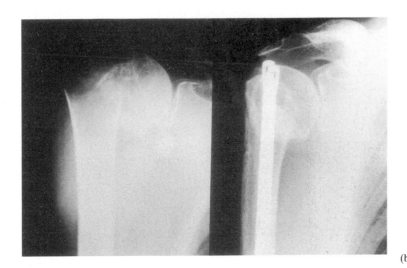

(b)

fixation is not uncommon (Figure 9.5a). Depending on the portion of the greater tuberosity that is ununited, there can be weakness of external rotation or elevation, or the fragment itself can block motion by abutting against the posterior rim of the glenoid or by causing subacromial impingement.

A chronically displaced greater tuberosity non-union is very difficult to treat. A deltoid-splitting superior approach with anterior acromioplasty provides the best exposure. The scarred retracted rotator cuff resists mobilization. The extensive subacromial and capsular scarring must be freed up. Reduction of the bone fragment to a normal

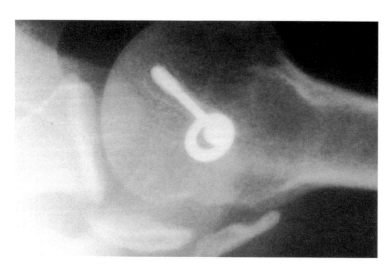

Figure 9.5 (a) The greater tuberosity displaced after initial fixation with a single screw. (b, c) The chronically displaced greater tuberosity was mobilized with the attached rotator cuff tendons and fixed to the humeral head with cerclage cables and heavy sutures

(a)

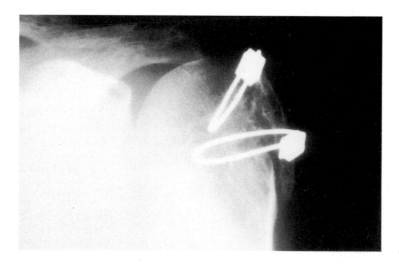

(b)

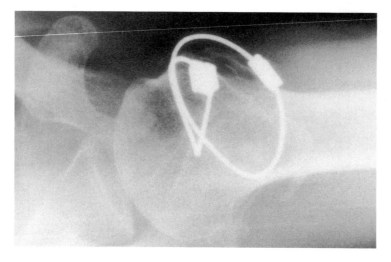

(c)

anatomical position may not be possible. In addition, motion may be limited after repair. We prefer to use multiple heavy non-absorbable sutures for fixation and have recently used cerclage cables (Figures 9.5b, c). Unfortunately, redisplacement is not uncommon.

Malunion

Malunion is limited to the minority of proximal humeral fractures that are displaced. The musculotendinous units that cross the glenohumeral joint generate deforming forces that determine the typical patterns of fracture displacement and malunion. The fact that adequate shoulder function can often be achieved with imperfect reduction has been used to rationalize non-operative treatment of displaced proximal humeral fractures. This is true to a great extent because factors other than the precision of reduction are important. Einarsson stated that 'union in anatomically correct position is, particularly in the case of juxtaarticular fractures, subordinate to the earliest possible training of function'[42]. Non-operative treatment, the mainstay of early fracture care, was based upon classification schemes that emphasized the level of fracture and did not give useful guidelines for treatment or prognosis. The risk of anaesthetic complications, limited operative experience and lack of reliable surgical techniques supported non-operative treatment. Nevertheless, early proponents of non-operative treatment recognized the suboptimal results that were obtained with malunited displaced fractures[42]. More recent work has specifically demonstrated that the results of non-operative treatment of displaced fractures are unsatisfactory[34,43,44]. This is especially true among active, though not necessarily younger patients.

Malunion is not limited to non-operatively treated fractures[45]. Inadequate reduction, and fixation failure with loss of reduction, are not uncommon[34,46,47]. Premature or overly aggressive range of motion exercises can easily disrupt tenuous fixation of well-reduced fractures if initiated prior to early healing.

The significance of malunion in terms of outcome relates to several factors. The initial displacement, accuracy of reduction, and fracture and soft tissue after-care, contribute to the degree of malunion. Several authors have noted the fact that range of motion and functional outcome correlate with the anatomical deformity. Displacement, in part, has a direct mechanical effect in limiting range of motion. Keene and co-workers noted poor results when there was greater than 55° of angulation or 1.5 cm of displacement[48]. Neer considered 1 cm of displacement and 45° of angulation as significant displacement[13]. These figures are somewhat arbitrary and have not been substantiated in the laboratory or well-designed clinical studies. For example, superior displacement of a greater tuberosity fracture of only 0.5 cm may lead to impingement. In our experience, the combination of the degree and direction of displacement determines the clinical significance.

Superior malunion of the greater tuberosity can cause subacromial impingement when the arm is abducted. Less commonly, the inferior facet of the greater tuberosity heals in a medial position and blocks external rotation by bumping against the posterior glenoid. Even with non-displaced or anatomically reduced fractures, impingement is not uncommon. Surgical treatment can be considered if there is persistent and disabling pain or mechanically limited motion that cannot be managed without surgery. Although removal of the prominent portion of the tuberosity is an appealing theoretical consideration, this could disrupt the insertion of the rotator cuff tendons. Subacromial decompression with anterior acromioplasty is a simple procedure that can improve impingement due to a superiorly displaced tuberosity in some cases.

Correction of significant malunion can only be accomplished by osteotomy. Unfortunately, this is a difficult procedure. The attached rotator cuff muscles subject the repair to repetitive tension and there is a high rate of redisplacement. Tanner and Cofield noted this problem when they combined greater tuberosity osteotomy with total shoulder arthroplasty[49]. Careful and secure fixation with multiple heavy sutures, wires or cables improves the success rate.

Surgical neck malunion is less likely to cause clinical problems. Relatively large degrees of angulation can be tolerated within a functional, though not full, range of motion. Excessive lateral and anterior angulation due to pull by the pectoralis major and rotational malunion are especially problematic. Surgical treatment should be entertained for pain or significant functional problems. Many older patients are able to tolerate significant angulation by limiting their functional demands. Occasionally, subacromial impingement caused by a prominent greater tuberosity secondary to a varus malunion can be treated with anterior acromioplasty.

In the most severe cases of surgical neck mal-

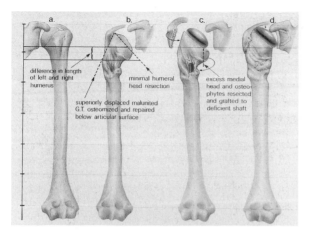

Figure 9.6 (a) Normal left humerus. (b) The right proximal humerus is shortened through the varus malunion of the shaft and collapse of the head. The greater tuberosity (GT) is malunited superiorly and medially over the head. A high cut on the head restores length. A biplanar GT osteotomy provides access to the medullary canal of the shaft. (c) The GT is lowered below the articular surface. Medial osteophytes are resected. (d) Humeral shaft deficiencies are grafted with the resected head and osteophytes. (From Watson[77], by permission)

union, proximal humeral osteotomy and prosthetic arthroplasty are the treatment options. The goals of these procedures and the potential risks and benefits must be carefully evaluated. Neither is simple or straightforward. Osteotomy is appropriate if there is isolated deformity at the surgical neck[50]. Careful surgical technique in exposing and osteotomizing the surgical neck, and in using internal fixation, are essential to avoiding avascular necrosis and other complications.

The most difficult cases with surgical neck malunion are those which occur after three- and four-part fractures. These may also involve greater tuberosity problems, avascular necrosis and post-traumatic arthritis (Figures 9.6a–d). Loss of humeral length can result in an apparent inferior glenohumeral instability. Humeral length can be assessed with scanograms[51]. In these cases, proximal humeral osteotomy alone is usually not an alternative and prosthetic arthroplasty is the only option other than glenohumeral arthrodesis. In some cases, osteotomy may be required to facilitate placement of the humeral implant (Figures 9.6a–d). Late shoulder arthroplasty after fracture is especially difficult. The incidence of complications is greater and outcomes are worse than arthroplasty for acute fractures[49,52–54].

Avascular necrosis

The vascular supply of the proximal humerus has important implications for the outcome of fracture treatment. Gerber and colleagues have recently performed vascular injection studies that confirm Laing's earlier findings[55,56]. The ascending branch of the anterior circumflex artery is the principal source of vascularity for the articular segment of the proximal humerus. There are also several extracapsular ascending posterior medial branches from the posterior circumflex artery. Vessels in the rotator cuff muscles and the capsule are probably only minor contributions to the blood supply of the proximal humerus. Brooks *et al.*[57] performed cadaveric injection studies that demonstrated that four-part fractures disrupt the perfusion of the humeral head. This work supports the clinical observation that avascular necrosis is more likely to develop in fractures with greater comminution and displacement, and when surgical technique disrupts the blood supply.

Post-traumatic avascular necrosis of the humeral head most commonly occurs after four-part factures. Open reduction and internal fixation clearly increase the risk of avascular necrosis. In Neer's series[34], collapse of the articular surface occurred in 2 of 30 three-part lesions treated by open reduction. Two of 20 three-part lesions treated closed had resorption of the humeral head. Among the four-part lesions, 3 of 11 treated closed and 6 of 8 treated open had avascular necrosis. Subsequent reports of open reduction and internal fixation of displaced proximal humeral fractures support the idea that the amount of soft tissue dissection required to obtain exposure to position implants such as T-plates predisposes to avascular necrosis[46, 58]. In contrast, Paavolainen *et al.*[47] did not observe avascular necrosis and Lee and Hansen[59] reported that avascular necrosis does not usually lead to resorption of the humeral head or have an impact on the result. In these two latter series the length of follow-up was too short for valid conclusions. The time from injury or treatment of fracture until humeral head resorption affects shoulder function is often at least 2 years[60]. In our experience with post-traumatic avascular necrosis, the initial injury is usually a four-part fracture. Less commonly, a two- or three-part fracture treated with open reduction and internal fixation will develop advanced avascular necrosis.

Early recognition and treatment is the key to successful management of avascular necrosis of the humeral articular segment. Nevertheless, most

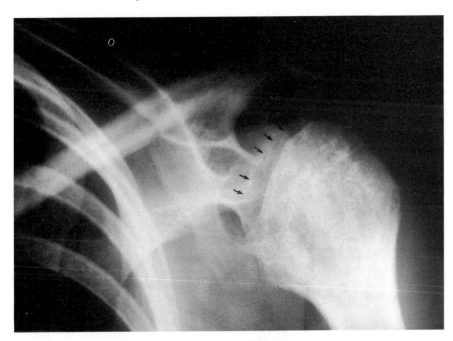

Figure 9.7 Flattening of the humeral head in avascular necrosis after a proximal humerus fracture

patients are referred for consultation after the articular segment has collapsed (Figure 9.7). As the soft tissues contract the humeral head is pulled medially and engulfs the glenoid. The net effect of this is a painful shoulder that has only scapulothoracic motion. Although prosthetic arthroplasty is difficult, we prefer it to glenohumeral arthrodesis. Arthroplasty can restore glenohumeral motion, give better function and avoid the potential problems associated with arthrodesis – including non-union due to poor bone quality and late scapulothoracic pain[61,62].

Hardware complications

The goal of operative treatment of proximal humeral fractures is accurate reduction and stable fixation that will permit early motion. In the past two decades, most reports have focused on a variety of operative techniques[1,20,34,37,40,46,47,58,63–71]. These include percutaneous internal and external fixation, wire, cable and suture fixation, screws with and without plates, intramedullary devices, and prosthetic replacement. Of all the major joints, the shoulder is probably the most notable for hardware complications[72,73]. Dramatic cases of intraspinal and intracardiac migration of hardware have been reported and appropriate caution has been advised. Internal fixation of proximal humeral

fractures is especially problematic. The combination of age- and activity-related osteopenia and the many deforming forces applied by the shoulder girdle muscles make it difficult to achieve and maintain reduction with internal fixation. Many types of internal fixation have been used to stabilize proximal humeral fractures. The proponents of the various techniques usually report good results and low complication rates. However, all forms of internal fixation have well known specific complications.

Unless the bone quality is excellent, screw fixation is likely to fail. Unrecognized articular penetration is disastrous and avoidable.[73] Transarticular fixation has no role in the management of glenohumeral problems (Figure 9.8). Plates require extensive soft tissue dissection to gain adequate exposure. This jeopardizes the already tenuous blood supply of the proximal humerus. Not infrequently, either by loss of reduction or malposition, plates extend above the greater tuberosity and impinge against the undersurface of the acromion. Similarly, most intramedullary devices do not have good purchase in the proximal or distal fragment and can migrate up to the undersurface of the acromion[34]. Supplemental fixation with interlocking devices, wires or sutures can improve fixation and prevent loosening and proximal migration. Proximal migration of Rush rods causing subacromial impingement is so common that

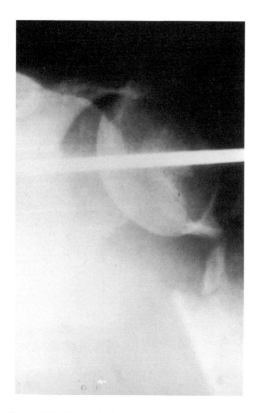

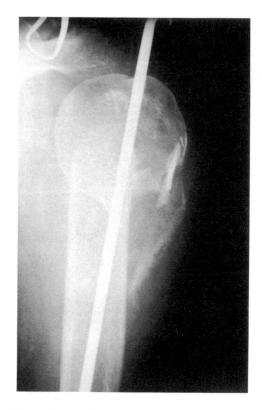

Figure 9.8 Transarticular fixation of the humeral head to the glenoid used to stabilize the humeral head in a surgical neck fracture

Figure 9.9 Proximal migration of a rush rod used to fix a surgical neck fracture

most advocates of this technique recommend early elective rod removal[68,71] (Figure 9.9).

Wire can achieve fixation with less extensive dissection. However, it must be applied carefully because tensioned wire can crush or cut through comminuted osteopenic bone. Motion at the fracture site can cause non-union, malunion or wire breakage. Suture fixation avoids some of the problems of wire. Pin fixation around the shoulder has been associated with dramatic complications due to migration[72]. Closed reduction and percutaneous pin fixation of proximal humeral fractures is gaining wider acceptance[67]. When attempted for three- or four-part factures, the reductions must be anatomical, or the procedure should be abandoned in favour of an open procedure (C. Gerber, personal communication, 1993). Care must be taken to avoid neurovascular structures and the pins should be left under the skin to prevent pin tract infection. The pins are removed as soon as fracture security permits.

As new devices and techniques to treat these injuries are introduced, there must be careful evaluation with biomechanical testing and clinical experience. Unfortunately, many new techniques have been heralded, only to turn out to be inadequate (Figure 9.10a, b).

Post-traumatic arthritis

Malunion, non-union and avascular necrosis can result in destruction of the articular surface of the humeral head. Long-standing joint incongruity, intra-articular hardware and stiffness eventually lead to destruction of the glenoid articular surface. Disabling pain is the best indication for surgical treatment. The options for reconstruction include resection arthroplasty, arthrodesis and prosthetic arthroplasty. Resection arthroplasty has little role as a reconstructive procedure and now remains as a rarely utilized salvage operation for infection[74]. The results of arthrodesis are considerably better but still limited compared to prosthetic arthroplasty[62,75].

Reconstruction of old trauma with gleno-

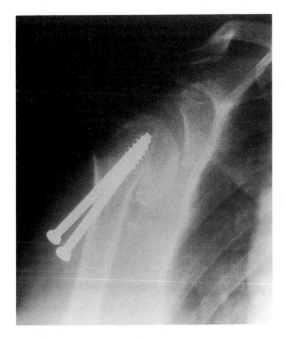

(a)

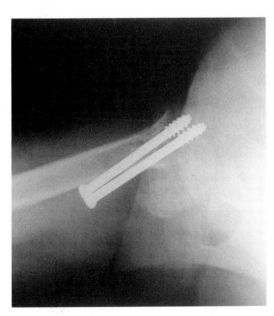

(b)

Figure 9.10 (a, b)   Errant percutaneous placement of cannulated screws led to early non-union of this two-part surgical neck fracture

humeral arthroplasty is difficult. Malunion, scarring, contracture, bone loss, rotator cuff deficiency and nerve injury offer formidable challenges for reconstructive surgery. Complex techniques, including tuberosity osteotomy, capsular release, subscapularis lengthening and humeral bone grafting, may be necessary.

The total reported experience of prosthetic arthroplasty for post-traumatic arthritis is fairly limited[49,52–54]. Pain relief is achieved in about 90% of cases. Improvements in range of motion are more modest. Active elevation averages about 100°. Functional gains are similarly modest. Poor results are generally associated with weakness due to either neurological or muscle deficits. The latter includes tuberosity and deltoid dehiscence, and rotator cuff deficiency. The idea that prosthetic arthroplasty can be used to salvage a good result from failed closed or open treatment that results in post-traumatic arthritis is incorrect. Late arthroplasty is much more technically difficult and the results are significantly worse than acute arthroplasty. Nevertheless, it is a satisfactory option and reliably provides good pain relief. However, function is generally fair, at best[54].

Stiffness

Loss of motion after proximal humeral fracture can be related to many of the factors discussed in the preceding sections. In addition, it can occur even when there has been accurate reduction and complete fracture healing if controlled range of motion exercises are not used early enough in post-injury or the postoperative period. Early motion can be safely initiated only if there has been enough healing or stable enough fixation for the entire proximal humerus to move as a unit. In some non-displaced fractures, passive pendulum motion can be initiated immediately. Other fractures treated non-operatively should be immobilized until the parts move together. This is usually not more than about 2–4 weeks. The rehabilitation of fractures treated open must be individualized according to the status of the reduction, soft tissue support and stability of the fixation.

Early stiffness can be effectively treated with passive stretching and active use of the shoulder. The physician or physiotherapist must ensure that the patient understands the difference between glenohumeral and scapulothoracic motion and that the former is preferentially emphasized. Manipulation, especially under anaesthesia, is risky. The osteopenic bone can fracture and early healing can be disrupted. When there is articular incongruity it only serves to further injure the delicate articular surfaces. Stiffness that does not respond to stretching is best treated with open releases and soft tissue or tendon lengthening. These steps are also an integral part of post-traumatic shoulder reconstruction[54].

Conclusion

Proximal humeral fractures are relatively common injuries. They usually occur in older individuals who tend to have poor-quality bone and whose functional demands are often underestimated. The majority are non-displaced, the management is usually straightforward and the risk of complications is relatively low. Treatment is more difficult in the minority of proximal humeral fractures that are displaced. The incidence of complications of treatment of these more severe fractures is greater. When complications occur, the outcome is usually unsatisfactory. The anatomical intricacies of the shoulder girdle, and the difficulties in rehabilitating soft tissue function, are relatively unforgiving obstacles in these difficult cases. Avoidance of complications requires careful clinical evaluation, appropriate and skilful management, and some degree of fortuity. Although a certain incidence of complications may be inevitable, it is far more rewarding to avoid complications than to treat them once they have occurred.

References

1. Norris, T.R. Fractures of the proximal humerus and dislocations of the shoulder. In *Skeletal Trauma* (eds B.D. Browner, J.B. Jupiter, A.M. Levine and P.G. Trafton), W.B. Saunders, Philadelphia (1992)
2. Hall, M.C. and Rosser, M. The structure of the upper end of the humerus with reference to osteoporotic changes in senescence leading to fractures. *Can. Med. Ass. J.* **88**, 290–294 (1963)
3. Horak, J. and Nilsson, B.E. Epidemiology of fracture of the upper end of the humerus. *Clin. Orthop. Rel. Res.* **112**, 250–253 (1975)
4. Rose, S.H., Melton, L.J. and Morrey, B.F. Epidemiologic features of proximal humerus fractures. *Clin. Orthop. Rel. Res.* **168**, 24–30 (1982)
5. Bigliani, L.U. Fractures of the proximal humerus. In *The Shoulder* (eds C.A. Rockwood and F.A. Matsen), W.B. Saunders, Philadelphia (1990)
6. Hawkins, R.J. and Angelo, R.L. Displaced proximal humerus fractures. Selecting treatment, avoiding pitfalls. *Orthop. Clin. N. Am.* **18**, 421–431 (1987)
7. Cofield, R.H. Comminuted fractures of the proximal humerus. *Clin. Orthop. Rel. Res.*, **230**, 49–57 (1988)
8. Muller, M.E., Allgower, M., Schneider, R. and Willenegger, H. *Manual of Internal Fixation* (ed. M. Allgower), Springer-Verlag, Berlin (1991)
9. Norris, T.R. History and physical examination of the shoulder. In *The Upper Extremity in Sports Medicine* (ed. E.B. Hershman), C.V. Mosby, St. Louis (1990)
10. Norris, T.R. and Green, A. Imaging modalities in the evaluation of shoulder disorders. In *The Shoulder: A Balance of Mobility and Stability* (eds F.A. Matsen, F.H. Fu and R.J. Hawkins), American Academy of Orthopaedic Surgeons, Rosemont, IL (1993), pp. 353–368
11. Castagno, A.A., Shuman, W.P., Kilcoyne, R.F. *et al.* Complex fractures of the proximal humerus. Role of CT in treatment. *Radiology* **165**, 759–762 (1987)
12. Hawkins, R.J., Neer, C.S., Pianta, R.M. *et al.* Locked posterior dislocation of the shoulder. *J. Bone Joint Surg.*, **69A**, 9–18 (1987)
13. Neer, C.S. Displaced proximal humeral fractures. Part I, Classification and evaluation. *J. Bone Joint Surg.*, **52A**, 1077–1088 (1970)
14. Sidor, M.L., Zuckerman, J.D., Lyon, T. *et al.* Neer classification of proximal humerus fractures. Assessment of inter- and intra-observer reliability. *J. Bone Joint Surg.*, **75A**, 1745–1750 (1993)
15. Siebenrock, K.A. and Gerber, C. The reproducibility of classification of fractures of the proximal end of the humerus. *J. Bone Joint Surg.*, **75A**, 1751–1755 (1993)
16. Blom, S. and Dahlback, L.O. Nerve injuries in dislocations of the shoulder joint and fractures of the neck of the humerus. *Acta Chir. Scand.*, **136**, 461–466 (1970)
17. Colachis, S.C., Strohm, B.R. and Brechner, V.L. Effects of axillary nerve block on muscle force in the upper extremity. *Arch. Phys. Med. Rehab.*, **50**, 647–654 (1969)
18. Howell, S.M., Imobersteg, A.M., Seger, D.H. *et al.* Clarification of the role of the supraspinatus muscle in shoulder function. *J. Bone Joint Surg.*, **68A**, 398–404 (1986)
19. Leffert, R.D. and Seddon, H. Infraclavicular brachial plexus injuries. *J. Bone Joint Surg.*, **47B**, 9–22 (1965)
20. Brockbank, W. and Griffiths, D.L. Orthopaedic surgery in the 16th and 17th centuries. *J. Bone Joint Surg.*, **30B**, 365–375 (1948)
21. Burkhead, W.Z., Scheinberg, R.R. and Box, G. Surgical anatomy the axillary nerve. *J. Shoulder Elbow Surg.*, **1**, 31–36 (1992)
22. Glousman, R.E., Seltzer, D. and Tibone, J.E. Anatomy of the axillary nerve and its relationship to deltoid splitting surgical approaches. Presented at the Closed Meeting of the American Shoulder and Elbow Surgeons, Williamsburg, VA (1993)
23. Flatow, E.L., Bigliani, L.U. and April, E.W. An anatomical study of the musculocutaneous nerve and its relationship to the coracoid. *Clin. Orthop. Rel. Res.*, **244**, 166–171 (1989)
24. Bach, B.R., O'Brien, S.J., Warner, R.F. *et al.* An unusual neurological complication of the Bristow procedure. *J. Bone Joint Surg.*, **70A**, 458–466 (1988)
25. Young, D.C. and Rockwood, C.A. Complications of a

failed Bristow procedure and their management. *J. Bone Joint Surg.*, **73A**, 969–981 (1991)

26. Henry, A.K. *Extensile Exposure*, Williams and Wilkins, Baltimore (1946), pp. 29–34

27. Narakais, A. Brachial plexus surgery. *Orthop. Clin. N. Am.*, **12**, 303–323 (1981)

28. Henson, G.F. Vascular complications of shoulder injuries. *J. Bone Joint Surg.*, **38B**, 528–531 (1956)

29. Lim, E.V.A. and Day, L.J. Thrombosis of the axillary artery complicating proximal humerus fractures. A report of three cases. *J. Bone Joint Surg.*, **69A**, 778–780 (1987)

30. Zuckerman, J.D., Flugstad, D.L., Teitz, C.C. *et al.* Axillary artery injury as a complication of proximal humerus fractures. Two case reports and a review of the literature. *Clin. Orthop. Rel. Res.*, **189**, 234–237 (1984)

31. LaFerte, A.D. and Nutter, P.D. The treatment of fractures of the humerus by means of a hanging plaster case: 'hanging cast'. *Ann. Surg.*, **114**, 919–930 (1941)

32. Stewart, M.J. and Hundley, J.M. Fractures of the humerus. Comparative study in methods of treatment. *J. Bone Joint Surg.*, **37A**, 681–691 (1955)

33. Winfield, J.M., Miller, H. and LaFerte, A.D. Evaluation of the 'hanging cast' as a method of treating fractures of the humerus. *Am. J. Surg.*, **155**, 228–249 (1942)

34. Neer, C.S. Displaced proximal humeral fractures. Part II Treatment of three-part and four-part displacement. *J. Bone Joint Surg.*, **52A**, 1090–1102 (1970)

35. Scheck, M. Surgical treatment of nonunions of the surgical neck of the humerus. *Clin. Orthop. Rel. Res.*, **167**, 255–259 (1982)

36. Norris, T.R., Bovill, D.F. and Turner, J.A. A review of 28 proximal humerus fractures leading to nonunion. In *Surgery of the Shoulder* (eds M. Post, R.J. Hawkins and B.F. Morrey), C.V. Mosby, St. Louis (1990), pp. 63–67

37. Hawkins, R.J., Bell, R.H. and Gurr, K. The three-part fracture of the proximal part of the humerus. Operative treatment. *J. Bone Joint Surg.*, **68A**, 1410–1414 (1986)

38. Janecki, C.J. and Barnett, D.C. Fracture-dislocation of the shoulder with biceps tendon interposition. Case report. *J. Bone Joint Surg.*, **61A**, 142–143 (1979)

39. Bigliani, L.U., Nicholson, G.P. and Pollock, R.G. Operative treatment of non-unions of the surgical neck of the humerus. Presented at the 9th Open Meeting of the American Shoulder and Elbow Surgeons, San Francisco, CA (1993)

40. Flatow, E.L., Cuomo, F., Maday, M.G. *et al.* Open reduction and internal fixation of two-part displaced fractures of the greater tuberosity of the proximal humerus. *J. Bone Joint Surg.*, **73A**, 1213–1218 (1991)

41. McLaughlin, H.L. *Trauma*, W.B. Saunders, Philadelphia (1959)

42. Einarsson, F. Fracture of the upper end of the humerus. *Acta Orthop. Scand.*, **Suppl. 32**, Chapters 4–13, pp. 70–161 (1957)

43. Leyshon, R.L. Closed treatment of fractures of the proximal humerus. *Acta Orthop. Scand.*, **55**, 48–51 (1984)

44. Stableforth, P.G. Four-part fractures of the neck of the humerus. *J. Bone Joint Surg.*, **66-B**, 104–108 (1984)

45. Norris, T.R., Boville, D.F. and Turner, J.A. Common prob-lems with proximal humerus fractures leading to malunion. A review of 27 cases. Presented at the American Shoulder and Elbow Surgeons' Fifth Open Meeting, Las Vegas (1989)

46. Kristiansen, B. and Christensen, S.W. Plate fixation of proximal humeral fractures. *Acta Orthop Scand.*, **57**, 320–323 (1986)

47. Paavolainen, P., Bjorkenheim, J.M., Slatis, P. *et al.* Operative treatment of severe proximal humeral fractures. *Acta Orthop Scand.*, **54**, 374–379 (1983)

48. Keene, J.S., Huizenga, R.E., Engber, W.D. *et al.* Proximal humeral fractures. A correlation of residual deformity with long-term function. *Orthopedics*, **16**, 173–178 (1983)

49. Tanner, M. and Cofield, R. Prosthetic arthroplasty for fractures and fracture-dislocations of the proximal humerus. *Clin. Orthop. Rel. Res.*, **179**, 116–128 (1983)

50. Solonen, V. Osteotomy of the neck of the humerus for traumatic varus deformity. *Acta Orthop. Scand.*, **56**, 79–80 (1985)

51. Green, A. and Norris, T.R. Imaging techniques for glenohumeral arthritis and glenohumeral arthroplasty. *Clin. Orthop. Rel. Res.*, **307**, 7–17 (1994)

52. Frich, L.H., Sojbjerg, J.O. and Sneppen, O. Shoulder arthroplasty in complex acute and chronic proximal humeral fractures. *Orthopedics*, **14**, 949–954 (1991)

53. Neer, C.S. Glenohumeral arthoplasty. In *Shoulder Reconstruction* (ed. C.S. Neer), W.B. Saunders, Philadelphia (1990), pp. 143–271

54. Norris, T.R., Green, A. and McQuigan, F.X. Late prosthetic arthroplasty for displaced proximal humerus fractures *J. Shoulder Elbow Surg.*, **4**, 271–280 (1995)

55. Laing, P.G. The arterial supply to the adult humerus. *J. Bone Joint Surg.*, **38A**, 1105–1116 (1956)

56. Gerber, C., Schneeberger, A. and Vinh, T.S. The arterial vascularization of the humeral head. *J. Bone Joint Surg.*, **72A**, 1486–1494 (1990)

57. Brooks, C.H., Revell, W.J. and Heatley, F.W. Vascularity of the humeral head after proximal humeral fractures. *J. Bone Joint Surg.*, **75B**, 132–136 (1993)

58. Sturzenegger, M., Fornaro, E. and Jakob, R.P. Results of surgical treatment of multifragmented fractures of the humeral head. *Arch. Orthop. Trauma Surg.*, **100**, 249–259 (1982)

59. Lee, C.K. and Hansen, H.R. Post-traumatic avascular necrosis of the humeral head in displaced proximal humeral fractures. *J. Trauma*, **21**, 788–791 (1981)

60. Fourrier, P. and Martini, M. Post-traumatic avascular necrosis of the humeral head. *Int. Orthop. (SICOT)*, **1**, 187–190 (1977)

61. Hawkins, R.J. and Neer, C.S. A functional analysis of shoulder fusions. *Clin. Orthop. Rel. Res.*, **223**, 65–76 (1987)

62. Cofield, R.H. and Briggs, B.T. Glenohumeral arthrodesis: operative and long-term functional results. *J. Bone Joint Surg.*, **61A**, 668–677 (1979)

63. Szyszkowitz, R., Seggl, W., Schleifer, P. *et al.* Proximal humeral fractures. *Clin. Orthop. Rel. Res.*, **292**, 13–25 (1993)

64. Green, A., Barnard, W.L. and Limbird, R.S. Humeral head

replacement for acute four part fractures. *J. Shoulder Elbow Surg.* **2**, 249–253 (1993)

65. Green, A. and Norris, T.R. Humeral head replacement for four-part fractures and fracture-dislocations. *Operative Techniques in Orthopaedics*, **4**, 13–20 (1994)

66. Hawkins, R.J. and Switlyk, P. Acute prosthetic replacement for severe fractures of the proximal humerus. *Clin. Orthop. Rel. Res.*, **289**, 156–160 (1993)

67. Jaberg, H., Warner, J.J.P. and Jakob, R.P. Percutaneous stabilization of unstable fractures of the humerus. *J. Bone Joint Surg.*, **74A**, 508–515 (1992)

68. Lentz, W. and Meuser, P. The treatment of fractures of the proximal humerus. *Arch. Orthop. Traumat. Surg.*, **96**, 283–285 (1980)

69. Mouradian, W.H. Displaced proximal humeral fractures. Seven years' experience with a modified Zickel supracondylar device. *Clin. Orthop. Rel. Res.*, **212**, 209–218 (1986)

70. Savoi, F.H., Geissler, W.B. and Vander Griend, R.A. Open reduction and internal fixation of three-part fractures of the proximal humerus. *Orthopedics*, **12**, 65–70 (1989)

71. Weseley, M.S., Barenfeld, P.A. and Eisenstein, A.L. Rush pin intramedullary fixation for fractures of the proximal humerus. *J. Trauma*, **17**, 29–37 (1977)

72. Lyons, F.A. and Rockwood, C.A. Current concepts. Migration of pins used in operations on the shoulder. *J. Bone Joint Surg.*, **72A**, 1262–1267 (1990)

73. Zuckerman, J.D. and Matsen, F.A. Complications about the glenohumeral joint related to the use of screws and stables. *J. Bone Joint Surg.*, **66A**, 175–180 (1984)

74. Jones, L. Reconstructive operation for non-reducible fractures of the head of the humerus. *Ann. Surg.*, **97**, 217–225 (1933)

75. Cofield, R.H. Total shoulder arthroplasty with the Neer prosthesis. *J. Bone Joint Surg.*, **66A**, 899–906 (1984)

76. Bigliani, L.U. (ed.) *Complications of Shoulder Surgery*, Williams and Williams, Baltimore, MD (1993)

77. Watson, M.S. (ed.) *Surgical Disorders of the Shoulder*, Churchill Livingstone, Edinburgh (1991)

10

Humeral diaphyseal fractures: their classification and epidemiology

M. McQueen, C.M. Court-Brown and C. Ulrich

The management of humeral diaphyseal fractures has a long pedigree. The first reference to a fracture of the humeral shaft is contained in the Edwin Smith papyrus published about 3000 BC[1]. The papyrus contains the first known references to fractures, open fractures and comminution. The author of the papyrus clearly recognized the severity and poor prognosis associated with open fractures. He suggested that closed humeral fractures had a good prognosis and that treatment should be instituted. However, the prognosis was so grave for open fractures that the author felt that treatment should be withheld! Since the time of the Edwin Smith papyrus the management of fractures has advanced considerably, although non-operative management of the humeral shaft fractures remained the only practical treatment option for about 5000 years. In the past 100 years, however, surgeons have had the option of using plates, intramedullary nails, external skeletal fixation devices and other methods of fixation when managing humeral diaphyseal fractures. All types of fixation have been recommended for the humerus, but before the relative merits of internal and external fixation are discussed it is important to adequately define the classification and epidemiology of humeral diaphyseal fractures.

Classification

As with all diaphyseal fractures, the major classification system for humeral shaft fractures is the AO classification[2]. Earlier classification systems were very rudimentary, separating fractures according to their location within the bone and their basic morphology. It was common practice for surgeons to categorize all long bone fractures by dividing them according to their location in the upper, middle and lower thirds of the diaphysis. An extension of this approach is the classification of Seidel[3], where the humerus is divided into six segments and the fracture is classified according to whichever segment it is in. This type of approach has a number of obvious drawbacks. The fracture may well occupy more than one-third or one-sixth of the diaphysis and the implication that the outcome is in any way based on fracture location is unproven. This type of classification is easy to use, although probably of very little value.

The AO classification combines the position of the fracture in the diaphysis with the morphology of the fracture. As in all the AO classifications the fractures are divided into 27 subtypes, some of which are further subdivided. By and large, the AO diaphyseal fracture classifications have proved to be successful. All of the common fracture variants are covered and the classification is relatively easy to use and allows surgeons to compare fractures fairly well. The principal disadvantage of the AO classification is that the state of the soft tissues is not taken into account in the principal classification, although a further rudimentary subclassification does exist. Since soft tissue damage is the main determinant of outcome, the AO classification is to all intents and purposes purely morphological. However, it is an improvement on previous classification systems.

The AO classification divides humeral diaphyseal fractures into three basic types: A, B and C.

Type A fractures (Figure 10.1) are simple fractures without any degree of comminution. Type B fractures are wedge fractures associated with intact or fragmented butterfly fragments (Figure 10.2). Type C fractures (Figure 10.3) are complex fractures with significant comminution or a segmental component.

Each AO fracture type is divided into three groups and each group into three subgroups. In type A fractures the A1 group consists of spiral fractures: the A2 group contains the oblique fractures and the A3 group all transverse fractures. The type B fracture is subdivided into B1 spiral wedge fractures, B2 bending wedge fractures and B3 fragmented wedge fractures. In the A and B

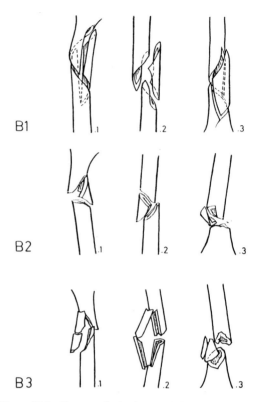

Figure 10.2 Humerus diaphysis (type B fractures): the subgroups and their qualifications

B1   wedge fracture, spiral wedge
   1   proximal zone
   2   middle zone
   3   distal zone
B2   wedge fracture, bending wedge
   1   proximal zone
   2   middle zone
   3   distal zone
B3   wedge fracture, fragmented wedge – (1) spiral wedge, (2) bending wedge
   1   proximal zone
   2   middle zone
   3   distal zone

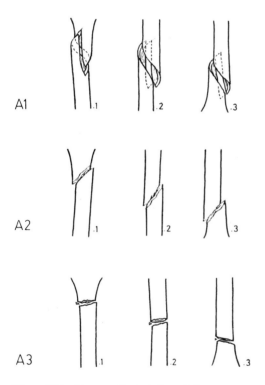

Figure 10.1 Humerus diaphysis (type A fractures): the subgroups and their qualifications

A1   Simple fracture, spiral
   1   proximal zone
   2   middle zone
   3   distal zone
A2   Simple fracture, oblique ($\geq 30°$)
   1   proximal zone
   2   middle zone
   3   distal zone
A3   Simple fracture, transverse ($<30°$)
   1   proximal zone
   2   middle zone
   3   distal zone

fracture types, the subgroups are defined by the position of the fracture within the diaphysis (Figures 10.1 and 10.2).

The type C fracture classification is more complex. The C1 group contains complex spiral fractures with varying numbers of intermediate fragments. The C2 group contains all segmental fractures, with further subdivision depending on the numbers of intermediate segments and their position within the bone. The C3 fracture group contains the extensively comminuted fractures (Figure 10.3).

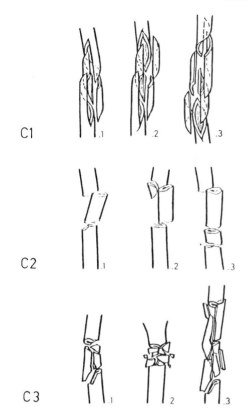

Figure 10.3 Humerus diaphysis (type c fractures): the subgroups and their qualifications

C1 Complex fracture, spiral – (1) pure diaphyseal, (2) proximal diaphysio-metaphyseal, (3) distal diaphysio-metaphyseal
    1 with two intermediate fragments
    2 with three intermediate fragments
    3 with more than three intermediate fragments
C2 Complex fracture, segmental
    1 with one intermediate segmental fragment – (1) pure diaphyseal, (2) proximal diaphysio-metaphyseal, (3) distal diaphysio-metaphyseal, (4) oblique lines, (5) transverse and oblique lines
    2 with one intermediate segmental and additional wedge fragment(s) – (1) pure diaphyseal, (2) proximal diaphysio-metaphyseal, (3) distal diaphysio-metaphyseal, (4) distal wedge, (5) two wedges, proximal and distal
    3 with two intermediate segmental fragments – (1) pure diaphyseal, (2) proximal diaphysio-metaphyseal, (3) distal diaphysio-metaphyseal
C3 Complex fracture, irregular
    1 with two or three intermediate fragments – (1) two main intermediate fragments, (2) three main intermediate fragments
    2 with limited shattering (<4 cm) – (1) proximal zone, (2) middle zone, (3) distal zone
    3 with extensive shattering (≥4 cm) – (1) pure diaphyseal, (2) proximal diaphysio-metaphyseal, (3) distal diaphysio-metaphyseal

While the AO group has devised classifications for open fractures and for the soft tissue injuries associated with closed fractures, in this chapter the more popular Gustilo[4,5] and Tscherne[6] classifications will be used. These have been extensively defined elsewhere, but basic definitions are contained in Tables 10.1 and 10.2.

Table 10.1 Gustilo classification of open fractures

Type I	Clean wound of less than 1 cm in length
Type II	Wound larger than 1 cm in length without extensive soft tissue damage
Type III	Wound associated with extensive soft tissue damage. Usually longer than 5 cm: Open segmental fracture Traumatic amputation Gunshot injuries Farmyard injuries Fractures associated with vascular repair Fractures more than 8 h old
Subtype IIIA	Type III wound with adequate periosteal cover
IIIB	Presence of significant periosteal stripping. Wound usually contaminated
IIIC	Vascular repair to revascularize leg

Table 10.2 Tscherne classification of closed fractures

Grade 0 closed fractures (C0). Soft tissue damage is absent or negligible. The fracture is caused by indirect violence and has a simple configuration. Torsion fractures of the tibia in skiers are typical of this category

Grade I closed fractures (CI). There is a superficial abrasion or contusion caused by fragment pressure from within. The fracture itself is of a mild to moderately severe configuration. A typical example is the pronation fracture-dislocation of the ankle joint, in which soft tissue lesions are caused by pressure from the fractured margin of the medial malleolus

Grade II closed fracture (CII). There is a deep, contaminated abrasion associated with localized skin or muscle contusion from direct trauma. Impending compartment syndrome is included in this category. Generally there has been direct violence producing a moderately severe to severe fracture configuration.

Grade III closed fracture (CIII). The skin is extensively contused or crushed, and muscle damage may be severe. Other criteria for this category are subcutaneous avulsions, decompensated compartment syndrome, and rupture of a major blood vessel associated with a closed fracture. The fracture configuration is severe or comminuted.

Epidemiology

Little has been written about the overall epidemiology of humeral diaphyseal fractures. What information there is in the literature is mainly skewed towards either those fractures treated non-operatively or fractures which have been internally or externally fixed. Since many surgeons have fixed views as to which treatment method is appropriate, any epidemiological analysis based on treatment method will be skewed towards the simple or more complex end of the spectrum of humeral shaft fractures.

The Edinburgh Orthopaedic Trauma Unit in the Royal Infirmary of Edinburgh is the only trauma unit for a population of 750 000 people. It takes in all humeral shaft fractures regardless of the severity, cause of the injury or the age of the patient. Thus an epidemiological analysis of data gained from the unit does give an indication of the types of humeral diaphyseal fractures that are present in the population as a whole.

In a 3-year period between April 1988 and April 1990, all adult inpatients and outpatients aged 12 years or over with a humeral diaphyseal fracture were included in a survey of the epidemiology of humeral shaft fractures. A diaphyseal fracture was defined according to the criteria of Muller *et al.*[2] excluding extra-articular fractures in the proximal and distal 5 cm of the bone. The fractures were classified using the AO system[2] to describe the morphology. The closed fractures were further classified using the Tscherne system[6]. The open fractures were also classified according to the Gustilo classification[4,5].

Six basic causes of injury were recorded. These were simple falls, falls from a height (irrespective of the height), sporting fractures, road traffic accidents, fractures resulting from direct blows or assaults and pathological fractures.

In the study period there were 143 humeral diaphyseal fractures treated in the unit on an inpatient or outpatient basis. The average age of the fracture group was 52.3 years (range 12–91 years), indicating that humeral diaphyseal fractures tend to occur in an older age group than either tibial or femoral diaphyseal fractures. Figure 10.4 shows the age distribution of the humeral fracture population. As with most fractures it shows a bimodal distribution with a relatively large number of patients presenting with humeral diaphyseal fractures over 60 years of age.

A breakdown of the fractures into their AO groups shows that 63% were simple type A fractures. A further 26.6% were type B wedge fractures and only 10.5% showed a complex type C fracture configuration. The incidence of the different AO groups is shown in Table 10.3. The commonest group encountered is the simple spiral (A1) fracture. Only this group and the simple transverse (A3) fracture occurred in more than 20% of patients. The A2 simple oblique, B1 spiral wedge and B2 bending wedge fractures occurred with approximately equal frequency of between 11% and 14%. The other groups were very much less common.

When the fractures are divided into their 27 AO

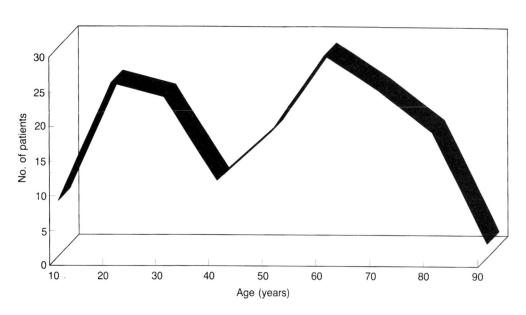

Figure 10.4 The bimodal distribution of humeral diaphyseal fractures

Table 10.3 Incidences of fractures in different AO fracture types and groups; average age of AO types also given

Type	Per cent	Average age
A1	29.4	
A2	11.9	
A3	21.7	
Total	63.0	56.2
B1	14.0	
B2	11.2	
B3	1.4	
Total	26.6	45.0
C1	5.6	
C2	3.5	
C3	1.4	
Total	10.5	57.4

Table 10.4 Relative incidence of fractures in the different AO subgroups

AO subgroups	A	B	C
1.1	6.3	4.2	4.2
1.2	21.0	8.4	1.4
1.3	2.1	1.4	–
2.1	2.1	0.7	2.8
2.2	8.4	10.5	–
2.3	1.4	–	0.7
3.1	2.8	1.4	0.7
3.2	18.9	1.4	–
3.3	–	–	0.7

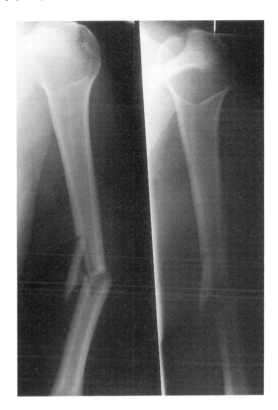

Figure 10.6 A B2.2 fracture. Table 10.3 illustrates that type B fractures occur in a younger population with better bone. This fracture occurred in a 42-year-old male in a fall from a height

subgroups (Table 10.4) it can be seen that only 3 fractures occur with a frequency of more than 10%. The simple mid-shaft spiral (A1.2) is the most common fracture configuration (Figure 10.5). This is followed by the mid-shaft transverse fracture (A3.2) and the mid-shaft bending wedge (B2.2). An illustration of this type B fracture is shown in Figure 10.6. Only 3 other fractures occurred with a frequency of more than 5%. These are the simple mid-shaft oblique fracture (A2.2), the mid-shaft spiral fracture (B1.2) and the proximal third spiral fracture (A1.2). Other fracture configurations are comparatively uncommon and a number of AO subgroups were not seen in this particular survey. Table 10.4 indicates the relative frequency of fractures occurring in the middle third of the diaphysis, with about 70% of the fractures occurring in this area.

There were 133 closed fractures, representing 93% of the whole group. The average age of these patients was 53.9 years. Table 10.5 gives a breakdown of the closed humeral fractures according to

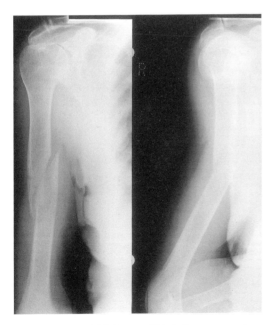

Figure 10.5 An A1.2 fracture. This is the commonest configuration of humeral diaphyseal fractures. The patient was a 76-year-old female who had had a simple fall

Table 10.5 Incidence and average age of the Tscherne closed fracture types. Correlation with the AO classification is demonstrated

Tscherne type	Incidence (%)	Average age (yr)	AO type (%) A	B	C
C0	21.1	63.8	87.5	12.5	–
CI	63.2	49.7	65.5	32.1	2.3
CII	12.8	58.6	5.9	41.2	52.9
CIII	3.0	40.2	–	–	100

their Tscherne types. The commonest were the C1 fracture (63.2%), followed by the C0 fracture (21.1%). The severe C3 fracture was only seen in 3% of cases. Interestingly, there did not appear to be a definite increase in fracture severity with age, as has been demonstrated in the tibia[7]. The relatively high age of the C0 fracture group is explained by the high number of pathological fractures in this group. There is a correlation between the Tscherne classification and the AO classification and Table 10.5 clearly shows an increasingly severe fracture morphology with increasing Tscherne fracture grading.

Of the 10 (7%) open fractures, 8 were Gustilo type 1 in severity, the remaining 2 being Gustilo type 3 fractures. One was a type 3A fracture and the remaining one a type 3B fracture. The average age of the open fracture group was 45.2 years. There was no significant difference in age or AO fracture morphology between the Gustilo type 1 and type 3 patients. Seven of the Gustilo type 1 patients had type A fractures and one had a type B fracture. Of the two more severe open fractures, one was AO type A and the other was type B.

An analysis of the causes of humeral diaphyseal fractures is presented in Table 10.6. By far the commonest cause is a simple fall occurring in an elderly patient. Over half of the fractures in the whole series occurred in this way. Table 10.6 refers to simple fall causing fractures in normal bone. Five further patients fractured through a

bone metastasis in a fall, making an overall incidence of 55.2% of fractures occurring secondary to a simple fall.

Road traffic accidents are the second commonest cause of humeral shaft fractures, followed by falls from a height. Sporting injuries and fractures following assaults or direct blows are comparatively rare. Sixteen patients (11.2%) presented with pathological fractures. Of these, 10 had no significant trauma, whereas 5 had had a simple fall and 1 had had a fall from a height. Of the whole group, 21 (14.7%) had had multiple injuries and a further 13 (9.1%) had other isolated orthopaedic injuries in addition to their humeral diaphyseal fractures.

Table 10.6 shows that the severe type C fractures (Figure 10.7) tend to occur in road traffic accidents and falls from a height. The relatively high incidence of 12.2% type C fractures associated with simple falls is, at first sight, a little surprising, but it must be remembered that the average age of this group is 62 years. There is an alteration of the biomechanical properties of bone with increasing age[8] and the association of increasing comminution with increasing age is commonly seen and certainly reported in other bones[7]. The other elderly group of patients presenting with humeral shaft fractures are those with metastases. All of these presented with AO type A morphology. This reflects the low-energy nature of most of these injuries. Other humeral diaphyseal fractures tend to occur in lower age groups.

Road traffic accidents

Further analysis of the data concerning road traffic accidents indicates that 33.3% of the diaphyseal fractures were in vehicle passengers, 29.2% occurred in pedestrians, 20.8% in vehicle drivers and 16.6% in motorcycle riders. Interestingly, the only AO type C fractures that occurred in the road traffic accident group involved pedestrians or

Table 10.6 Incidence of fractures associated with different causes. Average age and incidence of AO types also given

Cause of injury	Incidence (%)	Average age (yr)	AO type (%) A	B	C
Non-pathological					
Fall	51.7	62.0	63.5	24.3	12.2
Fall (height)	11.2	46.0	50.0	43.8	6.2
Sport	5.9	21.4	50.0	50.0	–
Road traffic accidents	16.8	47.9	45.8	33.3	20.8
Assault/direct blow	3.5	35.8	80.0	30.0	–
Pathological	11.2	70.0	100	–	–

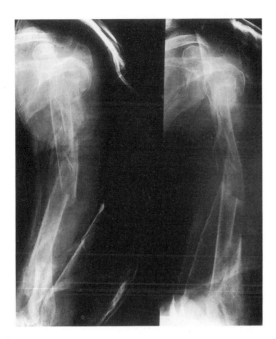

Figure 10.7   A C3.3 fracture. This represents the 'ultimate' C3.3 diaphyseal fracture, extending from the proximal to distal metaphyses. It occurred in a multiply injured 78-year-old female who was a pedestrian hit by a car

vehicle passengers, where the type C fractures made up 42.8% and 25%, respectively, of the open fractures. The morphology of the fractures in drivers and motorcycle riders was comparatively simple. The reason for the relatively high incidence of type C fractures in pedestrians may well be that the pedestrians tend to be older. The average age of the pedestrian subgroup was 47.9 years compared with 32.2 years for vehicle drivers, 21.5 years for motorcycle riders and 29.5 years for vehicle passengers.

Sports injury

Sports-related humeral diaphyseal fractures are comparatively uncommon (Table 10.6). As with all sporting injuries they occur in a young age group. There were no type C fractures, all showing an AO type A or B morphology. No one sport dominated. There were two fractures caused by soccer and cycling and one each were seen in rugby, skiing, horse-riding and parachuting accidents.

References

1. Breasted, J.H. The Edwin Smith papyrus, Chicago (1932)
2. Muller, M.E., Nazarian, S., Coch, P. and Schatzker, J. *A Comprehensive Classification of Fractures of Long Bones*, Springer-Verlag, Berlin (1990)
3. Seidel, H. Behandlung mit dem Humerus Verriegelungsnagel. In *Die Plattenosteosynthese und ihr Konkurrenzverfahren.* (eds D. Volter and W. Zimmer), Springer-Verlag, Berlin (1991), pp. 158–166
4. Gustilo, R.B. and Anderson, J.T. Prevention of infection in the treatment of one thousand and twenty five open fractures of long bones: retrospective and prospective analysis. *J. Bone Joint Surg.*, **58A**, 453–458 (1976)
5. Gustilo, R.B., Mendoza, R.M. and Williams, D.N. Problems in the management of type III (severe) open fractures: a new classification of type III open fractures. *J. Trauma*, **24**, 742–746 (1984)
6. Oesterne, H.-J. and Tscherne, H. Pathophysiology and classification of soft tissue injuries associated with fractures. In *Fractures and Soft Tissue Injuries* (eds H. Tscherne and L. Gotzen), Springer-Verlag, Berlin (1984), pp. 1–8
7. Court-Brown, C.M. and McBirnie, J. The epidemiology of tibial fractures. *J. Bone Joint Surg.*, **77B**, 417–421 (1995)
8. McCalden, R.W., McGeough, J.A., Barker, M.B. and Court-Brown, C.M. Age related changes in the tensile properties of cortical bone: relative importance of change in porosity, mineralisation and microstructure. *J. Bone Joint Surg.*, **75A**, 1206–1213 (1993)

11

Surgical treatment of humeral diaphyseal fractures

C. Ulrich

Operative treatment of fractures of the humeral diaphysis was introduced because some surgeons were dissatisfied with the existing non-operative treatment methods. As with the treatment of other fractures, surgeons are not always rational in their choice of treatment methods[1], but there is some evidence that the surgical stabilization of a humeral diaphyseal fracture confers benefit to the patient.

Until relatively recently the surgical methods employed in humeral diaphyseal fractures were adapted from the equivalent operations in the lower limb. As a result of this, the surgeons who advocated humeral fracture fixation frequently based their indications for operative stabilization on those that they utilized in other areas. They often rationalized that the success of one particular treatment method in one body area meant that it would be successful in other areas and they based their choice of treatment modality on this type of logic rather than on the analysis of prospective studies of the management of humeral diaphyseal fractures. In addition, the evolution of many of the surgical stabilization techniques has occurred relatively recently. Modern anaesthetic techniques have rendered surgery safer and this has led many surgeons to have more interest in surgical techniques than in the natural history of the fractures that they are treating.

Plate osteosynthesis

The first report of open reduction and internal fixation of a diaphyseal fracture using a metal plate and screws was by Hansmann in 1886[2]. He dealt with 21 cases and in the final sentence of his report he states that 'Apparently the procedure neither protects against necrosis, nor is it particularly propitious or conducive to its development. Some cases remained necrosis-free'. Following Hansmann's work, other orthopaedic surgeons became interested in the use of metal plates and Arbuthnott Lane[3] advocated the procedure for the management of humeral fractures under certain conditions. However, diaphyseal plating was finally popularized by the work of the AO group. This group advocated rigid plating of diaphyseal fractures to promote fracture stability and union[4]. They promoted the potential advantages of primary bone healing and showed in a series of animal experiments that this could be achieved by rigid internal fixation using bone plates. Callus was referred to as irritation-callus and the group preferred to see callus-free X-rays. Allgower referred to these as 'a reward for having precisely adhered to the principles of internal fixation'. Since the early work of the AO group there has been much debate about the clinical usefulness of callus, but in recent years the emphasis has turned away from rigid internal fixation and consequent callus suppression to the use of more flexible fixation techniques that encourage callus formation.

Open reduction and internal fixation using bone plates requires that not only the fracture be opened but also the bone ends be exposed. Inevitably this is associated with soft tissue stripping from the bone, thus interfering with the normal bone vascularization. This additional trauma to tissues already damaged by the injury has led to a worry-

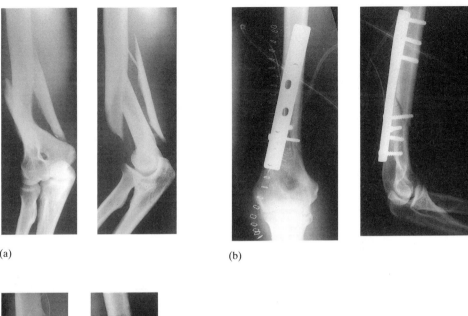

(a) (b)

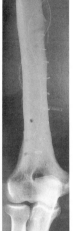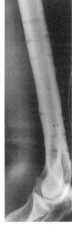

(c)

Figure 11.1 An AO B1 humeral shaft fracture: (a) it is not uncommon for there to be a butterfly fragment in distal diaphyseal humeral fractures; (b) the fracture has been stabilized with an interfragmentary screw and by the application of an AO dynamic compression; (c) after union the plate has been removed

ing incidence of non-union, infection and other complications. As a result of this, surgeons have tended to use techniques other than open reduction and plate osteosynthesis for diaphyseal fractures, reserving these techniques mainly for metaphyseal fractures. Currently most diaphyseal fractures are fixed using intramedullary nailing techniques, but these techniques have been least successful in the management of humeral diaphyseal fractures and some surgeons regard the anatomical conditions of the humerus as a contraindication to the use of intramedullary nailing[5].

In 1965 Böhler[6] strenuously promoted non-operative management of humeral diaphyseal fractures. In the same year, Bandi[7] advocated the use of plate osteosynthesis. At the time it was accepted that there were two major advantages of this technique in that the biomechanics of humeral plating were understood and the surgeon could directly visualize the fracture and its subsequent treatment. However, it was also accepted that these operations required extensive soft tissue dissection and bone exposure. Additionally, surgeons argued about the merits of removal of the fracture haematoma and opponents of the technique pointed out that the patients required a second operation to remove the plate. There is no doubt that excellent results can be obtained if the method is properly performed (Figure 11.1). This has been illustrated by a large number of publications. However, as with all surgical techniques, the clinical research pointing out the benefits of the technique has to be tempered with reports dealing with its failures.

A trial carried out by the ASIF group in their constituent clinics led to a report on the results of plate osteosynthesis in humeral shaft fractures by Schweiberer *et al.*[5]. In 225 patients with humeral diaphyseal fractures treated by plate fixation, 12% of the diaphyseal fractures were located in the proximal third, 53% were in the middle third and the remaining 27% were in the distal third of the diaphysis. Inadequate reduction, primary radial nerve palsy and delayed fracture healing were common indications for plate fixation. Eighteen per cent of the cases were said to have a number of surgical indications. Postoperative complications were relatively high, with 37.5% of patients having a radial nerve palsy and 6.8% showing evidence of a pseudarthrosis. A further 4.9% of patients had osteitis and 4.5% of cases showed evidence of soft tissue infection. It is of interest that 3.6% of the cases that presented with a primary radial nerve palsy had a complete palsy at final follow-up and a further 7.1% of the cases had an incomplete radial nerve lesion. Thus a policy of open reduction and internal fixation of humeral shaft fractures did not bring about uniform improvement in the incidence of radial nerve palsy. Despite these various complications the authors reported that the functional results at final follow-up were satisfactory in 96% of cases.

In the same year, Van der Griend *et al.*[8] presented their results of open reduction and plate osteosynthesis of humeral diaphyseal fractures in 36 seriously injured patients. Ten of the patients had at least one additional injury in the arm and many of the remaining cases were either open fractures or associated with poly-trauma. Nine of the patients showed evidence of a primary radial nerve palsy. Postoperatively, the authors noted two superficial wound infections and one temporary radial nerve lesion. Apparently there was unsatisfactory function in 6 cases and they concluded that non-operative management should be the treatment of choice for closed fractures of the humeral diaphysis.

In 1987, Hall and Pankovich[9] presented a meta-analysis of 146 humeral shaft fractures dealt with by plate osteosynthesis. This paper detailed a 10.2% incidence of pseudarthrosis (4.8 times higher than with non-operative management) as well as a 6.9% incidence of osteomyelitis (23.7 times higher than with non-operative management). They also reported a 16% incidence of postoperative radial nerve palsy, this being 1.7 times higher than that associated with non-operative management. These figures were corroborated by those of Giebel *et al.*[10].

Rommens *et al.*[11] presented a series of 78 humeral diaphyseal fractures of which 71 had been stabilized by plate osteosynthesis. In 16 of the fractures (20.6%) a primary radial nerve palsy was noted and in 10 patients (12.8%) a radial nerve palsy was noted postoperatively. In this series there were no pseudarthroses or deep infection, but in 2 cases the osteosynthesis had to be repeated due to implant loosening. Nine (56.2%) of the 16 preoperative radial nerve palsies and 6 (60%) of the 10 postoperative palsies showed complete resolution.

A number of authors stated that plate osteosynthesis was particularly useful in the management of the poly-traumatized patient for the obvious reason that osteosynthesis offered the advantages of anatomical reduction and immediate mobilization. The added advantage of its use in the poly-traumatized patient was the avoidance of any form of traction. The advantages of plate fixation in the poly-traumatized patient were detailed by Bandi[7], but subsequently Bleeker[12] also suggested that humeral fractures in poly-traumatized patients were an indication for plate fixation. He examined 58 patients with humeral diaphyseal fractures who had an Injury Severity Score of more than 18. He noted a low incidence of delayed union after plating compared to an equivalent group whose diaphyseal fractures were treated non-operatively. Rogers *et al.*[13] treated 19 patients with floating elbows, these patients having concomitant ipsilateral fractures of the humerus in the forearm. Those patients that were treated without open reduction and internal fixation had a high incidence of non-union. The authors advocated the use of open reduction and internal fixation for both the humerus and forearm fractures. Nast-Colb[14] analysed 170 fractures stabilized by plate osteosynthesis and observed a 10% incidence of operation-induced radial nerve palsy but no other complications were referred to.

An analysis of the various papers suggests that the incidence of complications associated with plate osteosynthesis of humeral diaphyseal fractures means that the indications for surgical treatment are exceptional. In addition, authors have noted that surgical treatments are associated with twice as many hospital bed days as needed for non-operative management. Overall the disadvantages of plate osteosynthesis outweigh the advantages. Most authors have highlighted a high incidence of pseudarthrosis, osteitis, soft tissue infection, radial nerve lesions and the requirement for secondary surgery to remove the plate. This latter procedure clearly exposes the radial nerve to further damage. If this technique is to be used, the orthopaedic traumatologist should realize that plating is the most demanding of all of the bone fixation techniques and should ideally only be used by those surgeons who are experienced in its use.

External skeletal fixation

Albin Lambotte was the first author to document the use of external fixation in the upper arm[15]. This method of fracture fixation has mainly been used for open fractures of the tibia. It has found less favour in humeral fractures and there is a higher incidence of pin-track infections associated with

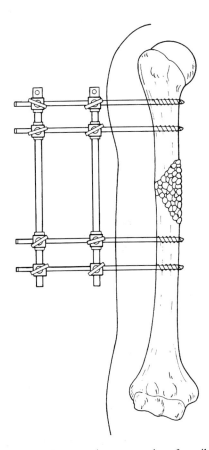

Figure 11.2 Diagrammatic representation of a unilateral frame applied to the humeral diaphysis. In this case there has been bone loss and the defect has been filled with corticocancellous graft

the relatively thick soft tissue envelope surrounding the humerus[16]. An early external fixator used to immobilize a humeral fracture is illustrated in Figure 11.2. Despite the fact that some of the early fracture surgeons achieved success using external fixation devices for humeral diaphyseal fractures, the method did not become popular because of the psychological barriers imposed on the surgeon and the patient by its method of management. There were, however, repeated reports, particularly in the French literature, about external fixation but it was left to Hoffmann[17] to popularize external skeletal fixation and to develop his own fixation device which is still in widespread use around the world. The use of the Hoffmann for humeral shaft fractures has been popularized by Burny and his co-workers[18–20] in particular.

Following the early work by Hoffmann, surgeons adopted two philosophies when recommending external fixation for humeral diaphyseal fractures. Workers such as Muller et al.[4] and Gustilo et al.[21] suggested that external fixation should mainly be reserved for the management of open fractures of the humeral diaphysis. An example of this is shown in Figure 11.3(a–c). Thus many of the publications regarding external fixation in the upper arm refer to severe open injuries often occurring under war conditions[22,23].

Burny[18–20] in Brussels was one of the few surgeons to employ external fixation for closed fractures of the humeral diaphyses. He was very enthusiastic about this method of fixation and he stated that the method had a number of advantages. He observed that it was a quick, easy and inexpensive operation. He also felt that the method was versatile and that one could use the same instruments for fractures in different parts of the body. Secondary correction of a fracture malposition was possible in contrast to plating or intramedullary nailing. He also pointed out that external skeletal fixation facilitated postoperative joint mobility as well as rapid periosteal callus formation. Lastly, he stated that the fixator could be removed in the outpatient clinic and the patient did not have to go through a second operative procedure. Burny did encounter a number of complications, however. He reported a 5% incidence of secondary temporary radial nerve palsy. He stated that 5.6% of his patients were intolerant of the fixator and he had a 5.1% incidence of pseudarthrosis. His malunion incidence was 3.2% and he documented a 3.8% incidence of refracture following fixator removal.

In 1980, Burny et al.[19] compared the use of the

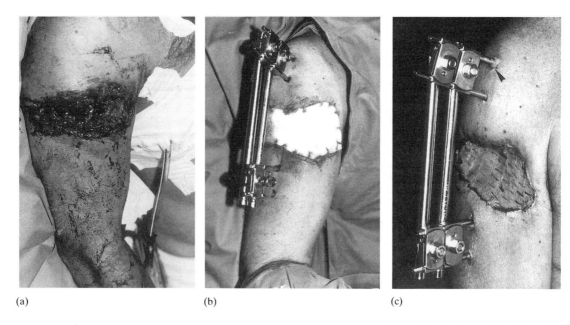

(a)   (b)   (c)

Figure 11.3   (a) Fracture of the proximal humeral diaphysis. (b) The fracture has been immobilized using a unilateral external fixator with two side bars. (c) A good result was obtained after split skin grafting. The arrow points to an infected pin track. Pin-track infection is not unusual in this location given the bulk of the soft tissue around the humerus

external fixator with both non-operative methods and operative intervention. He undertook a meta-analysis of 921 cases treated by non-operative means and 689 cases in which the fracture had been treated operatively. He pointed out that good and very good results were obtained after non-operative management in nearly 90% of cases, which was exactly the percentage he attained using the Hoffmann external fixator. In 1984, Burny and colleagues undertook a meticulous functional follow-up examination of 164 patients whose closed humeral diaphyseal fractures had been treated with the Hoffmann fixator[20]. They found that abduction, internal rotation and particularly external rotation all showed impaired mobility. This lack of movement was attributed to the necessity of inserting the fixation pins through the triceps in order to minimize radial nerve damage. The restriction of mobility was accepted as an inevitable by-product of this technique.

In 1984, De Bastiani *et al.*[24] presented a new unilateral external fixation device which allowed micro-movement at the fracture site, a phenomenon referred to as dynamization. De Bastiani advanced the same arguments as Burny and used the technique extensively in humeral shaft fractures. Brug *et al.*[25] also advocated the use of external skeletal fixation in humeral shaft fractures

and used it in situations where previously he would have used a plate. Brug pointed out, however, that the presence of transfixion pins limited the procedure to fractures of the middle third and, since many of these fractures are simple transverse fractures, he had treated a number of straightforward fractures which might well have been satisfactorily treated non-operatively. He felt, however, that the advantages of the procedure compared with non-operative management were improved comfort, better hygiene and enhanced mobility. It showed specific advantages when compared with plate osteosynthesis in that there was no requirement for an invasive procedure, the external fixator mounting was simple, there were few complications and it was at least theoretically possible to carry out a secondary correction for a fracture malposition. One disadvantage of external fixation of the humerus is that because of the comparatively thick layer of soft tissue present in the upper arm, pin-track infections, while frequently transitory and harmless, often result in unsightly scar formation (Figure 11.3c). It was Brug's view that external skeletal fixation could only be recommended for fractures in the middle third of the diaphysis in poly-traumatized patients or for open fractures where the pins could be placed outside the damaged area. He advocated the use of func-

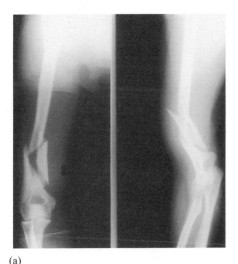

(a)

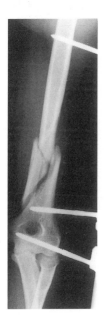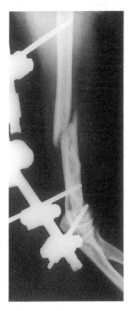

(b)

Figure 11.4 (a) An AO B1 fracture of the distal humeral diaphysis. (b) The fracture has adequately fixed with a unilateral external frame. Care must be taken to avoid the radial nerve and to avoid a significant fracture malposition

tional bracing in all situations where this technique was possible.

It is clear that external fixation of closed humeral diaphyseal fractures is only performed by a few traumatologists who are particularly enthusiastic about the technique. More surgeons accept that external skeletal fixation is useful where there

is a humeral fracture associated with a severe soft tissue injury or a subtotal amputation. However, the technique can be used for a wide variety of humeral fractures and its use in a low diaphyseal fracture is illustrated in Figure 11.4.

Intramedullary nailing

Intramedullary nailing of the humerus was advocated by the Rush brothers[26], who used their elastic nails to particularly good effect in proximal diaphyseal fractures. The principle of the nail is that it allows for three-point fixation in the intramedullary canal. Insertion is either performed in an antegrade manner through the proximal humerus outside the insertion of the rotator cuff or in a retrograde manner from the distal humerus (Figure 11.5).

Initial reports of the use of Rush nails were enthusiastic and the technique found widespread use in North America and Europe[27]. The problem that was initially encountered was that of impingement secondary to proximal nail projection, but no other significant complications were detailed. Later authors, however, did begin to experience some problems, mainly finding that the technique did not confer sufficient stability on the fracture to allow the patients to mobilize without an additional splint.

Stern et al.[28] analysed the technique of flexible pinning using Rush pins and Ender nails in 1984. They followed up 60 humeral fractures, finding that 8.3% of the cases developed pseudarthrosis. A further 15% showed delayed union and 5% had deep infection. These complications were more common in open fractures and following open reduction of closed fractures. Stern also considered that brace or plaster fixation for the first two postoperative weeks was indicated. He pointed out that there might well be a detrimental effect on shoulder function, as in 56% of his cases he documented a painful adhesive capsulitis of the shoulder. All of these patients had had an antegrade nail insertion. It is interesting to observe that in 9 patients who had a retrograde nailing of the humeral fracture, elbow function was not significantly impaired. The authors pointed out that the morbidity could be reduced with proper surgical technique and emphasized the importance of correct pin selection and placement as well as the importance of proper three-point fixation. They also advocated early removal of the pins to reduce the risk of shoulder stiffness.

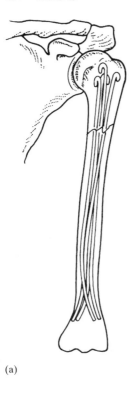

(a)

Figure 11.5 (a) Diagrammatic representation of a proximal humeral fracture immobilized using antegrade insertion of multiple Rush nails. Note the distal spreading of the nails to facilitate rotational control of the fracture. (b) A retrograde insertion of multiple Rush nails to treat a mid-diaphyseal humeral fracture. The arrow represents the point of insertion of the nail

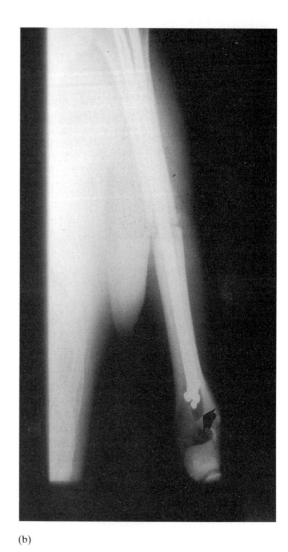

(b)

Brumback *et al.*[29] also examined the use of flexible nailing in humeral shaft fractures. They stated that antegrade insertion of the nails caused fewer problems than retrograde insertion, provided that rotator cuff integrity was preserved. If an impingement syndrome developed, they advocated removal and replacement of the nails. They demonstrated bone healing in 94% of their cases and excellent results in 62%. In 1987, Hall and Pankovich[9] reported on the use of Ender nails for the management of humeral shaft fractures. In 89 fractures that received functional treatment postoperatively they only encountered 1 case of pseudarthrosis. There were no infections and no cases of malunion. All their postoperative radial nerve palsies resolved spontaneously. In 8 patients, one

of the Ender nails broke necessitating revision in 5 cases.

Analysis of elbow function showed excellent results, with an average loss of extension of 4° and an average flexion of 132° being achieved. Shoulder abduction averaged 91°, with 54° of external rotation and 68° of internal rotation. The authors concluded that intramedullary Ender nailing was a safe and effective technique when performed in selected cases of humeral shaft fractures. They also stated, however, that non-operative functional bracing should remain the standard method of management.

At the same time as the Rush brothers were developing their concept of flexible intramedullary nailing, Kuntscher[30] was developing his technique

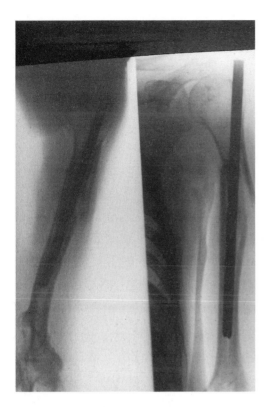

Figure 11.6 A Küntscher nail used to immobilize a
proximal humeral diaphyseal fracture. Note the varus
malposition and the proximal prominence of the nail leading
to an impingement syndrome

using a single larger intramedullary nail (Figure
11.6). Kuntscher's technique was essentially
adapted from his earlier successful techniques of
femoral and tibial intramedullary nailing, but there
were a number of disadvantages when these techniques were adapted for the humerus. One of the
main problems was fracture site distraction and
this was shown to be a major cause of pseudarthrosis in humeral shaft fractures[6,31–34]. The anatomical configuration of the intramedullary canal
of the humerus is not uniform and therefore a
Kuntscher type of nail does not easily fit into the
canal. In addition, the elastic locking which was
postulated to occur with the Kuntscher nail cannot
occur because of the lack of an adequate fit
between the nail and the endosteal surface of the
intramedullary canal. Additionally, the Kuntscher
nail requires a large fenestration to be made in the
bone to permit insertion and this fenestration facilitates the formation of an iatrogenic fracture.

Few series of the management of humeral shaft
fracture with Kuntscher nails were reported. Chris-

tensen[35] reported the management of 13 pseudarthroses with the Kuntscher nail, 7 of which had
initially been operated on using a Rush nail. One
of the remaining fractures had been treated by cer-
clarge wire and the remaining 6 had been managed
non-operatively. He found that only 7 of the 13
pseudarthroses healed after Kuntscher nailing.
Concern was expressed about the development of
an impingement syndrome secondary to proximal
prominence of the nail and Christensen suggested
that a specially designed humeral nail might be
required.

Vander Griend et al.[36] discussed the management of 18 humeral fractures which were stabilized with Kuntscher nails. Six of the fractures
were pathological and 12 were fresh fractures in
poly-traumatized patients. All fractures united and
the authors concluded that in certain selected
cases Kuntscher nailing could be a successful
procedure.

The next development in intramedullary nailing
of humeral fractures was by Hackethal[37]. He
developed the stacked nailing method which was
felt to combine the best aspects of Kuntscher
nailing and flexible nailing. Hackethal nails were
usually inserted in a retrograde manner (Figure
11.7) and Hackethal believed that using his
method he could achieve adequate elastic locking
in many humeral diaphyseal fractures. The disadvantages of the technique, namely inadequate
stability on loading and a requirement for peroper-
ative radiation, were apparently outweighed by the
advantages, these being a relatively easy operative
technique, few instruments and a short operation
time. As is often the case, the technique was used
in inappropriate complicated humeral fractures
and pseudarthrosis, infection and malunion inevitably occurred. The method became less popular,
although it remains in use by surgeons familiar
with it[38].

In 1976, Brug et al.[39] reported on 108 humeral
fractures treated with Hackethal nails. Three of
them developed a postoperative radial nerve palsy
and 13 patients developed a pseudarthrosis, 10 of
which were successfully managed by further surgery. The authors pointed out that the method
required appropriate experience and suggested that
only particular fractures were suitable for stacked
nailing. In comminuted fractures and in cases
involving nerve and vascular lesions, they advocated the use of plate osteosynthesis or an external
fixator.

Durbin et al.[40] also reported their results using
Hackethal stacked nails in 30 humeral shaft frac-

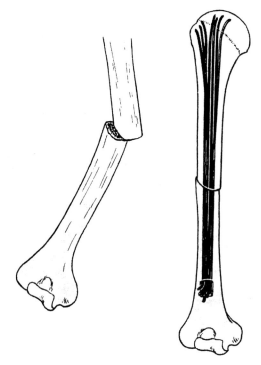

Figure 11.7　Diagrammatic representation of stacked Hackethal nails used to immobilize a mid-diaphyseal fracture. These have been inserted in a retrograde fashion

the fresh fractures and the pathological fractures but the patients with non-unions did not have satisfactory results. However, they reported that the technique was relatively simple with shoulder stiffness being a preventable complication.

Kuntscher's principle of a single large intramedullary nail was developed further by Seidel[42]. His nail was based on the detensor nail suggested by Kuntscher in 1968. He developed a locked intramedullary nail which was shaped to fit the humeral shaft. The nail is illustrated in Figure 11.8. It is an unslotted nail which achieves proximal locking with screws and distal locking by means of fins which are expanded using a spreading bolt.

In his first report[42] on 80 humeral shaft fractures stabilized with this implant, Seidel described a union rate of 100% with only minimally reduced mobility of the shoulder. In 1991 he reported on 160 fractures stabilized with the Seidel nail, finding only 1 pseudarthrosis and 2 infections. There was no postoperative radial nerve lesion among his patients, but Seidel did advocate that the presence of a preoperative radial nerve lesion meant that the nerve should be opened and explored before nailing. He also advocated that the nail

tures. They felt that the technique was relatively simple, resulting in only minor blood loss and a low incidence of radial nerve palsy. They detailed a bone union rate of 92%, but did have a 14% incidence of reoperation. They described a number of complications, including local bone damage at the insertion site, heterotopic calcification and extension loss in the elbow. They also pointed out that nail loosening occurred, but felt that this was not a serious problem. Baranowski and Brug[38] reported on 53 patients who had had stacked Hackethal nails used for their humeral fractures. They also reported a relatively low morbidity with only one pseudarthrosis, 5 cases of limited mobility and no infection.

Christensen's earlier suggestion that specially adapted nails might diminish the problems encountered with Kuntscher nailing of the humerus was explored by Gallagher *et al.*[41] in 1988. They reported on 12 patients in which they had used a special nail with a strong proximal thread. Six of the cases involved fresh fractures, 3 had pathological fractures and the remaining 3 cases had pseudarthroses. They reported good results with

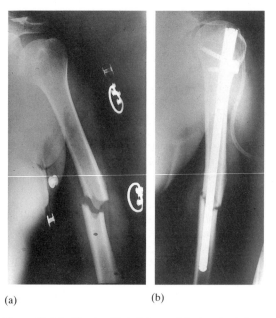

(a)　　　　　　　　　　(b)

Figure 11.8 (a, b)　A mid-shaft humeral fracture treated initially by the application of a functional brace. The fracture has subsequently been immobilized using a Seidel nail which has been locked proximally and distally. The tight fit of the nail inside the intramedullary canal has prevented much spreading of the distal fins. Note the slight fracture distraction postoperatively

Table 11.1 Indications for fractures surgically stabilized with a Seidel nail (*n*=83)

Distraction of fragments	27
Transverse fractures	22
Metastatic destruction	14
Patient's request	12
Additional fractures in same extremity	8

should not be driven forcefully into the intramedullary canal in order to avoid cortical damage. The main problem reported was that of a minor impingement syndrome in 40% of the patients. Similar results were gained by Haberneck and Orthner[43].

A contrary view was taken by Robinson *et al.*[44], who reported on 30 humeral fractures stabilized with the Seidel nail. They encountered a number of technical problems, particularly with the locking mechanisms. They found proximal nail migration secondary to inadequate locking, which caused impingement syndrome and they also demonstrated in other patients that even where there was no proximal nail migration there was impaired shoulder function secondary to rotator cuff damage. In their 30 patients, 21 secondary operations were required. They took the view that unlike femoral and tibial intramedullary nailing they could not recommend this procedure as a standard method of management for humeral diaphyseal fracture. Jensen *et al.*[45] were more enthusiastic about the technique. They examined 16 patients, demonstrating impingement in 4 patients, but they felt that this was a manifestation of proximal nail projection and they advocated that the nail needed to be driven into the proximal humerus. In 1993, Evans *et al.*[46] pointed out in a cadaveric study that the proximal locking of the Seidel nail might produce axillary nerve damage as well as damage to the biceps tendon.

In the period between June 1987 and October 1992, 83 humeral shaft fractures were surgically stabilized using a Seidel nail at our clinic. The average age of the patients was 63.2 years, with a range of 25–98 years. The indications for surgery are shown in Table 11.1. There were 22 transverse fractures, 14 short oblique fractures, 29 long oblique fractures, 4 comminuted fractures and 14 pathological fractures. The average time to union was 10 weeks. Two patients showed evidence of osteomyelitis which was successfully eradicated with appropriate treatment.

Fifty-five of the patients were adequately fol-lowed up. All the patients were X-rayed and their shoulder function was assessed. In addition, sonography of the rotator cuff was performed to assess any damage.

Restricted shoulder movement was found in 9 patients (16.4%) and subacromial calcification in a further 10 patients (18%). Without exception, sonography showed the presence of scar tissue and adhesions in the gliding tissues of the rotator cuff. There was, however, no functional correlation with 80% of the cases showing no evidence of functional impairment. The remaining 20% had difficulty in moving their shoulders. Ten patients (18%) reported pain and X-rays showed that in a further 8 cases there was evidence of distal screw loosening. In 12 cases, proximal nail projection caused painful impingement which necessitated nail removal.

In 6 cases there was bony damage during drilling and in 2 further cases an undisplaced additional fracture was created in the distal fragments. These iatrogenic fractures, however, healed completely without the need for further surgical intervention. In 3 cases there was evidence of fracture site distraction (see Figure 11.8). However, in all cases this was less than 1 cm and did not apparently disturb the healing process.

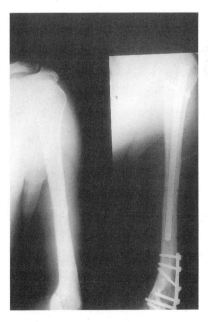

Figure 11.9 A combined fracture of the humeral diaphysis and distal metaphysis treated by proximal intramedullary nailing and distal plate osteosynthesis. The patient achieved a good result

It was felt that the technique was useful as it minimized discomfort and facilitated mobilization. It was particularly useful in the elderly and in poly-traumatized patients. It was also found to be useful for the rare combination of fractures involving a diaphyseal fracture and a distal intra-articular fracture. In these cases intramedullary nailing can be used for the proximal fracture and conventional plate osteosynthesis for the distal fracture (Figure 11.9).

Work continues in designing new intramedullary nails for the humerus. Unfortunately, however, there is little clinical experience with new nail designs. It is recognized that humeral nailing is somewhat unsatisfactory compared with tibial and femoral nailing and at the moment only the Seidel locking nail can be recommended.

Operative techniques

Plate osteosynthesis

When applying a plate to the humeral shaft four surgical approaches are possible, these being the anterior, lateral, medial and dorsal approaches.[47] The choice of the approach depends on a number of factors, but is particularly determined by the location of the fracture and the extent of any co-existing soft tissue injury.

Anterior approach

The anterior approach provides excellent access for proximal and middle third fractures of the humeral shaft. However, due to the shape of the humerus, plating is less easy to perform on the anterior aspect of the bone compared with the dorsal or lateral aspect. Thus if the anterior approach is used, it is recommended that the plate is applied laterally. In this approach the origins of the deltoid muscle and brachialis muscle must be elevated.

It is also recommended that the patient be recumbent, with a pillow placed under the shoulder and the upper arm adducted. The main incision begins distal to the tip of the coracoid process and runs distally along the deltopectoral groove lateral to the biceps muscle, ending in the midline near the elbow. Initially the subcutaneous layer and fascia are incised and the deltoid muscle and cephalic vein mobilized laterally.

The surgeon should then locate the insertion of the pectoralis major muscle on the humerus and it may be necessary to incise part of the pectoralis muscle attachment (Figure 11.10). Careful traction of the biceps muscle in a medial direction exposes the underlying brachialis muscle. The muscle is split longitudinally, approximately one finger-breadth lateral to the midline. The surgeon should incise through the muscle, aiming towards the middle of the shaft to preserve the supply of the brachialis muscle. Subperiosteal exposure of the bone is performed, care being taken when mobilizing the tissues in the area of the radial nerve. To this end, it is recommended that lever retractors are not used in the area of the nerve.

The incision can be extended proximally to the area of the shoulder joint. If the surgeon requires to do this, it is recommended that the fascia over-

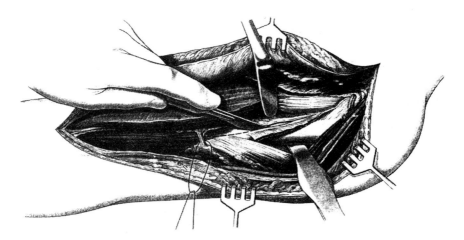

Figure 11.10 Diagrammatic representation of the anterior approach to the humerus

lying the bicipital groove is opened with blunt dissection medial to the short head of the biceps and the coracobrachialis muscle. Again, traction exerted on the coracobrachialis muscle must be applied carefully in order to avoid injuring the musculocutaneous nerve. The theoretical advantage of the anterior approach lies in the fact that the complete humerus can be exposed, from the shoulder joint to the elbow.

Treatment of the humeral fracture is only possible after adequate fracture visualization. The surgeon and assistant should employ indirect reduction as much as possible. Direct reduction with excessive bone handling results in further periosteal stripping. Humeral shaft fractures are frequently associated with the presence of long butterfly fragments and the surgeon may choose to stabilize these with interfragmentary screws in the manner advocated by the AO group. However, if interfragmentary screws are used the surgeon must remember that by themselves they do not produce adequate fixation and fracture stability[4]. The implant of choice is a broad 4.5 mm dynamic compression plate. The plate should be applied with at least six cortices being transfixed above and below the fracture. To this end the plate should have at least seven holes. In the case of long oblique fractures, additional interfragmentary screws applied, if possible, through the plate should be used. Preliminary prestressing of the plate is obligatory. Wherever possible the new generation of low contact plates should be chosen. The surgeon should always remember that it is important that the screws should not be placed in a row, but slightly obliquely towards the medial or lateral sides of the bone, depending on the position of the hole in the plate. In areas of comminution it is advisable to use primary corticocancellous bone grafting.

It is recommended that the wound be closed in layers over subfascial and subcutaneous drains. Ideally, muscular sutures should be avoided and only the fascial and tendinous attachments that have been detached should be reinserted. It is recommended that the plates be left *in situ* for at least one year and only be removed if there are clinical indications.

Lateral approach

In this approach it is recommended that the patient is again recumbent, but that the arm is in a degree of abduction. The elbow should be free and the forearm and hand contained in a sterile towel. The incision begins two finger-breadths proximal to the deltoid attachment and is continued in the midline to just above the elbow. After the skin and fascia have been incised, the dissection is continued between brachialis muscle anteriorly and the triceps and brachioradialis muscles posteriorly (Figure 11.11). Prior to exposing the humeral shaft the radial nerve is located and protected. Once this has been done, the periosteum is incised in front of the lateral intermuscular septum (Figure 11.12). If necessary, the incision can be continued distally to expose the distal third of the humerus and the elbow joint. This is done by following the bra-

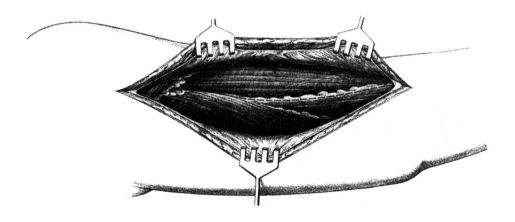

Figure 11.11 Diagrammatic representation of the lateral approach to the humerus. The skin and fascia have been incised and space between the brachialis muscle anteriorly and the triceps and brachioradialis muscles posteriorly is about to be incised

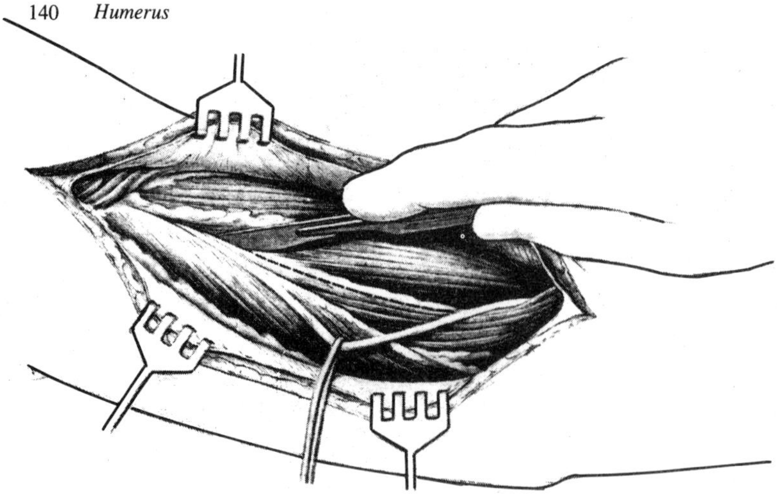

Figure 11.12 Once the space between the muscles has been opened and the neurovascular bundle protected, the periosteum can be incised and the fracture site exposed

chialis muscle distally as far as the elbow. If this is done the surgeon must be careful to avoid damage to the radial nerve.

Medial approach

The medial approach is rarely used because of the potential damage to neurovascular structures. It allows access to the middle third of the humerus and if the surgeon wishes to perform this approach it is recommended that the patient be placed supine with the arm in 90° of abduction. The incision is made from the axilla to the ulnar epicondyle and the fascia is split in the usual way. Access is gained between the muscles of the flexor and extensor compartments and care must be taken when mobilizing the ulnar nerve. Once the bone has been exposed the periosteum is elevated in the usual way and a plate applied using the techniques already discussed. There are few indications for selecting the medial approach to the humerus, the most obvious of which is the presence of pre-existing soft tissue damage to other parts of the upper arm.

Dorsal approach

If the surgeon wishes to use the dorsal approach to the humeral shaft, the patient can be placed in one of three ways: either prone or lateral with the arm adducted, or prone with the arm abducted resting on an arm roll.

The incision begins three finger-breadths distal to the acromion and is continued to the tip of the olecranon (Figure 11.13). Subcutaneous tissue and fascia are incised and the triceps muscle is mobilized between the long and lateral head using blunt dissection. If the surgeon finds that it is impossible

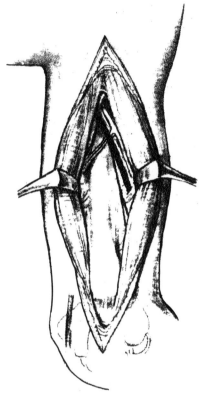

Figure 11.13 Diagrammatic representation of the dorsal triceps-splitting approach to the humerus. Great care must be taken to protect the radial nerve, but if this approach is done excellent exposure can be achieved

to separate the muscle bellies without dissection, the muscle bellies should be lifted upwards with a finger at the point where they unite. This then allows sharp dissection to be carried out safely. The surgeon must take great care in incising the triceps muscle in the area of the radial nerve as damage is relatively easy. Once the neurovascular bundle has been located, it should be mobilized from the bone and carefully retracted. The upper humeral shaft can then be exposed by incising the triceps and retractors or levers can be inserted to facilitate plate placement.

The surgeon will find that fracture reduction is easier than with the lateral approach. The plate should be applied using the previously described technique, but the surgeon must be careful not to allow the bone plate to encroach onto the olecranon fossa. Care must also be taken to ensure that after the plate has been applied the radial nerve lies on the plate without any tension. It is also strongly recommended that the area at which the radial nerve crosses the implant is carefully recorded in the notes as this may help plate removal if this becomes necessary. Following plating, the wound is closed in layers over subfascial and subcutaneous drains.

Postoperative regimen

Rest the arm on a pillow and start limited active exercises without axial or bending load.

Intramedullary nailing of the humerus

Antegrade insertion

It is recommended that the patient be placed in a sitting position with the upper body raised by at least 30°. The trunk is draped in a manner which allows free exposure of the shoulder and upper arm and the patient should be placed such that the

arm extends beyond the operating table to allow for adequate visualization by the C-arm of the image intensifier. The forearm should rest on a support and the C-arm is placed vertically beside the patient (Figure 11.14). The skin incision is a short sabre cut 3–5 cm in length, running from the anterior to posterior aspects of the humeral head. This type of approach allows for an extension to permit exposure of the humeral head if this is required. The deltoid muscle is incised subcutaneously distal to its acromial attachment. The rotator cuff is incised longitudinally and a curved bone awl is inserted into the medullary canal from the tip of the greater tuberosity. The fracture is reduced under X-ray control and a guidewire placed across it. The nail length is then computed and the medullary canal is reamed in steps of 0.5 mm up to 11 mm. The reaming guidewire is exchanged for the nail guidewire and the nail is then inserted over the second guidewire.

If a Seidel nail is used, the proximal screwdriver is used to open the distal spreading bolt and a proximal jig is used to facilitate proximal screw placement. It is important that hammering of the intramedullary humeral nail should be kept to a minimum to reduce the risk of bone damage and fracture site distraction.

Retrograde insertion

If the surgeon is contemplating retrograde humeral nailing, it is recommended that the patient be placed in a prone position. As with the dorsal approach for plate osteosynthesis, the abducted arm is placed on an arm pulley so that the proper

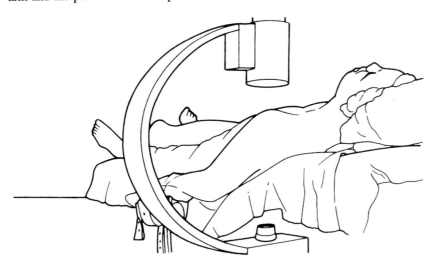

Figure 11.14 The patient position for antegrade nailing of the humeral diaphysis

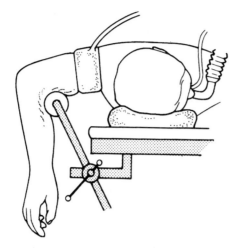

Figure 11.15 The patient positioning for a retrograde nailing of the humeral diaphysis

access to the humeral head can be maintained and the C-arm can be moved (Figure 11.15). The skin is incised longitudinally, starting about one finger-breadth proximal to the tip of the olecranon and carrying the incision proximally for a further 4 or 5 cm. The triceps is split longitudinally and the dorsal aspect of the distal humerus exposed. Fenestration must be performed very carefully as the risk of iatrogenic fracture is much greater distally than proximally. It is recommended that the fenestration be performed by initially drilling four screw holes and then joining these with a sharp osteotome. The window must be positioned over the distal intramedullary canal, but slightly to the ulnar side of the diaphysis. In this area the radial side of the distal humerus is broadened by a broad compact flange of bone.

Reaming should be carried out as in the manner described for antegrade nailing. Once the nail has been inserted and locked distally and proximally, the incision can be closed.

Postoperative regimen

Isometric exercises can be started on the first day after surgery and all the joints slowly mobilized.

Table 11.2 **Postoperative regimen for intramedullary nailing of the humerus**

Postoperatively	Treatment	Recommendation
1–2 weeks	Active function	No rotation
3–6 weeks	Free movement	No rotation
6–12 weeks	Dynamization	
6–12 months	Removal of nail	

It is recommended that during the first two postoperative weeks no rotatory movements should be performed. A possible postoperative regimen is given in Table 11.2.

External skeletal fixation

If the surgeon wishes to immobilize a humeral shaft with an external fixation device, it is recommended that the patient be once again placed in a sitting position with the upper part of the body raised by at least 30°. As with humeral nailing, it is important that the patient be placed so that the upper arm extends beyond the operating table, as it is essential that the C-arm reaches all parts of the arm. The forearm rests on a support and initially the C-arm is sited in the vertical plane.

The exact mode of insertion of the external fixation device depends on the device that is chosen. Usually a unilateral frame will be selected and two or three pins must be introduced proximally and distally. It is vital that the surgeon understands the anatomy of the radial nerve when placing the pins. Proximal pin placement should also avoid the long biceps tendon and the circumflex nerve.

The technique of pin placement is the same as for the application of an external fixator to other sites. After skin incision, the tissues are dissected using blunt scissors down to the bone. A tissue protector is inserted and the bone is predrilled. The pins are inserted and the external fixator applied, the fracture being reduced under image intensifier control. Postoperatively, the pin sites are dressed and the subsequent treatment is similar to that for plate osteosynthesis.

References

1. Apley, A.G. and Rowley, D.I. Fixation is fun. *J. Bone Joint Surg.*, **74B**, 486–487 (1992)
2. Hansmann, C. Eine neue Methode der Fixierung der Fragmente bei complicierten Frakturen. *Verl. Dtsch. Ges. Chirg.*, **15**, 134 (1886)
3. Lane, W.A. *The Operative Treatment of Fractures*, Med Publish Co., London (1913)
4. Müller, M.E., Allgöver, M., Schneider, R. and Willenegger, H. *Manual of Internal Fixation*, Springer, New York (1991)
5. Schweiberer, L., Betz, A., Krüger, P. and Wilker, D. Bilanz der konservativen und operativen Knochenbehandlung – obere Extremität. *Chirurg*, **54**, 226 (1982)
6. Böhler, L. Conservative treatment of fresh closed fractures of the shaft of the humerus. *J. Trauma*, **5**, 464–468 (1965)
7. Bandi, W. Indikation und Technik der Osteosynthese am Humerus. *Helv. Chir. Acta*, **31**, 89 (1964)

8. Van der Griend, R.A., Tomasin J., and Ward, E.F. Open reduction and internal fixation of humeral shaft fractures. *J. Bone Joint Surg.*, **68A**, 430

9. Hall, R.F. and Pankovich, A.M. Ender nailing of acute fractures of the humerus. *J. Bone Joint Surg.*, **69A**, 558–567 (1987)

10. Giebel, G., Tscherne H. and Reißmann, K. Die gestörte Frakturheilung am Oberarm. *Unfallchirurg*, **89**, 353–360 (1986)

11. Rommens, P.M. Vansteenkiste, F.P., Stappaerts, K.H. and Broos, P.L.O. Indikationen, Gefahren und Ergebnisse der operativen Behandlung von Oberarmschaftfrakturen. *Unfallchirurg*, **92**, 565–570 (1989)

12. Bleeker, W.A. Nijsten, M.W.N., ten Duis, H.-J. Treatment of humeral shaft fractures related to associated injuries. *Acta Orthop. Scand.*, **62**(2), 148–153 (1991)

13. Rogers, J.F., Bennett, J.B. and Tullos, H.S. Management of concomitant ipsilateral fractures of the humerus and forearm. *J. Bone Joint Surg.*, **66A**, 552–556 (1984)

14. Nast-Kolb, D.C. *Der Oberarmschaftbruch. Ergebnisse einer AO- Sammelstudie.* Hefte zur Unfallheilkunde 222 (eds P. Habermeyer and L. Schweiberer), Springer, Berlin (1992), pp. 62–65

15. Lambotte, A. *Le traitement des fractures*, Masson, Paris (1907)

16. Brooker, A.F. and Edwards, C.C. (ed.) *External Fixation – The Current State of the Art*, Williams and Wilkins, Baltimore (1979)

17. Hoffmann, R. *L'osteotaxis. Osteosynthèse transcutanée par fiches et rotules*, Gead Pub., Paris (1951)

18. Burny, F. Principles of external fixation in the upper extremities. *Eur. Forum Orthop. Sci.*, 103–107 (1985)

19. Burny, F. Hinsenkamp, M. and Donkerwolcke, M. External fixation of the fractures of the humerus. Analysis of 100 cases. *7 émes Journées Internationales: la Fixation Extérne* d'Hoffmann, Montpellier 1980, Diffinco SA Pub., Geneve (1980), pp. 191–202

20. Burny, F., Hinsenkamp, M., Andrianne, Y. *et al.* External fixation of the humerus, a review of 164 cases. Monograph presented at the American Academy of Orthopedic Surgeons, 51st Annual Meeting, Atlanta, 9–14 February (1984)

21. Gustilo, R.B., Mendoza, R.M. and Williams, D.N. Problems in the management of type III (severe) open fractures: a new classification of type III open fractures. *J. Trauma*, **24**, 742 (1984)

22. Kamhin, M., Michaelson, M. and Waisbrod, H. The use of external skeletal fixation in the treatment of fractures of the humeral shaft. *Injury*, **9**, 245 (1978)

23. Rich, N.M., Metz, C.W., Hutton, J.E., Baugh, J.H. and Hughes, C.W. Internal vs external fixation of fractures with concomitant vascular injuries in Vietnam. *J. Trauma*, **11**, 463–673 (1971)

24. De Bastiani, G., Aldegheri, R. and Renzi-Brivio, L. The treatment of fracture with the dynamic axial fixateur. *J. Bone Joint Surg.*, **66B**, 538–545 (1984)

25. Brug, E. Bündelnagelung- nur bei Oberarmfrakturen? *Unfallchirurgie*, **2**, 113–117 (1976)

26. Rush, L.V. and Rush, H.C. Intramedullary fixation of fractures of the humerus by longitudinal pin. *Surgery*, **27**, 268 (1950)

27. Gelbke, H. Die 'dynamische Osteosynthese' nach Rush, eine wertvolle Vervollständigung der Küntscher Nagelung. *Chirurg*, **26**, 529–534 (1955)

28. Stern, P.J., Mattingly, D.A., Pomeroy, D.L. *et al.* Intramedullary fixation of humeral shaft fractures. *J. Bone Joint Surg*, **66A**, 639–646 (1984)

29. Brumback, R., Bosse, M.J. and Poka, A. Intramedullary stabilization of humeral shaft fractures in patients with multiple trauma. *J. Bone Joint Surg.*, **68A**, 960 (1986)

30. Küntscher, G. Intramedullary surgical technique and its place in orthopedic surgery – my present concept. *J. Bone Joint Surg*, **47A**, 808 (1965)

31. Bircher, J.L. Complications following fractures. *Reconstr. Surg. Traumatol.*, **16**, 1 (1978)

32. Böhler, L. *Die Technik der Knochenbruchbehandlung*, Band 1: Oberarmbrüche, Wilhelm Mandrich, Wien, XIII. Auflage (1929), pp. 2638 ff.

33. Böhler, L. *Die Technik der Knochenbruchbehandlung*, Ergänzungsband, Wilhelm Mandrich, Wien (1977), pp. 644 ff.

34. Tscherne, H. Primäre Behandlung der Oberarmfrakturen. *Langenbecks Arch. Chir.*, **332**, 379 (1972)

35. Christensen, N.O. Küntscher intramedullary reaming and nail fixation for non union of the humerus. *Clin. Orthop.*, **116**, 222 (1976)

36. Van der Griend, R.A., Ward, E.F. and Tomasin, J. Closed Küntscher nailing of humeral shaft fractures. *J. Trauma*, **25**, 1166 (1985)

37. Hackethal, K.H. (1961) *Die Bündel-Nagelung*, Springer, Berlin (1961)

38. Baranowski, D. and Brug, E. Aktuelle Indikationen zur Bündelnagelung. *Unfallchirurg.*, **92**, 486–492 (1989)

39. Brug, E.W., Klein, S. and Winckler, S. Fixateur-Externe-Behandlung. In *Die Plattenosteosynthese und ihre Konkurrenzverfahren* (eds D. Wolter and W. Zimmer), Springer Verlag, Berlin (1991), pp. 167–171

40. Durbin, R.A., Gottesmann, M.J. and Saunders, K.C. Hackethal stacked nailing of humerus shaft fractures. Experience with 30 patients. *Clin. Orthop.*, 169–174 (1983)

41. Gallagher, J.E., Keogh, P. and Black, J. Humeral medullary nailing – a new implant. *Injury*, **19**, 254–256 (1988)

42. Seidel, H. Humeral locking nail – a preliminary report. *Orthopedic*, **12**, 129 (1989)

43. Habernek, H. and Orthner, E. A locking nail for fractures of the humerus. *J. Bone Joint Surg.*, **73B**, 651–653 (1991)

44. Robinson, C.M., Bell, D.M., Court-Brown, C.M. and McQueen, M.N.M. Locked nailing of humeral shaft fractures. Experience in Edinburgh over a two-year period. *J. Bone Joint Surg.*, **74B**, 558–562 (1992)

45. Jensen, C.H., Hansen, D. and Jorgensen, U. Humeral shaft fractures treated by interlocking nailing: a preliminary report on 16 patients. *Injury*, **23**, 234–236 (1992)

46. Evans, P.D., Conboy, V.B.L. and Evans, E.J. The Seidel humeral locking nail: an anatomical study of the complications from locking screws. *Injury*, **24**(3), 175–176 (1993)

47. Bauer, R., Kerschbaumer, F. and Poisel, S. *Operative Zugangswege in Orthopädie und Traumatologie*, Georg Thieme, Stuttgart (1986), pp. 237–250

12

Non-operative management and selection of treatment method for humeral diaphyseal fractures

C. Ulrich

Development of non-operative management techniques

Over the years most authors have advocated that uncomplicated humeral shaft fractures are most appropriately managed by non-operative·means[1–23]. As with all non-operatively treated fractures, the surgeon must expect to encounter some cases of malunion. However, in the humerus minor degrees of malunion rarely present a problem because of the ability of the shoulder girdle and upper extremity to compensate for alteration of humeral length as well as rotatory and angular deformities. In addition, simple humeral diaphyseal fractures are distinguished from more complex fractures by the absence of static strain and the presence of normal functioning antagonistic muscle groups[19]. This tends to minimize the incidence of significant malunion.

The history of non-operative management of humeral diaphyseal fractures shows that a multiplicity of different treatment methods have been employed. Historically, no one method of treatment stands out from all the others. Treatment methods employed in the past included the sling and swathe method (Figure 12.1). This is essentially a sling with a component that passes around the body and is not dissimilar from many of the slings in vogue today. In addition, reversed sugar tong splints, thoracobrachial spica casts and plaster Velpeau dressings were also employed. Surgeons also made use of abduction splints or casts and, if the humeral fracture was associated with multiple injuries, lateral or overhead traction was occasionally employed[9]. These treatment methods

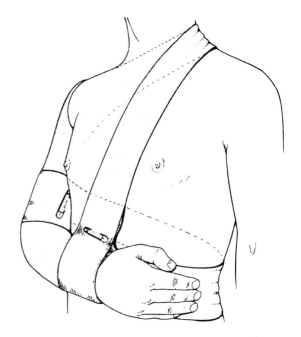

Figure 12.1 The classical sling and swathe method of immobilization. The principle behind this method of immobilization is still in active use today and provides for excellent immobilization of the shoulder and humerus

often immobilized the shoulder and elbow joints for considerable periods and consequently were associated with joint stiffness and impaired function for a prolonged period.

The introduction of the hanging cast by Caldwell[4] and the Rush brothers[18] at approximately the same time marked a turning point in the management of humeral diaphyseal fractures. The principle of the hanging cast is straightforward in that the humeral diaphysis is subjected to continuous traction using gravity. Surgeons found the technique to be particularly useful in the management of shortened angulated mid-diaphyseal fractures. An early example of the hanging cast is shown in Figure 12.2. There is no doubt that although Caldwell devised and used the hanging cast, he recognized the importance of returning the patient to full function through early joint mobilization. He felt that prolonged immobilization decisively weakened the arm musculature and he believed that this was an important factor in the development of humeral pseudarthrosis.

This interest in early function return following humeral shaft fracture was also stimulated by the work of Esmarch and later of Poelchen[16]. They emphasized the importance of maintaining early function through active exercise during the healing period. Poelchen did not use supporting dressings or casts for humeral shaft fractures.

Early results of the management of humeral shaft fractures by hanging casts were published by La Ferte and Nutter in 1941[11]. They analysed the results of 37 cases of humeral shaft fracture which had healed with good or excellent results. As with other early literature, the assessment of outcome is deficient and it is likely that the first patients did encounter a number of problems. These authors certainly documented that a number of patients preferred to sleep in a sitting position to ease the discomfort at the fracture site. Stewart[21] stated that

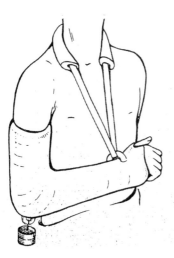

Figure 12.2 A hanging arm cast. Rarely are weights now applied to such a cast, but the general principle of applying a heavy cast to the arm to facilitate reduction is still used extensively

the incidence of pseudarthrosis had fallen since the introduction of a hanging cast. (Interestingly, however, he pointed to the important therapeutic factor being the surgeon's adherence to a standardized protocol in the management of these injuries. It was his view that the excellent vascularity of the humeral shaft should ensure bone union, provided that the surgeons attended to 'minor details' and did not deviate from the correct surgical protocol. He also believed in the maintenance of early joint function and stated that 'the method of treatment which permits consistent active exercise, therefore, is the one most conducive to early and firm union'. Using the hanging cast, Stewart achieved good and excellent results in 93% of his cases compared with 89% using the abduction splint and 71% using the upper arm cast method. He did, however, document 3 cases of pseudarthrosis using the hanging cast, a problem that he did not encounter with the abduction splint[21].

The use of the hanging cast stood the test of time, and Epps and Grant[8] continue to advocate its use for many closed fractures. They state that with attention to detail anterior and posterior bowing and varus and valgus deformity can be corrected. They advocate its use in many closed humeral shaft fractures. Other surgeons point to complications associated with the use of a hanging cast. As already stated, Stewart had encountered some cases of pseudarthrosis. In addition, Charnley[6] and Mast *et al.*[12] also documented a relatively high incidence of pseudarthrosis associated with the use of a hanging cast. Ciernek *et al.*[25] pointed out that many patients also had impaired shoulder mobility as a result of this method of management.

In the 1960s and 1970s there was still considerable debate about the type of non-operative management that should be employed. Bohler[2] analysed the use of non-operative management in 1019 humeral diaphyseal fractures treated under his care since 1946. He had used a number of different treatment methods including the abduction splint, U-shaped plaster splint and Desault cast. He documented only 4 cases of pseudarthrosis which he attributed to excessive fracture distraction. Mast *et al.*[12] analysed the different non-operative methods of management statistically and showed that the overall incidence of pseudarthrosis was 5%. However, they demonstrated no statistical difference between the various treatment methods. They suggested that non-operative treatment produced excellent or satisfactory results in 96% of cases. In 1977, Sarmiento and Latta[19] introduced a

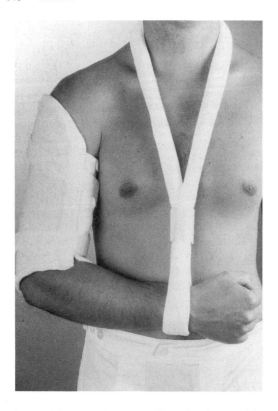

Figure 12.3   A Sarmiento brace, illustrating the use of the collar and cuff and the close fit of the brace sleeve

method of early functional treatment of humeral shaft fractures by means of a standardized plaster splint. They pointed out that the advantages of this method of bracing were maintenance of joint mobility and muscular activity. They observed that not only were minor degrees of non-union not associated with any significant functional deficit, but they were cosmetically insignificant. Humeral shaft shortening was observed in very few cases and was also not of any clinical importance. Rotatory malunions were fairly minor and were compensated for by glenohumeral mobility.

As with previous authors Sarmiento and Latta[19] demonstrated that allowing the arm to hang often permitted the fracture to reduce to an acceptable position due to the effect of gravity and the correcting force of the extensor and flexor muscles. With the introduction of modern bracing techniques, Sarmiento's functional casts gave way to functional braces which were easier for the patient to use. An example of a Sarmiento humeral functional brace is shown in Figure 12.3. There is no doubt that Sarmiento's enthusiastic advocacy of the functional humeral brace has altered the man-

agement of the humeral diaphyseal fractures. Many surgeons now use more restrictive methods of immobilization for a period of only 10–14 days and follow this by the application of a functional brace. Sarmiento's results are very good. He reports that in 85 fractures there was only one pseudarthrosis and that all cases of radial nerve palsy resolved during treatment. He documented some minor skin problems associated with the use of the brace and only one asymptomatic malunion. The average time to union was 10 weeks. One of his cases showed significant functional impairment of the shoulder joint. Others showed minor degrees of impairment which were considered to be of little functional significance.

The use of prefabricated humeral braces was explored further by Zagorski *et al.*[23] They had initially used humeral bracing as described by Sarmiento with primary plaster splintage, followed by secondary use of a humeral brace. However, in 1981, they started to use a functional brace as primary treatment. Initially they used a prefabricated brace over cast padding, the padding being removed approximately 1 week after injury and being substituted by a double layer of cotton stockinet. The patient was instructed in pendulum exercises at 1 week, and active function of the hand, wrist, elbow and shoulder was encouraged. The patient was allowed to remove the brace for hygiene purposes and the use of the brace was continued until there were clinical and radiographic signs of union. Open and closed fractures were treated in the same manner, although the open fractures were admitted for operative exploration, irrigation and debridement. Wounds were left open to heal by secondary intention and bracing was begun at the first change of dressing 2–3 days after injury.

The authors detailed an average time to union of 9.5 weeks for the closed injuries and 13.6 weeks for the open fractures. They found that fractures in the middle third of the humeral diaphysis were the slowest to unite. Ninety per cent of their patients showed no more than 8° of varus or valgus angulation and 85% had no more than 8° of anterior or posterior bowing. Their proximal third diaphyseal fractures showed significantly less residual angulation in all planes than fractures at other levels.

Measurement of shoulder and elbow function showed that 95% of the patients had an excellent functional result, with essentially a full range of motion at the shoulder and elbow. There were few complications. Three patients developed non-union, all being successfully treated. Two patients showed minor skin problems and one patient had a refracture. A further three patients showed significant varus angulation and it is of interest that all three of these patients were obese women whose ipsilateral breast acted as a fulcrum around which the fracture angulated. Camden and Nade[5] also examined the usefulness of humeral fracture bracing and compared this method with U-slab immobilization. Outcome was measured by estimation of union time, incidence of delayed union and non-union and measurement of elbow and shoulder function. They found no significant difference in time to union or in the incidence of delayed union and non-union. They did, however, find differences in joint mobility. They demonstrated elbow extension to be significantly greater in the brace group, although the degree of elbow flexion showed no significant difference and they advocated the use of functional bracing. In a second study, they analysed the results of early application of a functional brace and showed that this was associated with an improved outcome. The conclusions were that early use of a functional brace was a cost-effective, satisfactory method of treating humeral diaphyseal fractures.

Technique of non-operative management

Reduction of humeral shaft fractures is usually straightforward. It is a mistake to strive for immediate closed reduction of a humeral shaft fracture as one is relying on gravity to undertake the reduction. To facilitate reduction, the cast or brace should be applied with the patient in the sitting position and the arm hanging. The elbow should be flexed at 90°. If a plaster is to be applied, care must be taken to adequately pad the cast to minimize the deleterious effects of soft tissue swelling. Surgeons have made much of the different types of casts or splints that can be primarily applied to a humeral diaphyseal fracture. In reality, one is relying on gravity to reduce the fracture and the use of the cast is mainly to stabilize the fracture, thereby reducing discomfort and minimizing the risk of further soft tissue damage.

Different types of casts are popular in different parts of the world. A surgeon may use a temporary well-padded U-plaster splint with plaster applied over the upper arm and around the elbow. The plaster should not be applied over the shoulder as this will prevent the fracture reduction effect of gravity. Some surgeons apply a Desault cast, this being a plaster reinforced body bandage applied around the arm, proximal forearm and body. While this certainly minimizes discomfort it is inconvenient to wear and there is no demonstrable advantage over a lighter temporary plaster support. A number of surgeons[5,23] now recommend the use of primary functional braces. If these are to be used, it should be stressed that adequate soft tissue padding is essential.

The technique of Sarmiento humeral fracture bracing

The surgeon must decide whether or not to use the Sarmiento brace primarily or after a period of cast immobilization. In either case the technique of application is similar, although in the use of secondary bracing the requirement for arm padding under the brace is less and indeed excess padding applied secondarily may effect fracture reduction. Figure 12.4 illustrates the essentials of brace application. It is suggested that the patient be provided with a collar and cuff which is of an appropriate length to allow the arm to hang by the patient's side. This facilitates the reduction of the fracture by gravity. If the collar and cuff is too short the arm will be drawn across the chest and the effect of gravity may be to cause a malunion. The sleeve must be tight fitting, but must not hinder venous return, this resulting in impairment of forearm and wrist function. Ideally the sleeve should be made of plastic and easily adjustable. To this end Velcro fasteners should be used. This type of sleeve is readily adaptable and as the swelling settles in the arm the sleeve can easily be tightened to maintain a close fit. The length of the brace is such that elbow flexion and extension should be possible (Figure 12.4b,c).

As soon as a sleeve is applied, pendulum movements of the shoulder are encouraged to prevent shoulder stiffness. In addition, forearm, wrist and hand activity is recommended. These exercises not only assist with the maintenance of joint mobility but accelerate resolution of arm swelling. With the sleeve applied, the arm should be taken out of the sling several times a day and elbow extension and flexion should be undertaken. Particular importance should be attached to restoring elbow extension, as this may take a considerable time. As soon as the fracture has developed callus, patients will be able to extend and flex their elbow more fully. At this point the sling can be discarded and the physiotherapy regimen for both shoulder and elbow joints accelerated.

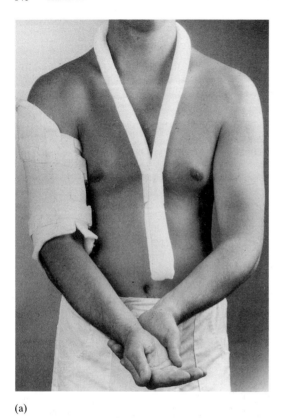

(a)

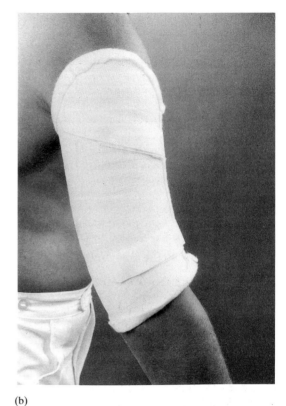

(b)

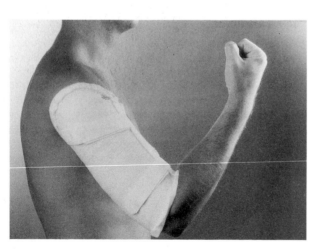

(c)

Figure 12.4 Sarmiento brace application. (a) The length of the collar and cuff is crucial. It must be applied so that the arm is held at about 90°, to facilitate the effect of gravity of fracture reduction. (b) The sleeve should be close fitting and Velcro fasteners should be used to facilitate brace tightening. The shoulder should be free to facilitate movement and elbow extension should be possible. (c) It is also important that the patient retains adequate elbow flexion

As with any treatment regimen there may be complications. The surgeon should be aware of the most common errors associated with non-operative management and take every precaution to avoid them. In the acute situation the most important problem is the avoidance of compartment syndrome secondary to an over-tight circumferential plaster cast. Thus it is recommended that every plaster cast be split down to skin and held with a bandage. Should there be any disturbance of circulation, sensation or joint function distal to the fracture, the patient should be told immediately to consult a doctor.

The surgeon should make certain that the state

of the radial nerve is examined on initial presentation and should remember that reduction of the fracture may cause radial nerve entrapment – the so-called Holstein–Lewis fracture (Figure 12.5). There are obvious legal implications in failing to determine the state of the radial nerve in the conscious patient before any treatment is undertaken. Once a primary cast or splint has been applied, radial nerve function should be re-examined and subsequently it should be examined at intervals over the first 2 weeks of non-operative management. If radial nerve function is normal before the application of a cast and abnormal after the cast is applied, the surgeon should not persevere with non-operative management but should open and fix the fracture with direct exploration of the radial nerve[26].

Fracture distraction is the most common cause of non-union in humeral diaphyseal fractures. This should be carefully looked for after the application of a U-slab or other heavy cast. If fracture distraction is present the cast should be changed. The surgeon should always bear in mind that a deltoid paralysis associated with a proximal third diaphyseal fracture may result in fracture distraction.

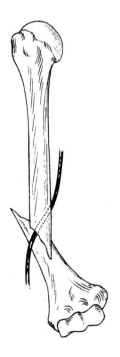

Figure 12.5 The Holstein–Lewis spiral fracture in which there may be radial nerve entrapment

Selection of treatment method

As with the management of all fractures, the surgical treatment of humeral features is frequently guided by fashion and new ideas of fracture management are often adopted for a short period to be replaced by other methods[24]. It is undoubtedly the case that surgeons adopted operative management for humeral shaft fractures in the 1970s and 1980s. However, considered examination of their results frequently led them to return to non-operative management. Operative procedures are undoubtedly associated with a higher incidence of major complications, but as with many fractures there are few prospective studies detailing the functional outcome of humeral shaft fractures after both non-operative and operative treatment. Only after these are done will we be able to say for certain which is the optimal treatment method for different types of humeral shaft fracture.

Bohler was an undoubted proponent of non-operative management of humeral shaft fractures. He attributed the increased incidence of pseudarthrosis, infection and radial nerve damage after humeral shaft fracture to fracture distraction but also, more importantly, to the use of internal fixation. He was of the opinion that humeral fractures were benign and easily treated non-operatively. Just as Sarmiento did at a later date, he stated clearly that minor degrees of angulation displacement and shortening were of no functional or cosmetic importance. This was not true of marked angulatory displacement or rotatory displacement. Mast *et al.*[12], in their retrospective study of 240 humeral shaft fractures, showed that in 100 patients treated non-operatively there were 5 non-unions and 15 delayed unions, whereas in 11 patients treated with primary internal fixation there were 3 non-unions and 2 delayed unions. The authors felt that non-operative functional treatment produced a 96% incidence of excellent or satisfactory results, whereas open reduction and internal fixation was associated with a 60% incidence of excellent or satisfactory results.

Hall *et al.*[27] undertook a meta-analysis of 52 publications dealing with the non-operative and operative methods of treatment of the humeral shaft. They showed that in the series of papers published between 1940 and 1984 involving the non-operative management of 2653 patients, the average incidence of pseudarthrosis was 2.1%. There was a 0.3% incidence of osteomyelitis and a 9% incidence of radial nerve paralysis. In their analysis of 574 operatively managed fractures, the pseudarthrosis rate was 8.3% with a 3.8% incidence of osteomyelitis and a 9.9% incidence of radial nerve lesions. The authors examined the results of both plate osteosynthesis and intramedullary nailing and showed that there was a higher incidence of pseudarthrosis and osteomyelitis after plate osteosynthesis than after intramedullary nailing. It was their conclusion that internal fixation was associated with a higher incidence of complications than non-operative management. The authors did, however, acknowledge that their literature concerning internal fixation was historical and they concluded that traumatologists still face a dilemma in selecting between operative and non-operative management, particularly for complicated humeral fractures.

Nast-Kolb[15] evaluated 302 patients with humeral shaft fractures. Of these patients, 170 had been treated operatively. In a follow-up of 173 patients, the functional results were very similar for both non-operatively and operatively treated fractures. Subjectively, however, 45% of the non-operatively treated patients had no complaints, whereas only 30% of the operatively treated group were complaint free. The most common problems encountered were sensitivity to changes in the weather, pain, generalized weakness and paraesthesia. No non-operatively managed patient complained of radial nerve palsy, but 12% of the patients that were internally fixed had evidence of radial nerve paresis at final follow-up. One of the problems with this study is that a large number of the patients that presented with primary radial nerve palsy were treated operatively. However Nast-Kolb still concluded that the incidence of radial nerve palsy secondary to internal fixation was unacceptably high when compared with the relatively low incidence associated with non-operative management.

It was the author's conclusion that operative intervention showed no significant benefit in terms of bone union. In addition, it was more expensive and associated with an unacceptable risk of postoperative paralysis of the radial nerve. It therefore seems reasonable that surgeons adopt particular indications for humeral diaphyseal fixation rather than adopt an overall policy of fixing all humeral shaft fractures.

It is not uncommon for surgeons who invent new surgical procedures to advocate the use of their techniques for a wide range of indications. They often believe that they have developed a treatment method which will cope with almost any clinical situation and they therefore frequently ignore the use of non-operative management. However, it is up to other users of these methods to perform prospective trials and to formulate protocols for the management of different types of humeral diaphyseal fractures. It is important that all traumatologists be experienced in all different types of management of humeral shaft fractures. The surgeon should be able to choose an appropriate method of management for the type of fracture that is being dealt with and to carry out the treatment method skilfully with knowledge as to how to treat the inevitable problems that will arise.

Unfortunately there is a paucity of information regarding absolute indications for operative management of humeral shaft fractures and their complications. However, examination of the literature suggests that there is some conformity in the views of surgeons as to when operative treatment is indicated.

Pseudarthrosis

There is little dissension from the view that humeral shaft pseudarthrosis should be treated operatively[7,14,19,22,27–36] Bircher[37] stated that there were three major reasons for the development of pseudarthrosis using non-operative management. These were inadequate immobilization, fracture distraction and soft tissue interposition. In addition, there are a number of reasons to explain the formation of a pseudarthrosis after operative treatment. These are inadequate fixation secondary to selection of the wrong implant, the use of an incorrect surgical technique or distraction of the fracture during fixation. In addition, the surgeon may have devitalized the bone peroperatively. This is a particular problem of plating, where extensive periosteal stripping may result in avascularity. If plating is performed in comminuted fractures in which there is already significant periosteal damage, bone avascularity may be a particular problem. Pseudarthroses may also occur if there is a bone defect or infection.

Pseudarthroses following non-operative management are more commonly seen with the use of a hanging cast or U-shaped splint than with a functional brace. Such pseudarthroses are usually hypertrophic and it is recommended that they are treated by an intramedullary procedure which does not cause additional periosteal damage. If an atrophic pseudarthrosis is encountered bone grafting will be essential and it is recommended that the surgeon undertakes rigid fixation by means of plate osteosynthesis. If the pseudarthrosis is infected the basic principles of the management of bone infection should be followed with bone being resected until vascular bone is encountered. Following this there should be adequate surgical stabilization and bone grafting.

Neurovascular injury

Fractures of the humeral shaft which are associated with vascular injuries are extremely rare[13]. However they do occur and if a vascular repair or vein graft is required it is suggested that the bone be fixed rigidly. Whether the humerus is fixed prior to vascular repair or whether the vascular repair is carried out primarily is a choice for the orthopaedic and vascular surgeons. However, the use of a vascular stent prior to plating can preserve the vascularity of the limb.

In contrast, humeral diaphyseal fractures show a high incidence of associated nerve lesions, these usually involving the radial nerve. It has been estimated that the incidence of primary and secondary radial nerve palsies averages 11%[12]. There is little controversy about the requirement for operative exploration in the case of secondary radial nerve palsies, but there is debate about the best method of management for primary paralysis of the radial nerve. Proponents of a non-operative regimen state that 80–90% of radial nerve lesions resolve spontaneously [1-3,38] and surgical exploration does not always lead to satisfactory results[39]. Advocates of surgical exploration point out that the non-operative approach may miss radial nerve entrapment and that some radial nerve lesions do improve following surgery. However, it must be understood that primary internal fixation associated with mobilization of the radial nerve involves the risk of damage to the nerve. The site of the fracture is of some importance, with spiral fractures of the distal zone of the diaphysis having a particular tendency to trap the radial nerve. This is referred to as the Holstein–Lewis lesion (see Figure 12.5)[36]. The most common area for radial nerve involvement is in the middle third of the diaphysis, where up to 30% of fractures may show radial nerve involvement. However in this area the lesion usually takes the form of a neuropraxia and has a good prognosis.

In summary, all humeral diaphyseal fractures associated with significant vascular injury that requires vascular surgery should be treated by internal fixation. If there is a primary radial nerve paralysis the associated fracture can be treated non-operatively unless there is a spiral fracture to the distal third in which operative intervention is advocated. All humeral fractures associated with secondary nerve palsies should be explored and fixed. If the surgeon decides to use an intramedullary nailing technique for a fracture associated with either a primary or secondary radial nerve paresis, the nerve should always be explored prior to reaming or nailing. There is some debate about the optimal time for exploration of a radial nerve which has not regained function after a fracture. The literature suggests that the time for exploration should be between 6 weeks[15] and 12 weeks[2,38].

Pathological fractures

There is little written in the literature regarding the optimal treatment of pathological fractures[40]. There is, however, some agreement that in pathological fractures fixation techniques offer distinct advantages over non-operative management in the provision of pain relief and maintenance of arm function. As illustrated in Chapter 10, dealing with classification and epidemiology of humeral shaft fractures, pathological fractures tend to have an AO type A morphology and can easily be treated by simple nailing techniques. This is a straightforward technique which can be applied in most cases without any significant morbidity. Open procedures with tumour resection are only indicated in the case of the solitary metastasis or for some rare primary tumours.

Open fractures, poly-trauma patients, floating elbow and bilateral humeral shaft fractures

There has been a modern tendency to regard open fractures in all bones as an indication for operative stabilization[34]. Some authors do report good results after local surgical debridement and non-operative management using a functional brace[23]. However, while this technique might be acceptable for Gustilo type 1 fractures, more severe open fractures are better treated by either internal or external fixation techniques.

The advantages of fixation for the poly-trauma patient have been pointed out by a number of authors[34,35,41-45]. Early fixation means that it is rela- There has been a modern tendency to regard open fractures in all bones as an indication for operative stabilization[34]. Some authors do report good results after local surgical debridement and non-operative management using a functional brace[23].

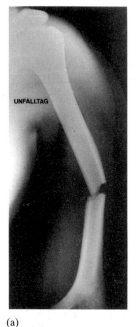
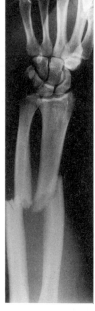
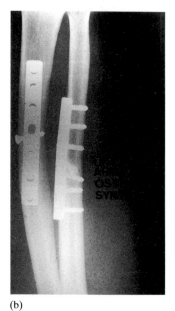
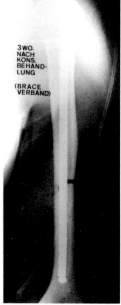

(a)

(b)

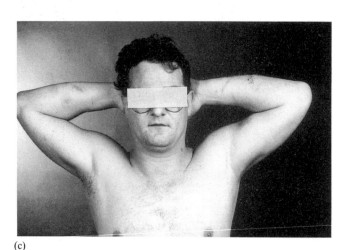

(c)

Figure 12.6   Internal fixation for the floating elbow complication. (a) Floating elbow with an ipsilateral midshaft humeral fracture and fractures of the radius and ulna. (b) The forearm fractures have been treated by internal fixation with AO plates and a Seidel nail has been used to treat the humeral diaphyseal fracture. This fracture was initially treated with a cast brace, but a significant malposition and fracture distraction was encountered and Seidel nail treatment was instituted. (c) Following internal fixation of both the humerus and the forearm the patient regained good function

However, while this technique might be acceptable for Gustilo type 1 fractures, more severe open fractures are better treated by either internal or external fixation techniques.

The advantages of fixation for the poly-trauma patient have been pointed out by a number of authors[34,35,41–45]. Early fixation means that it is relatively easy to nurse the patient and any pulmonary complications that occur following injury can be treated without having to consider the problem of the humeral fracture. Internal fixation is also recommended for both the humerus and forearm if there is a floating elbow problem (Figure 12.6).

It is also recommended that bilateral humeral diaphyseal fractures be treated operatively.

The surgeon should be aware of the advantages and disadvantages of all the treatment options that are available. Non-operative management may be associated with a malunion, pseudarthrosis and some restriction of joint mobility, although it is frequently difficult to correlate the radiographic findings with the subsequent clinical outcome (Figure 12.7). It is a truism that any complications encountered following operative intervention of a fracture may be more severe than those encountered with non-operative intervention, and the sur-

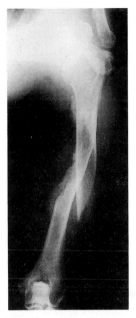
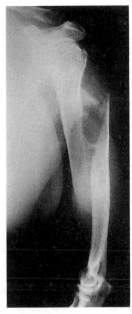

(a)

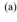

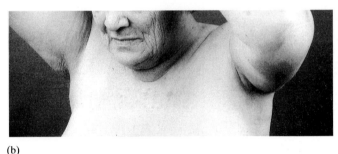

(b)

Figure 12.7 A non-operatively managed midshaft spiral fracture: (a) this has gone on to heal with shortening and a degree of varus angulation; (b) despite the apparent malunion the patient had excellent function

geon who is a proponent of fracture fixation must be aware of what salvage procedures are available should complications arise. Such a problem is illustrated in Figure 12.8.

The primary aim of the surgeon must be to restore function, but in selecting the optimum treatment method the surgeon must take into account not only the fracture morphology and the associated soft tissue injury but also the patient's overall general condition and physical state. When selecting the optimal treatment the surgeon should bear in mind that the non-operative treatment method using a Sarmiento type functional brace is probably the least complicated method and offers the advantage of outpatient treatment. Early functional therapy is relatively straightforward and this method is the treatment of choice for most humeral shaft fractures.

Plate osteosynthesis has the advantage of exact bone fragment reduction as well as permitting inspection of soft tissue damage. However, the incidence of radial nerve damage is higher and any open bony procedure with its associated periosteal stripping increases the incidence of union problems. Although superficially attractive this method of fixation is in fact the most technically challenging for the surgeon. Intramedullary nailing is an easier technique which allows for callus formation, but to date the implants that are available to the surgeon do not confer the same stability as plate osteosynthesis. There is still debate about whether the nailing should be antegrade or retrograde and also whether antegrade nailing causes significant rotator cuff damage. At the moment it can only be recommended in the hands of an experienced trauma surgeon.

External skeletal fixation has a number of potential complications. Its use is essentially restricted

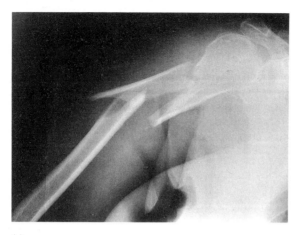

Figure 12.8 A complication of humeral fracture fixation. (a) An AO type B proximal humeral diaphyseal fracture. (b) This fracture has been stabilized with a Seidel nail. (c) Unfortunately the proximal nature of the fracture made nailing very difficult and it is clear that the nail has come out of the proximal humeral fragment. This provides a difficult situation for the surgeon, as any form of subsequent internal and external fixation will be extremely difficult

(a)

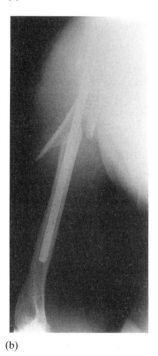

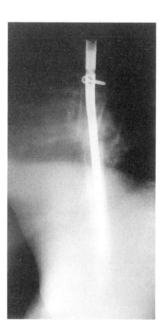

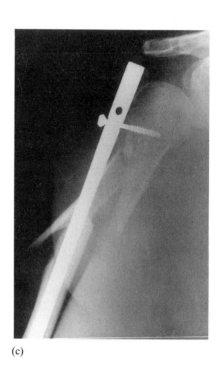

(b)   (c)

to fractures in the middle zone of the diaphysis. Care must be taken in pin placement to avoid damage to the radial nerve. The main indication is probably for open fractures, but as has been demonstrated in Chapter 10, severe open fractures of the humerus are relatively rare and it is unlikely that most traumatologists will have much experience of external fixation of the humerus. One potential use for this technique is in the polytraumatized patient, where the surgeon may wish to stabilize the humerus relatively quickly.

References

1. Böhler, L. *Die Technik der Knochenbruchbehandlung*, Band 1: Oberarmbrüche, Wilhelm Mandrich, Wien, XIII. Auflage (1929), pp. 2638 ff.
2. Böhler, L. Conservative treatment of fresh closed fractures of the shaft of the humerus. *J. Trauma*, **5**, 464–468 (1965)
3. Böhler, L. *Die Technik der Knochenbruchbehandlung*, Ergänzungsband, Wilhelm Mandrich, Wien (1977), pp. 644 ff.
4. Caldwell, J.A. Treatment of fractures of the shaft of the humerus by hanging cast. *Surg. Gynecol. Obstet.*, **70**, 42 (1940)
5. Camden, P. and Nade, S. Fracture bracing the humerus. *Injury*, **23**(4), 245–248 (1992)

6. Charnley, J. *The Closed Treatment of Common Fractures*, E. and S. Livingstone, Edinburgh (1959), p. 51

7. Christensen, S. Humeral shaft fractures: operative and conservative treatment. *Acta Chir. Scand.*, **133**, 455 (1967)

8. Epps, C.H. and Grant, R.E. Fractures of the shaft of the humerus. In *Fractures in Adults* (eds C.A. Rockwood Jr, D.P. Green and R.W. Bucholz), J.B. Lippincott, Philadelphia (1991), pp. 843–869

9. Holm, C.L. Management of humeral shaft fractures. *Clin. Orthop.*, **77**, 132 (1970)

10. Key, J.A. and Conwell, H.E. *Management of Fractures, Dislocations and Sprains*, 6th edn. C.V. Mosby, St. Louis (1956), p. 419

11. La Ferte, A.D. and Nutter, P.D. Treatment of fractures of humerus by means of hanging plaster cast – 'hanging cast.' *Ann. Surg*, **114**, 919 (1941)

12. Mast, J.W., Spiegel, P.G., Harvey, J.P. and Harrison, C. Fractures of the humerus shaft – a retrospective study of 240 adult fractures. *Clin. Orthop.*, **112**, 254 (1975)

13. Muhr, G., Tscherne, H. and Zech, G. Konservative oder operative Behandlung der Oberarmschaftbrüche. *Monatsschr. Unfallheilk*, **76**, 128 (1973)

14. Nast-Kolb, D. Wandel und Fortschritt in der Frakturenbehandlung des Oberarmschaftes. *Orthopäde*, **18**, 208–213 (1989)

15. Nast-Kolb, D.C. *Der Oberarmschaftbruch. Ergebnisse einer AO-Sammelstudie*, Hefte zur Unfallheilkunde 222 (eds P. Habermeyer and L. Schweiberer), Springer, Berlin (1992), pp. 62–65

16. Poelchen, R. Die Selbstinnervationsbehandlung der Fraktur der oberen Extremität. *Monatsschr. Unfallheilk.*, **41**, 176–185 (1934)

17. Rüedi, T., Moshfegh, A., Pfeffer, K.M. and Allgöwer, M. Fresh fractures of the shaft of the humerus – conservative or operative treatment? *Reconstr. Surg Traumat.*, **14**, 65–74 (1974)

18. Rush, L.V. and Rush, H.C. Intramedullary fixation of fractures of the humerus by longitudinal pin. *Surgery*, **27**, 268 (1950)

19. Sarmiento, A. and Latta, L.L. *Closed Functional Treatment of Fractures*, Springer, Berlin (1981), pp. 497 ff.

20. Schweiberer, L., Betz, A., Krüger, P. and Wilker, D. Bilanz der konservativen und operativen Knochenbehandlung – obere Extremität. *Chirurg*, **54**, 226 (1982)

21. Stewart, M.J. and Hundlay, J.M. Fractures of the humerus. A comparative study in methods of treatment. *J. Bone Joint Surg.*, **37A**, 681–692 (1955)

22. Tscherne, H. Primäre Behandlung der Oberarmfrakturen. *Langenbecks Arch. Chir.*, **332**, 379 (1972)

23. Zagorski, J.B., Latta, L.L., Zych, G.A. and Finnieston, A.R. Diaphyseal fractures of the humerus; treatment with prefabricated braces. *J. Bone Joint Surg.*, **70A**, 607–610 (1988)

24. Ward, E.F., Savoie, F.M., Hughes, J.L. Fractures of the diaphyseal humerus. In *Skeletal Trauma* (eds B.D. Browner, J.B. Jupiter, A.M. Levine and P.G. Trafton), W.B. Saunders, Philadelphia (1992), pp. 1177–1200

25. Ciernik, I.F., Meier, L. and Hollinger, A. Humeral mobility after treatment with hanging cast. *J. Trauma*, **31**, 230 (1991)

26. Brumback, R., Bosse, M.J. and Poka, A. Intramedullary stabilization of humeral shaft fractures in patients with multiple trauma. *J. Bone Joint Surg.*, **68A**, 960 (1986)

27. Hall, R.F. and Pankovich, A.M. Ender nailing of acute fractures of the humerus. *J. Bone Joint Surg*, **69A**, 558–567 (1987)

28. Bandi, W. Indikation und Technik der Osteosynthese am Humerus. *Helv. Chir. Acta*, **31**, 89 (1964)

29. Christensen, N.O. Küntscher intramedullary reaming and nail fixation for non union of the humerus. *Clin. Orthop*, **116**, 222 (1976)

30. Durbin, R.A., Gottesmann, M.J. and Saunders, K.C. Hackethal stacked nailing of humerus shaft fractures. Experience with 30 patients. *Clin. Orthop.*, **179**, 169–174 (1983)

31. Van der Griend, R.A., Ward, E.F. and Tomasin, J. Closed Küntscher nailing of humeral shaft fractures. *J. Trauma*, **25**, 1166 (1985)

32. Healy, W.L., White, G.M., Mick, C.A., Brooker, A.F. and Weiland, A.J. Nonunion of the humeral shaft. *Clin. Orthop.*, **219**, 206–214 (1987)

33. Gallagher, J.E., Keogh, P. and Black, J. Humeral medullary nailing – a new implant. *Injury*, **19**, 254–256 (1988)

34. Müller, M.E., Allgöver, M., Schneider, R. and Willenegger, H. *Manual of Internal Fixation*, Springer, New York (1991)

35. Rogers, J.F., Bennett, J.B. and Tullos, H.S. Management of concomitant ipsilateral fractures of the humerus and forearm. *J. Bone Joint Surg.*, **66A**, 552–556 (1984)

36. Holstein, A. and Lewis, G. (1963) Fractures of the humerus with radial nerve paralysis. *J. Bone Joint Surg.*, **45A**, 1382 (1963)

37. Bircher, J.L. Complications following fractures. *Reconstr. Surg. Traumatol.*, **16**, 1 (1978)

38. Pollock, F.H., Drake, D., Bovill, E.G., Day, L. and Tafton, P.G. Treatment of radial neuropathy associated with fractures of the humerus. *J. Bone Joint Surg.*, **63-A**, 239–243 (1981)

39. Böstmann, O., Bakalim, G., Vainionpää, S., Pätiälä, O., and Rokkanen, P. Immediate radial nerve palsy complicating fracture of the shaft of the humerus; when is early exploration justified? *Injury*, **16**, 499–502 (1985)

40. Flemming, J.E. and Beals, R.K. Pathologic fracture of the humerus. *Chir. Orthop.*, **203**, 258–260 (1986)

41. Bell, M.J., Beauchamp, C.G., Kellam, J.K. and McMurtry, R.Y. The results of plating humeral shaft fractures in patients with multiple injuries: the Sunnybrook experience. *J. Bone Joint Surg.*, **67B**, 293–296 (1985)

42. Bleeker, W.A., Nijsten, M.W.N., ten Duis, H.-J. Treatment of humeral shaft fractures related to associated injuries. *Acta Orthop Scand.*, **62**(2), 148–153 (1991)

43. Rommens, P.M., Vansteenkiste, F.P., Stappaerts, K.H. and Broos, P.L.O. Indikationen, Gefahren und Ergebnisse der operativen Behandlung von Oberarmschaftfrakturen. *Unfallchirurg*, **92**, 565–570 (1989)

44. Ulrich, Chr., Burgis, H., Teubner, E. and Muth, W. Der Verriegelungsnagel nach SEIDEL am Humerus – klinische Ergebnisse. *Hefte zu der Unfallchirurg*, **230**, 840–842 (1993)

45. Van der Griend, R.A., Tomasin J. and Ward E.F. Open reduction and internal fixation of humeral shaft fractures. *J. Bone Joint Surg.*, **68A**, 430 (1986)

13

Fractures of the distal third of the humerus

P.M. Rommens

Injuries of the distal part of the humerus can badly influence the normal functioning of the elbow joint, which is indispensable for the activity of the whole upper limb. Injuries vary from simple to complex fractures, dislocations or a combination of those and can be combined with mild to severe soft tissue damage. The prognosis of lesions in the lower part of the humerus not only depends on the localization and complexity of the fracture, but also on the accuracy of the clinical and radiological evaluation, the condition of the patient and not least on the skill and ability of the surgeon. Inappropriate conservative treatment can lead to malalignment or non-union with disastrous functional results. On the other hand, surgery of the elbow joint is also a challenge and demands appropriate preoperative investigations, a thorough knowledge of the topographical anatomy, meticulous care of the soft tissues and an individualized careful after-treatment. Potential complications such as infection, heterotopic ossification, neurological damage or failure of fixation should be kept in mind and must be treated promptly and properly. Nevertheless, anatomical restoration and stable fixation of the fractures can give excellent functional results with little or no disability.

Topographical anatomy

In its distal third, the humeral shaft can be compared with a cylindrical tube, composed of a thick cortical wall and a small endomedullary canal. More distally, this tube flattens out to become a triangular structure with thinner cortical walls. An anteromedial and an anterolateral surface can be distinguished, both separated from the dorsal surface by distinctly pronounced margins: the medial and lateral supracondylar crest. In the metaphyseal region, the flatter humerus widens out into a medial and a lateral triangular column: the medial and lateral condyles. Both these columns form an angle of 40–45° to the frontal plane at the anterior side. They are separated by the olecranon fossa, a single deeper groove on the posterior surface, and by the smaller radial and coronoid fossae on the anterior side. Between the olecranon fossa and the coronoid fossa there is only a thin cortical bone plate. When the fossae are very deep, it may even be non-existent.

Both condyles contain *non-articulating portions* and *articulating surfaces*[1,2]. The non-articulating part of the medial condyle contains the medial epicondyle, situated at the distal end of the medial supracondylar ridge. It is more prominent than the lateral epicondyle and directed distally but not anteriorly. It serves as the origin of the flexor muscles of the forearm. In its posterior and inferior part, the medial epicondyle is smooth as it forms a sulcus for the ulnar nerve. The non-articulating part of the lateral condyle contains the lateral epicondyle, which is smaller than its medial homologue. It is situated at the distal end of the lateral supracondylar ridge, being thinner and sharper than the medial epicondylar crest. The lateral epicondyle, from which the superficial extensor muscles of the forearm originate, is curved in an anterior direction. The articulating surfaces of the medial and lateral condyles are in continuity with each other. The articulating surface of the medial

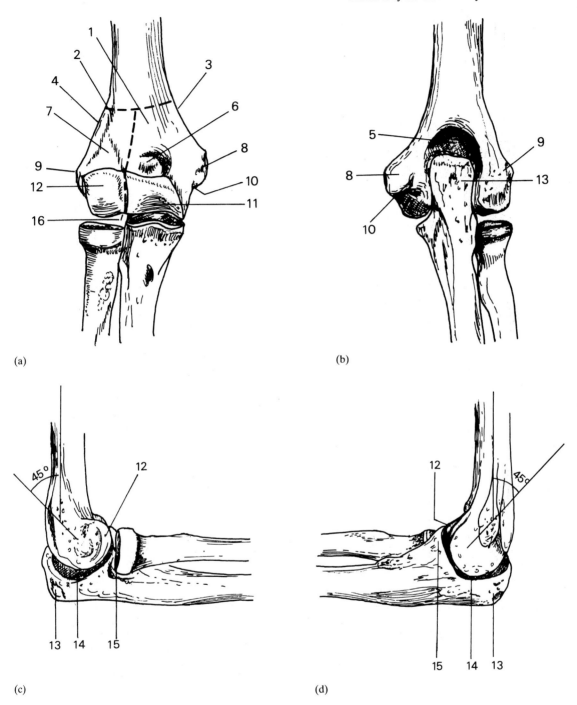

(a)

(b)

(c)

(d)

Figure 13.1 Bones of the elbow joint: (a) right elbow: anterior view in extension; (b) right elbow: posterior view in extension; (c) right elbow: lateral view in 90° flexion; (d) right elbow: medial view in 90° flexion (1, Medial condyle; 2, lateral condyle; 3, medial supracondylar crest; 4, lateral supracondylar crest; 5, olecranon fossa; 6, coronoid fossa; 7, radial fossa; 8, medial epicondyle; 9, lateral epicondyle; 10, sulcus for the ulnar nerve; 11, trochlea; 12, capitulum; 13, olecranon; 14, trochlear notch; 15, coronoid process; 16, capitellotrochlear sulcus)

condyle is called the *trochlea* and has a pulley-like shape. A central groove, situated between and in continuity with the medial and lateral ridge articulates with the trochlear notch of the proximal ulna. The articular surface of the trochlea runs from the coronoid fossa to the olecranon fossa over nearly 300°. The medial ridge is somewhat more prominent than the lateral ridge; in its posterior portion the central groove is directed slightly laterally. Both produce the so-called 'carrying angle' of the elbow, when it is extended. The articulating surface of the lateral condyle is called the *capitulum* or little head. It can only be seen at the anterior side of the distal humerus and has a hemispherical form. It articulates with the proximal concavity of the radial head. On its medial side, the capitulum is in continuity with the lateral ridge of the trochlea. The groove between capitulum and trochlea is called the capitello-trochlear sulcus. It is the transition between the medial and lateral condyle, its articular surface being in permanent contact with the peripheral ridge of the radial head.

Proximal to the capitulum and the trochlea, the radial and coronoid fossae can be recognized. They receive the peripheral ridge of the radial head and the coronoid process of the ulna when the elbow is in flexion. The olecranon fossa receives the tip of the olecranon, when the elbow is extended. The anterior and posterior fossae form bony boundaries for the flexion–extension movement of the elbow joint (Figure 13.1a-d). Occasionally a cortical spur or process can be found at the medial supracondylar crest. It is attached to the medial epicondyle with fibrous tissue, thus forming a channel for the median nerve and/or the brachial artery[3].

Collateral ligaments improve the intrinsic stability of the bony structures of the elbow joint. The medial or ulnar collateral ligament is fan-shaped and originates at the medial epicondyle. It is thicker and stronger than the lateral collateral ligament and consists of three portions. The upper band or anterior portion attaches to the medial part of the coronoid process and the posterior band attaches to the medial side of the olecranon. The oblique band contains transverse fibres, strengthening and connecting the anterior and posterior portions. The lateral or radial collateral ligament is also fan-shaped, but thinner than its medial homologue. Its anterior portion radiates into the annular ligament of the radial head. Its posterior portion attaches to the ulna, proximal to the origin of the annular ligament (Figure 13.2a,b).

The capsule of the elbow joint contains an outer

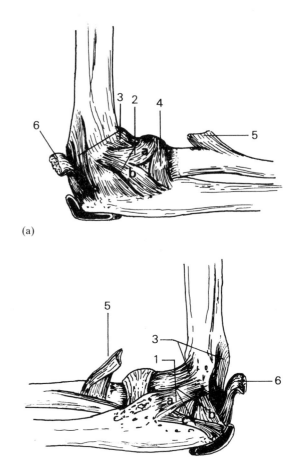

(a)

(b)

Figure 13.2 Ligaments of the elbow joint: (a) right elbow: lateral view in 90° flexion; (b) right elbow: medial view in 90° flexion (1, Medial collateral ligament – **a** anterior portion, **b** posterior portion, **c** oblique band; 2, radial collateral ligament – **a** anterior portion, **b** posterior portion; 3, capsule of the elbow joint; 4, annular ligament; 5, biceps brachii tendon; 6, triceps brachii tendon)

fibrous layer and an inner synovial layer. They have slightly distinct attachments to the distal humerus. The fibrous capsule emerges from the upper part of the floor of the olecranon, coronoid and radial fossae; the synovial layer extends deeper from the floor of these fossae. This means that the upper parts of the different fossae are situated extra-articularly. Distally, both capsular layers attach to the margin of the trochlear notch of the proximal ulna and to the annular ligament around the radial head. There is a sack-like protrusion of the capsule around the radial head, allowing movements in the proximal radio-ulnar joint (Figure 13.3a,b). The anterior side of the cap-

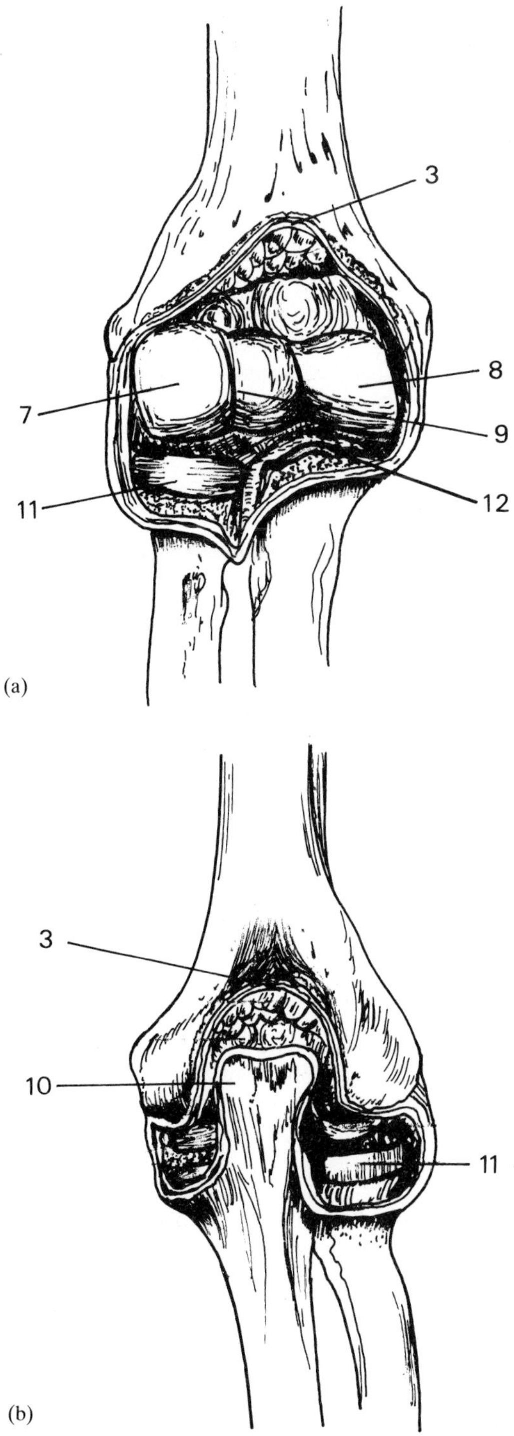

Figure 13.3 The elbow capsule: (a) right elbow: anterior view in extension; (b) right elbow: posterior view in extension (3, capsule of the elbow joint; 7, cartilage of the capitulum; 8, cartilage of the trochlea; 9, capitello-trochlear sulcus; 10, olecranon; 11, cartilage of the radial head; 12, coronoid process)

sule is strengthened by an oblique anterior ligament, the posterior side by a posterior ligament.

Functional anatomy

The elbow joint or cubital articulation has only one synovial cavity, but has functionally two distinct movements and is composed of three different bones, articulating with each other in three different joints. The flexion–extension movement takes place in the humero-ulnar and humero-radial joint, the pro-supination in the proximal radio-ulnar joint. The humero-ulnar connection is the largest articulation in the elbow and has also the greatest intrinsic stability. It is remarkable that both the medial and lateral collateral ligaments attach to the proximal ulna! Together with the medial and lateral ridge of the trochlea, they guarantee the medial and lateral stability of the elbow joint[4]. Furthermore, they can be compared with tension wires, pushing together the trochlea with the trochlear notch[5]. Deformities in the humero-ulnar joint or loosening of one of the collateral ligaments can lead to loss of stability and loss of contact between the articulating surfaces, with a negative influence on the joint mobility.

The centres of rotation of the humero-ulnar and humeroradial joint are the same. They lie on a nearly horizontal line running from medial to lateral through both condyles. This line is not perpendicular to the longitudinal axis of the humeral shaft, but shows an open angle of 10–15° to the medial side. This *carrying angle* is the physiological valgus angulation of the elbow joint and is most obvious when the elbow is extended and the forearm supinated. A malalignment of both condyles after trauma involves the separation into two centres of rotation of the humero-ulnar and humeroradial joints, respectively, which has a disastrous influence on the flexion–extension of the elbow[6].

On the anterior side, both humeral condyles form an angle of 40–45° to the frontal plane. As a result, the centre of rotation of the flexion–extension movement is also situated before this frontal plane. The trochlear notch is directed upward and also forms an angle of 45° to the same frontal plane. This construction promotes extreme flexion of the forearm. The tip of the coronoid process and the peripheral margin of the radial head only reach their respective fossae in extreme flexion; as a result, the interposition of muscle bellied between forearm and arm becomes possible[5]. Malreduction of one or both condyles in a different angle to the humeral shaft will have a negative influence on the flexion–extension range of the elbow.

It was mentioned earlier that the different fossae of the distal humerus form bony boundaries for the flexion–extension of the elbow joint. Changes in the form or depth of these fossae, the presence of fibrous tissue, calcifications or small fracture fragments will hinder free movements and full range of motion.

Definition and classification systems

The distal end of the humerus is separated from the shaft by the top of a square, the sides of which have the same length as the widest part of the epiphysis[7]. Fractures within this skeletal part can vary from simple, undisplaced epicondylar lesions to complex, displaced supracondylar and intracondylar fractures. They can involve one single humeral condyle, the articular surface or be totally extra-articular. They only account for a few per cent of all skeletal fractures in adults and the great majority of them are intra-articular. The fractures are equally distributed between males and females, though males form the younger patient population, while females more often appear among the older patient group.

Several authors have proposed a classification system for all or some of the spectrum of distal humerus fractures. Horne[8] classified all lesions into three groups without further differentiation. The first group contains 'simple condylar' fractures. These fractures run through the medial or lateral condyle, involving the articular surface of the trochlea or capitulum. The second group contains all 'extra-articular' fractures in the supra-

condylar region. The fractures can be transverse, oblique, spiroid or even comminuted. The third group includes all 'T' or 'Y' distal humeral fractures. These fractures consist of a vertical fracture component running through the articular surface and two diverging fracture lines, running horizontally (T-fracture) or oblique and proximally (Y-fracture), separating the two condyles from each other and from the humeral shaft. The advantage of the Horne classification is that it makes a distinction between extra-articular, partial articular and complete articular fractures as does the AO classification system. Major disadvantages are that epicondylar fractures and fractures of the capitulum are not included and that the three groups are not divided into simple fractures and comminuted types which have a totally different treatment regimen and prognosis.

Riseborough and Radin[9] divided the intra-articular fractures into four types (Figure 13.4). They distinguish undisplaced fractures (type I), fractures with displaced but not rotated condyles (type II), fractures with displaced and rotated condyles (type III) and fractures with significant intracondylar comminution (type IV). This classification system is well known in North America. It is, however, incomplete as extra-articular and unicondylar fractures are not considered. A further disadvantage is that a clear distinction between bicondylar fractures with or without rotation cannot always be made. For that reason, the Orthopaedic Trauma Association[10,11] slightly modified the Riseborough and Radin classification and brought type II and type III fractures together in one group. But a distinction between fractures with extra-articular or intra-articular comminution is not made in both systems. The Orthopaedic Trauma Association also classified the unicondylar fractures in seven subgroups (Figure 13.5). Frac-

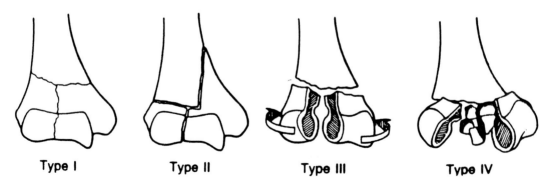

Type I   Type II   Type III   Type IV

Figure 13.4   Riseborough and Radin classification of bicondylar distal humeral fractures. (After Riseborough and Radin[9])

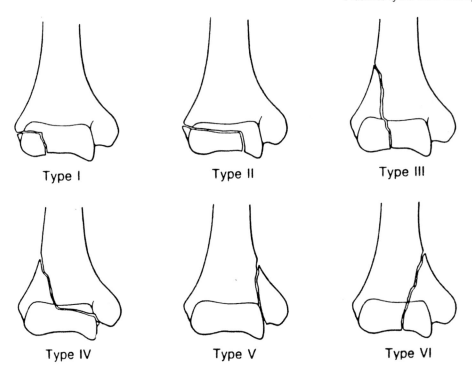

Figure 13.5 The Orthopedic Trauma Association classification of unicondylar intra-articular fractures. (After National Orthopaedic Trauma Registry[11]). The six basic fracture styles are shown. The seventh type represents combined fractures

tures of the capitulum are considered as the first type, fractures of the capitulum with a part of the trochlea as the second type, lateral condylar fractures as the third type, latero-medial fractures as the fourth, extra-articular medial condylar fractures as the fifth, intra-articular medial condylar fractures as the sixth and combined fractures as the seventh type. This classification of condylar fractures seems comprehensive, but it does combine complete extra-articular, complete intra-articular and partial intra-articular fractures with different prognoses into one subgroup.

The most recent and most complete classification system is that of the AO group[12] (Figure 13.6). The system divides the fractures into three main groups: The A group contains extra-articular fractures, the first subgroup epicondylar, the second subgroup simple and the third subgroup complex supracondylar fractures. The B group comprises vertical fracture types, the first subgroup lateral condylar, the second subgroup medial condylar and the third subgroup capitellar shear fractures. The C group contains bicondylar T- or Y-fractures, the first subgroup with a simple condylar and a supracondylar fracture pattern, the second sub-

group with a simple condylar and a comminuted supracondylar and the third subgroup with a complex condylar and supracondylar fracture pattern. Each subgroup is further subdivided into three subgroups. This classification system is both comprehensible, thorough, difficult and complex. Nevertheless it allows each fracture pattern to be designated and enables complete documentation and scientific comparison among different patient populations. Schatzker and Tile[13] do not completely agree with the AO classification, because it combines fracture patterns with different treatment problems and prognoses in one group, such as the A1 fractures with the A2 and A3 or the B3 fracture together with the B1 and B2. They only distinguish simple lesions such as epicondylar and condylar fractures and complex supracondylar and intracondylar lesions.

Treatment alternatives

Numerous techniques, varying from closed reduction or skeletal traction, to limited open reduction and open reduction with rigid internal fixation

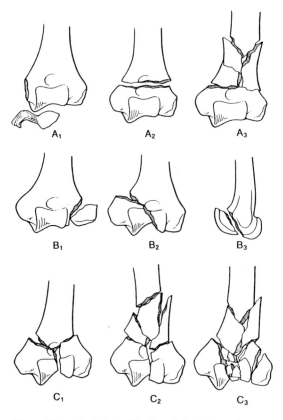

Figure 13.6   The AO classification of distal humeral fractures. (After Müller *et al.*[12])

were advocated during the past decades. The defenders of conservative treatment felt that operative dissection and internal fixation resulted in a high complication rate and that the functional end results were quite unsatisfactory[8,14,15]. It must be admitted that the early materials used for fracture fixation were not always adequate. Many fractures were not anatomically reduced or sufficiently stabilized and needed postoperative plaster cast immobilization, leading to irreversible joint stiffness. In the past, inappropriate surgery has led to worse functional results than inappropriate reduction by conservative means. The advocates of operative treatment clearly stated that anatomical reduction cannot be obtained without surgical intervention[16–23]. Malalignment and malunion lead to stiffness, osteoarthritis and pain. Closed reduction is always followed by plaster cast immobilization of at least 6–8 weeks, with an irreversible limitation of elbow mobility. Neither skeletal traction or limited open reduction were considered as optimal treatment alternatives. Although the posi-

tion of displaced fracture fragments may improve, an anatomical restoration of the articular surface is seldom obtained. Limited open reduction never gives adequate stability, and necessitates immobilization, so that the disadvantages of closed and open methods are combined. An anatomical reduction and stable fixation of the fracture fragments can only be obtained by surgery. With the implants and techniques recommended by the AO group[22], it was possible to obtain these therapeutic objectives. Stable fixation makes postoperative immobilization superfluous, so that active motion of the elbow can be started.

The author strongly advocates the principles of anatomical reduction, stable fixation and early active motion recommended by the AO group and is convinced that only these treatment methods can lead to optimal functional recovery of the sometimes very complicated lesions of the distal humerus. The different AO implants, approaches and operative techniques in relation to the different fracture types are discussed below. Other treatment modalities are included, if appropriate.

Extra-articular lesions (type A)

Fractures of the epicondyles (type A1)

The extensor muscles of the forearm originate from the lateral epicondyle and the superficial flexor muscles from the medial epicondyle. Epicondylar fractures mostly occur as a result of an avulsion, less frequently from direct trauma. Lateral epicondylar fractures are rare lesions, medial fractures being much more common. The latter fracture is often combined with an elbow dislocation. The fracture fragment may vary in size and displacement. If the fragment is undisplaced or in an anatomical position after reduction of the elbow dislocation, it can be treated by conservative means[15]. Plaster cast immobilization for 4–6 weeks with the elbow in 90° flexion is advised. If the fracture fragment is displaced or entrapped in the joint, an open reduction and fixation should be performed[22,24,25]. The approach is lateral or medial. In the case of a medial incision, the ulnar nerve should be identified and protected before manipulation of the fracture fragment is started. The fragment is fixed with a 4.0 mm cancellous screw or a 3.5 mm cortical screw (Figures 13.7a,b). In the case of comminution of the avulsed fragment, fixation with sutures or a cancellous screw with a soft tissue washer is possible. The ulnar nerve is replaced at the end of the opera-

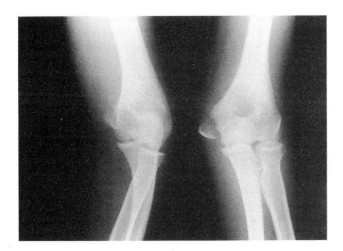

Figure 13.7(a) Avulsion fracture of the medial epicondyle

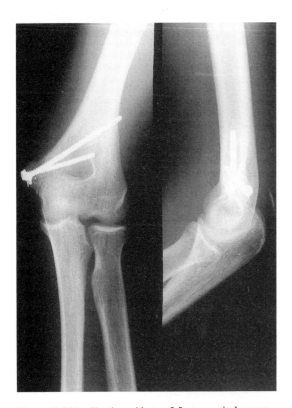

Figure 13.7(b) Fixation with two 3.5 mm cortical screws

tion. If fracture fragments or implants disturb its anatomical position, it can be transposed anteriorly.

Supracondylar fractures (types A2 and A3)

Supracondylar fractures are typical childhood lesions. In adults, they occur less commonly than epicondylar, unicondylar or intracondylar fracture types. The fracture pattern may be transverse, oblique (type A2) or comminuted (type A3). Kocher originally subdivided the transverse fractures into extension-type injuries (dorsal displacement of the epiphyseal part) and flexion-type injuries (ventral displacement of the epiphyseal part)[26]. The fractures are caused by a fall on the outstretched hand, less commonly by direct trauma. The clinical examination reveals an angulation just above the elbow joint and a shortening of the arm by proximal displacement of the distal fragment. In the extension-type injury, the force of the triceps muscle on the olecranon displaces the distal fragment in a proximal direction; in the flexion-type injury the same is done by the biceps and brachialis muscles. The bicondylar distance does not change because the medial and lateral condyles are not separated from each other. On X-ray examination, the fracture line runs through the fossae just above the articular capsule. Oblique and comminuted fractures may extend more proximally into the shaft. In the case of a transverse fracture, the lateral X-ray reveals an oblique fracture line: it runs from anterior distally to posterior proximally in the extension-type injuries, whereas it runs in the opposite direction in the flexion-type injuries. The sharp end of the proximal fragment may damage surrounding soft tissues such as the triceps, the biceps or even the brachial artery or median nerve. The elbow is always markedly swollen and a compartment syndrome should be excluded! A thorough neurovascular examination is always necessary.

Supracondylar fractures are very unstable and are difficult to maintain after closed reduction. The

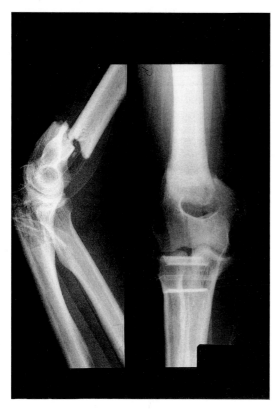

Figure 13.8(a)   Supracondylar fracture

reason for this instability is well known: the biceps and triceps muscles tend to displace the fragment proximally, while the flexor and extensor muscles of the forearm tend to rotate the condyles. This can lead to partial loss of the condylar angulation, resulting in decreased flexion or extension after consolidation, to a varus or valgus deformity in the elbow or to non-union. Overhead or side-arm olecranon pin traction has been advocated in the past[27,28], but is very uncomfortable for the patient. It should be maintained for 4–6 weeks and the patient must remain in the hospital during the whole period. Skeletal traction allows early and limited active motion, but has generally been replaced by stable internal fixation. Closed or limited open reduction and Kirschner wire fixation[29] is a well-known treatment for supracondylar fractures in children, but it does not provide sufficient stability to allow after-treatment with early active motion without plaster cast immobilization. Moreover, the percutaneous technique is very risky for the ulnar nerve on the medial side. This technique is not recommended for supracondylar fractures in adults.

The most appropriate technique for the stabilization of supracondylar fractures is open reduction and internal fixation. To obtain sufficient stability, two plates should be implanted. To obtain stable fixation, screws alone are not sufficient. Small fragment dynamic compression plates

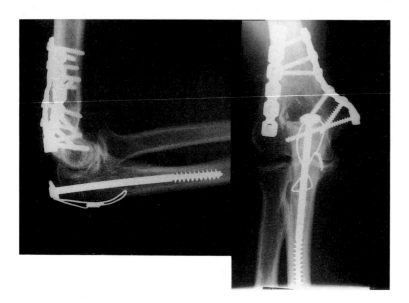

Figure 13.8(b)   Internal fixation with two small fragment reconstruction plates. The plate on the medial column is placed along the epicondyle; on the lateral column the plate is placed dorsally. The supracondylar fracture was approached through an osteotomized olecranon. The olecranon is repaired with a 6.0 mm cancellous screw and a cerclage wire

(DCP), small fragment low contact dynamic compression plates (LC-DCP), small fragment reconstruction plates, semitubular or one-third tubular plates can be used. One plate is placed on the medial column and one on the lateral column (Figures 13.8a, b). The anatomy of the distal humerus does not allow careless positioning of the implants. On the medial side, the plate can be placed along the broad epicondyle. On the lateral side, where the epicondyle is too small and sharp, the plate should be placed along the dorsal surface of the condyle, which is free of cartilage. It can also be placed at the lateral supracondylar crest and lateral epicondyle. The screws should neither perforate the articular surface of trochlea and capitulum nor pass through the fossa. On the medial side, care should also be taken not to damage the ulnar nerve, which passes the medial epicondyle dorsally and inferiorly. If the fracture runs more proximally, the plate can be placed on the dorsal side of the humerus.

The most suitable approach for this procedure is a dorsal one. Therefore, the patient is positioned in a lateral decubitus position or prone with the upper arm in horizontal position, the elbow flexed and a free-hanging forearm (Figures 13.9a, b). A rolled-up sheet is placed under the arm and elbow. The free forearm can be manipulated by an assistant for reduction. Before starting the operation, a tourniquet is placed as far proximally as possible around the upper arm. It reduces intraoperative blood loss and facilitates the surgical exposure. The incision starts in the distal part of the humeral shaft at the centre of the arm and runs in an S-shaped curve to the proximal part of the ulnar shaft, some 10 cm distally to the olecranon. Using an S-shaped incision, one can avoid a painful scar at the tip of the olecranon. The incision can run medially or laterally to the olecranon. The author prefers the medial way, because the ulnar nerve should always be exposed before reducing and stabilizing distal humeral fractures and because this part of the scar is well covered when the arm is hanging down[13,30].

To expose the olecranon fossa and the supracondylar region, the triceps muscle can be divided in its distal part or the olecranon can be osteotomized. The approach through the olecranon is preferable for the exposure of the trochlea and capitulum and will be discussed together with the management of intra-articular fractures. When the approach through the triceps is chosen, the aponeurosis of the triceps muscle is isolated from the muscle fibres by a V-shaped incision with its top

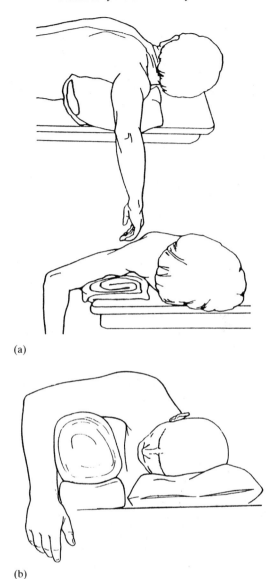

(a)

(b)

Figure 13.9 Stabilization of supracondylar fractures by the open reduction and internal fixation technique: (a) prone position; (b) lateral position – the upper arm lies horizontally, the elbow is flexed at 90° and the forearm hangs down free

proximal and its base on the olecranon; the underlying fibres are split longitudinally and retracted medially and laterally. All fragments of comminuted fractures which are recognized on the X-rays should be carefully identified and the main fracture line exposed from medial to lateral. It is very important to handle the soft tissue attachments of all larger and smaller fragments carefully, to avoid sequestration, which can lead to bone-healing disturbances or even infection. Larger fracture fragments in the supracondylar region should be fixed to the humeral shaft with isolated lag screws. They achieve interfragmentary compression, enhance stability and facilitate reduction and fixation of the main fracture. The main fracture can temporarily be fixed with two crossed Kirschner wires, inserted from the epicondyles in a proximal direction. The main fracture should then be fixed under interfragmentary compression with small fragment plates. The implants must, of course, be curved so that they fit perfectly to the bony structures to which they belong[22,31].

After definitive fixation, the elbow joint must be carefully examined in the anteroposterior and lateral direction under the image intensifier in order to control the correct position of plates and screws. In case there should be any doubt, intraoperative X-rays should be taken. Before wound closure, the elbow joint should also be mobilized from full extension to full flexion and from pronation to supination to ensure the free mobility of the operated joint.

Partial articular lesions (type B)

Unicondylar fractures (types B1 and B2)

Schatzker and Tile[13] classify these fractures as simple because of their straightforward treatment and good prognosis. In adults, they are less common than bicondylar lesions. While medial epicondylar fractures are more common than lateral epicondylar fractures, lesions of the lateral condyle occur more frequently than those of the medial condyle. The great majority of them are intra-articular lesions, although extra-articular lesions are theoretically possible. The Orthopaedic Trauma Association subdivided the unicondylar lesions into seven types, of which only one was extra-articular[10,11]. Milch subdivided condylar fractures into a medial and lateral group with a type I and a type II in each group. In his opinion, the lateral trochlear ridge is the keystone for the medio-lateral stability of the elbow joint[4]. When the lateral trochlear ridge is a part of the fractured condyle (type II in each group), the medio-lateral stability is no longer guaranteed and dislocation may occur.

With regard to bicondylar fractures, the mechanism of injury is a fall on the outstretched hand. In addition to the indirect forces applied to the elbow through the radius and ulna, abduction and adduction forces also exist. Direct force to the

elbow is less common. The most obvious clinical signs are swelling and tenderness in the region of the fractured condyle. The contralateral side of the joint may also be swollen and painful, when its collateral ligament is torn or ruptured. Instability and crepitus may occur, but should not be looked for. Loss of motion is always present. In medial condylar fractures, the ulnar nerve may be damaged. A neurovascular examination must always be done!

On X-ray examination, the fracture line usually runs from the articular surface in an oblique and proximal direction to the supracondylar crest. In general, the fractured fragment is rotated in the frontal and/or sagittal plane, due to the traction of the forearm muscles. Subluxation or dislocation of the radius and ulna may be present.

Nearly all condylar fractures will need open reduction and fixation, because the displaced fracture needs perfect reduction for the anatomical reconstruction of the articular surface[32]. Only undisplaced or minimally displaced fractures can be treated conservatively with a plaster cast. Immobilization is necessary for 4–6 weeks[4]. If open reduction and internal fixation is carried out, a medial or lateral approach is recommended. In the case of a very large or comminuted condylar fragment, a dorsal approach with or without olecranon osteotomy is preferable. For all approaches, the patient is best positioned supine or in a lateral decubitus position. Before manipulation of the medial condyle, the ulnar nerve must be isolated and protected. As many soft tissue attachments as possible must be preserved to maintain the vascularity of the fractured condyle while reducing the fragment. After reduction, the surgeon must control the anatomical reconstruction of the articular surface through the arthrotomy. Flake fractures or articular damage of the radial head, capitulum, trochlea or trochlear notch should be detected. Kirschner wires can be used for provisional stabilization of the reduced fragment. Small fragment 4.0 cancellous screws or 3.5 cortical bone lag screws are used to provide definitive fixation (Figures 13.10a, b). One screw runs through the condyles and the other runs proximally in the direction of the opposite supracondylar crest. It may not cross the olecranon fossa. Additionally, a small fragment buttress plate can be placed on the medial or lateral supracondylar crest to prevent minimal displacement of the fragment (Figures 13.11a, b and 12a, b)[22,31]. Although they may sometimes be used, Kirschner wires are not a good alternative to small fragment screws for

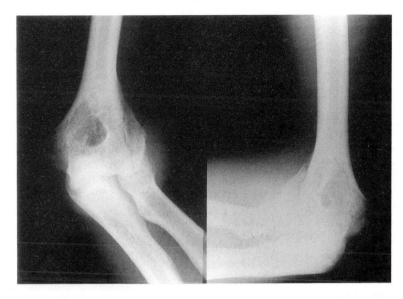

Figure 13.10(a)　Lateral condylar fracture

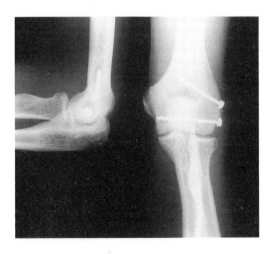

Figure 13.10(b)　Reduction and fixation with two 4.0 cancellous screws with washer

fracture fixation. They do not provide the necessary fracture stability to allow early postoperative motion. We do not recommend them for the fixation of condylar elbow fractures in adults. After fixation, the elbow joint must be washed out to evacuate small intra-articular fracture fragments, which can interfere with normal elbow motion. Before closing the arthrotomy, the correct position of the implants must be controlled under the image intensifier in both directions. Finally, the normal mobility and stability of the elbow joint are verified. If instability remains, due to rupture of the contralateral collateral ligament, an operative

repair may be considered. This issue will be discussed further in relation to elbow dislocations.

Fractures of the capitulum or trochlea (type B3)

These fractures run in the frontal or coronal plane, parallel to the anterior side of the humerus. The fracture fragment consists of articular cartilage of the capitulum and/or trochlea and of a varying amount of subchondral bone. As it has no soft tissue attachments, the fracture fragment lies free in the elbow joint. The fracture is caused by indirect compressive and shearing forces applied

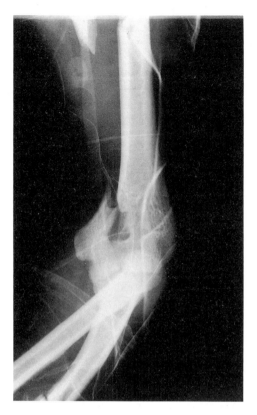

Figure 13.11(a) Medial condylar fracture in a patient with an open type II humeral shaft fracture and a closed ulnar fracture

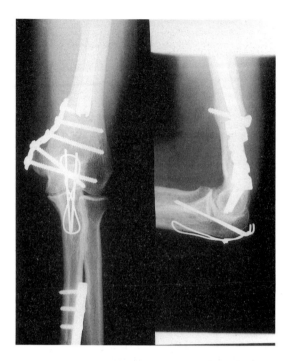

Figure 13.11(b) Retrograde nailing of the humeral shaft. Open reduction and fixation of the medial condyle through an olecranon osteotomy. Plate and screw fixation of the ulnar shaft

through the radial head on the flexed elbow. It may also be caused by a direct blow to the fully flexed elbow[33,34]. These fractures are rare, accounting for less than 1% of all elbow lesions. On clinical examination, there is little swelling, because the haematoma is held by the articular capsule. There is no joint instability. But there is significant pain, sometimes bone crepitus and always severely limited motion or locking of the elbow joint.

In older literature these lesions are divided into two types. The first or Hahn–Steinthal type[35,36] involves the capitulum with a varying portion of the articular cartilage of the trochlea and a large amount of subchondral bone. The second or Kocher–Lorenz type[35,37] mainly contains articular cartilage of the capitulum with very little subchondral bone. The AO classification subdivides the type B3 lesions into lesions of the capitulum, lesions of the trochlea and lesions of the capitulum and trochlea[12].

On X-ray examination it is seen that the free fracture fragment is almost always displaced. It lies anteriorly within the radial fossa and sometimes can be dislocated posteriorly. X-rays can be misleading in underestimating the real size of the fragment, because a big part consists of cartilage. On the antero-posterior view, the normal contour of the distal humerus can give a false impression to the inattentive observer that there is no bony lesion. The displaced fragment can best be seen on the lateral X-rays, but the involvement of the trochlea is more easily discovered on the AP view. Bony lesions of the radial head should be excluded.

Only undisplaced fractures can be treated conservatively with a posterior splint for at least 3 weeks. Even in those cases, a secondary displacement can be expected in some patients, because of the upward directed force of the radial head. All displaced fractures must be treated operatively. For open reduction, a posterior approach with olecranon osteotomy is recommended[13,22]. The osteotomy gives a good view of the inferior part of the humeral epiphysis. The free fragment is then identified. It can mostly be found in the radial fossa, from where it can be dislodged with the elbow in full flexion and under varus stress. Occasionally, it will appear on the dorsal side when retracting

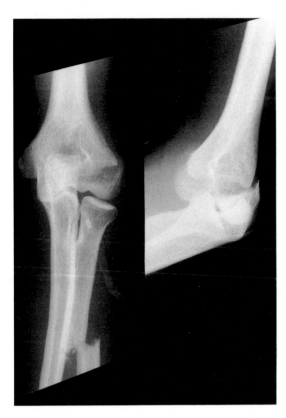

Figure 13.12(a) Lateral condylar fracture running to the trochlea

the olecranon proximally after osteotomy. It is cleaned carefully and the amount of subchondral bone is appreciated. If there is only a flake of cartilage with a minimal piece of bone, the chances of this fracture of being stabilized safely is minimal and the piece should be removed. If the fracture fragment is larger, it should be reduced anatomically. It can be difficult to hold the fragment correctly in place, because it always tends to migrate proximally. The fragment can be held with a small forceps or with a hook and fixed temporarily with a Kirschner wire. After meticulous control of its position, the fragment should be fixed with 4.0 small fragment cancellous screws or with mini-fragment screws inserted from posterior to anterior without perforating the anterior cartilage. When a fracture of the trochlea is reduced, the screws must be drilled through the articular cartilage. The screw heads must be countersunk in order to provide undisturbed mobility. Sufficient stability can only be obtained when more than one screw is inserted. The stability of the fixation should be carefully checked in mobilizing the elbow joint under direct view of the fracture.

Complete articular lesions (types C1–C3)

Although they only account for 1% of all skeletal lesions, these fractures represent the great majority

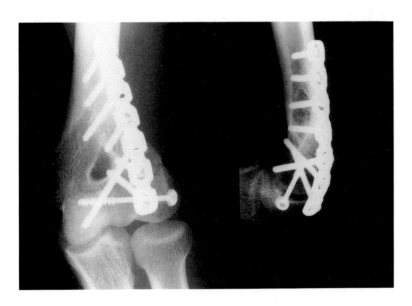

Figure 13.12(b) Reduction and fixation with small fragment reconstruction plate and one cancellous screw

of all distal humerus fractures in adults. They are the most difficult fractures of the distal humerus to treat. For this reason, Schatzker and Tile[13] designed them as 'complex fractures' together with supracondylar extra-articular fractures. They are also called T- or Y-shaped fractures, because of the intercondylar and supracondylar fracture pattern. Riseborough and Radin[9] and the Orthopaedic Trauma Association[10,11] subdivide these lesions depending on the displacement and comminution of the fracture fragments; the AO classification makes a distinction between simple lesions without comminution (type C1), lesions with supracondylar comminution (type C2) and lesions with supra- and intracondylar comminution (type C3).

These fractures are caused by a high energy force directed against the condyles of the elbow. This force is conducted through the proximal ulna, its trochlear notch or coronoid process acting as a wedge to split the condyles. This can occur with the elbow in extension or in flexion. The forces can be indirect, as in the case of a fall on the outstretched hand, or direct, as in motor vehicle injuries[38]. Due to the high energy forces and the displacement of the fracture fragments, these complete articular lesions are often associated with severe soft tissue damage. This can influence the primary management of the injury. Not only the trauma-related forces, but also the muscles of the upper arm and forearm help to displace the fragments. The biceps and triceps tend to pull the proximal ulna proximally, while the flexor and extensor muscles tend to rotate the condyles.

Clinical examination reveals significant swelling of the elbow and major instability in all directions. The distance between both condyles is larger than on the opposite side and their normal relation to the tip of the olecranon disappears. A meticulous neurovascular examination of the arm should be done: compartment syndrome, lesion of the brachial artery and neurological damage to the ulnar, radial or even median nerve are not exceptional[21,30,39].

Antero-posterior and lateral views of the elbow joint will always reveal the distal humeral fracture. It may however be difficult to interpret the pictures so that the origin of all fracture fragments can be understood. If it is impossible to obtain an AP X-ray of good quality because the patient is unable to bring the joint in extension, a second X-ray can be obtained in the operation theatre with the patient under anaesthesia and with light longitudinal traction on the arm[13,38].

As mentioned before, several treatment modalities have been proposed in the literature. They range from the 'bag of bones' technique, include closed reduction and plaster cast immobilization, skeletal traction, Kirschner wiring, open reduction and internal fixation. The closed techniques have the major disadvantage that an anatomical reduction of the fracture fragments can almost never be obtained and can never be maintained. Moreover immobilization is usually required, leading to malalignment, joint stiffness and pain. The same can be said for skeletal traction, although active motion can be started earlier. Kirschner wiring does not provide stable fixation and therefore immobilization is needed after operation. This also leads to unsatisfactory functional results. In the past decades there has been growing enthusiasm for open reduction and internal fixation of these difficult lesions. Many authors are convinced that only anatomical reconstruction of the elbow joint together with stable internal fixation and early active motion can lead to excellent functional results[13,16–23,30,31].

The operative procedure must be planned by the surgeon. Making a drawing of the fractured distal humerus is recommended[30]. To do so, an outline of the reversed AP X-ray of the opposite, non-traumatized distal humerus is made. On this drawing, all main fracture fragments are placed in their anatomical position and the implants, necessary to ensure stable fixation, are added.

The patient must be positioned in a lateral or prone position with an abducted shoulder joint, the upper arm lying on a radiolucent side-table, a flexed elbow joint and a free-hanging forearm (see Figures 13.9a, b). A tourniquet is placed as far proximal as possible. The optimal approach is a dorsal one. The incision is the same as for the supracondylar fractures: it is S-shaped with medial or lateral deviation around the tip of the olecranon. In the author's view, an olecranon osteotomy is always necessary as it provides excellent exposure of the dorsal and inferior surfaces of trochlea and of the inferior surface of the capitulum. Several types of osteotomy can be performed. The extra-articular osteotomy (distal to the trochlear notch) has the advantage that the whole trochlear notch remains intact and can be used as a template for the reconstruction of the condyles. The intra-articular osteotomy gives a better exposure of the distal humerus with its articular surfaces. It can be transverse or V-shaped. In the author's experience, it is easier a obtain a precise anatomical reduction of the olecranon after a V-shaped osteotomy. The rotational stability of the olecranon fixation is also higher with a V-shaped osteotomy than with a transverse osteotomy. A high-speed oscillating saw is used to cut the cortex and underlying bone opposite the trochlear notch. The articular cartilage and subchondral bone are finally divided with an osteotome. This 'manual osteotomy' causes little indentations in the cartilage, which makes a perfect reduction easier. Before the osteotomy, the ulnar nerve must be identified and protected. Predrilling and tapping of the proximal ulna makes the fixation of the olecranon easier[13,31,40].

The reconstruction of the distal humerus is carried out in different steps. As with all other intra-articular fractures, the articular surface must be reconstructed first. In manipulating the condyles, as many soft tissue attachments as possible should be preserved, to secure the vascularity of the bone fragments. The smaller fracture fragments should be handled very carefully, so that none of them falls from the operative field. They are cleaned of clotted blood and fitted together until an anatomical articular surface is obtained. Only very small and completely loose fragments may be removed. Kirschner wires can be used for temporary fixation. They must be replaced by 4.0 mm cancellous screws or 3.5 mm cortical screws. At least two of these are necessary to avoid rotational instability of the condyles (Figure 13.13a, b). If there is no condylar comminution, they can be used as lag screws. When comminution exists, the screws must maintain the correct distance between the lateral and medial ridge of the trochlea. When the trochlea is too small, it will no longer allow free flexion–extension of the elbow joint. It is helpful to drill the first Kirschner wire before condylar reduction from inside to outside in the radial condylar fragment to ensure its correct position. This wire can then be drilled from lateral to medial after reduction. The screws should also be inserted from the lateral to medial parallel to the Kirschner wire. If placed medial to lateral the screwhead lies in the sulcus of the ulnar nerve and may provide an obstruction (Figure 13.13c). Only when the radial fragment is too small or comminuted may the screws be inserted in the opposite direction. Their screwheads are then countersunk and they will never be removed to avoid damage to the ulnar nerve (Figures 13.14a–c).

When the articular surface is reconstructed, the humeral epiphysis must be fixed to the metaphysis and shaft. For temporary fixation, crossed Kirschner wires, which are drilled from both condyles proximally and oblique, can be used (Figure 13.13d). They have to be replaced by plates and screws, because they do not afford sufficient stability for early postoperative active motion. It was mentioned earlier that the fracture pattern must be made as simple as possible before plating, by fixing smaller fracture fragments with lag screws to the humerus. Care should be taken not to place these lag screws in such a way that they disturb the optimal position of the plates. Here the preoperative drawing of the fracture with the implants can be helpful. In general, two small fragment plates are necessary to provide sufficient stability. As in supracondylar fractures, several types of plate can be used. On the lateral side, the plate is placed on the dorsal surface of the condyle and runs proximally upon the lateral and dorsal border of the humerus. On the medial side, the plate is best applied on the medial supracondylar crest to run down to the medial epicondyle[41] (Figure 13.13e). At least two screws in each plate must pass into the condyles. None of the screws should perforate the articular surface or the fossae! In young patients with very good bone quality and large fracture fragments, only one plate may be inserted, while the other condyle is stabilized with one or two lag screws (Figure 13.13f). After reduction and stabilization, the position of plate and screws is controlled in the AP and lateral direction under the image intensifier. In case of any doubt, intraoperative X-rays must be taken.

Finally, the ostetomized olecranon is refixed. There are two alternatives: one is the tension-band wire with a 6.0 mm cancellous screw placed intramedullary, the other is the tension-band wire with two Kirschner wires, also used in the fixation of olecranon fractures. The channel of the cancellous screw is best drilled before the osteotomy, so that it easily finds its correct position afterwards[31]. The use of one cancellous screw without a tension-band wire or the use of a tension-band wire alone is not recommended: these types of fixation are unable to resist the traction of the triceps muscle on the olecranon and end up with loosening, dislocation or non-union (Figures 13.14a–c).

Finally, the ulnar nerve is replaced in its sulcus. If the sulcus is filled up with a screw head or if another obstacle exists, it should be transferred anteriorly.

Postoperative care

After wound closure, the arm is splinted in a posterior plaster slab with the elbow in 60–70° flexion

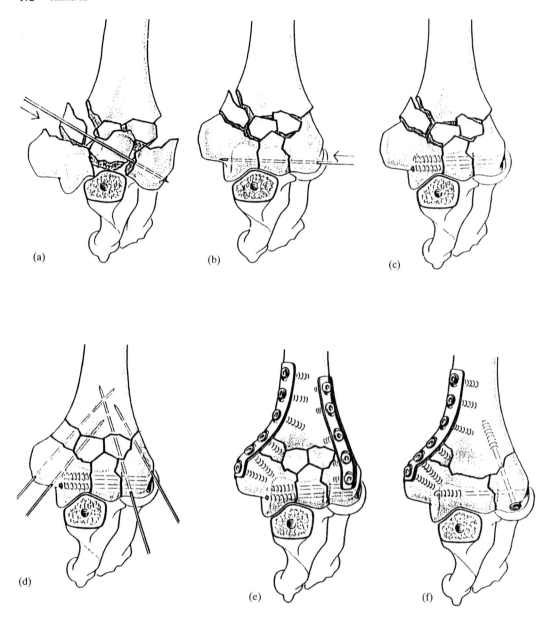

Figure 13.13(a–f) Operative technique for open reduction and internal fixation of type C condylar fractures of the humerus. (After Heim and Pfeiffer[31]) See text for explanation

and elevated in a sling for the first 2 days. The suction drain is removed on the second postoperative day, on condition that it produced less than 20 ml during the last 24 h. Active and active-assisted flexion–extension exercises of the elbow joint can be started after drain removal[42]. It is the surgeon and not the radiologist who assesses the stability of the fixation and gives permission to start the exercises. The splint normally remains for a few more weeks, but can be removed for exercises. In some patients, the fixation of the fracture is not safe enough to allow free joint movements. In these cases a brace for the elbow is manufactured, which allows a limited mobility of the joint under protection[13,30].

Passive mobilization of the elbow joint is very

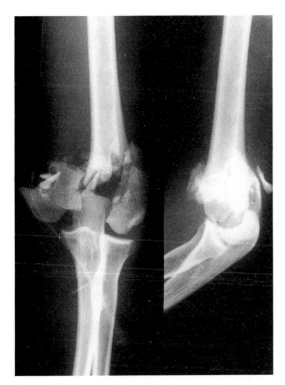

Figure 13.14(a) Type C2 condylar fracture of the distal humerus

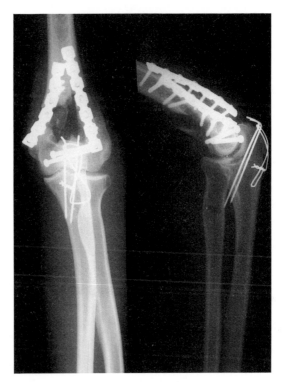

Figure 13.14(b) Open reduction and internal fixation through a dorsal approach with olecranon osteotomy. The two reconstruction plates are placed dorsally and the two small fragment screws are inserted from medially, their screwheads being countersunk. Fixation of the olecranon has been performed with K-wires and cerclage wiring

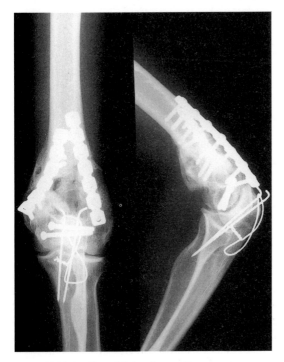

Figure 13.14(c) Consolidation 1 year after surgery– excellent functional result

dangerous. It can lead to more soft tissue and capsular damage and end up with extra-articular ossification, limited range of motion and pain. It is therefore forbidden in our trauma centre. Early continuous passive motion, as advocated by Salter *et al.*[43], can be considered in patients with secondary, elective interventions on the elbow joint. In our view, the advantages in patients with fresh fractures of the distal humerus do not exceed the possible disadvantages. Again, it is our strong conviction that the most important factors which influence the functional end result are the anatomical reconstruction of the elbow joint, its stable fixation and early active motion.

Emergencies

Open reduction and internal fixation of fractures of the distal humerus is a surgical challenge. It should be performed in optimal conditions for the surgeon and patient. A careful examination of the injury, together with preoperative planning, may take several hours. These injuries can be treated as delayed emergencies, when no contraindication exists to postpone surgery. However, the articular surface of intra-articular lesions should be reconstructed as early as possible. Therefore, the ideal time to perform the procedure may be between the first and third day after trauma. In some conditions, the injury must be seen as an emergency and should be treated as soon as possible.

In the case of an *open fracture* or a fracture with *extensive soft tissue damage* there is an indication for urgent surgery[44]. In comminuted and/or severely displaced fractures, open or closed soft tissue damage is not uncommon. In closed fractures, this can evolve in a compartment syndrome. The elbow joint is extremely swollen and in a lightly flexed position; the forearm is also swollen and painful. Paraesthesia and even pulselessness may occur distal to the injury. The last can be caused by compression of the brachial artery, when it passes the rigid lacertus fibrosus just distal and anterior to the elbow joint. In open fractures, an urgent debridement and lavage of the wound is mandatory. The best prevention of secondary infection of the wound and the elbow joint is stable fixation of the fracture fragments with a minimal amount of implants. At least the articular surface should be reconstructed. When osteosynthesis is delayed until the soft tissues are healed and safe, the only chance of obtaining a functioning anatomical elbow joint has been lost. Even in the case of infection, the fixed fracture fragments will heal better than when they are unstable.

In the case of extensive closed soft tissue damage, a preventive fasciotomy of the compartments of the forearm, together with the transection of the lacertus fibrosus, is recommended[45]. Fixation of the fracture fragments must follow the fasciotomies. When wounds have to be left open or when the soft tissue coverage of plates and screws is not safe, a bridging external fixator with the elbow in 90° of flexion is used temporarily. The fixator is replaced by implants when the soft tissues are healed after one or a few weeks.

Fractures combined with a *vascular lesion* are also emergency cases[46,47]. A stable fixation of the whole fracture must be performed first to protect the vascular sutures and to minimize infection. Fasciotomies of the forearm compartments are also necessary. Two different approaches are used for the osteosynthesis and the vascular repair. For the latter, the patient is best in dorsal decubitus,

but the prone position is best for the former. In simple fracture patterns, both procedures can be carried out with the patient in dorsal decubitus and the arm on a radiolucent side-table.

Patients with multiple trauma need urgent stabilization of all skeletal lesions. Highly unstable fractures such as femoral shaft fractures and pelvic ring fractures must be fixed as emergencies. The meticulous reconstruction of distal humerus fractures or other intra-articular lesions can be postponed to the second operative phase, which takes place after the primary operative phase and the haemodynamic stabilization of the patient.

Contraindications

Although we strongly advocate the open reduction and internal fixation following the principles of the AO, there are contraindications to surgery. Nowadays, the scope of anaesthesiology is such that even sick patients with several medical problems can be anaesthetised. Instruments and implants are developed to such a degree that they can be easily adjusted to the specific demands of each individual patient or fracture. The main problems and possible contraindications for operative treatment are the poor quality of the fractured bone and the complexity of the articular lesion[13,38]. Poor quality of the bone means poor holding power of the screws, less stable fixations and the impossibility of early active motion. Poor bone quality is generally caused by significant osteoporosis, but can also be seen in patients with bone diseases. Osteoporosis is common in the elderly population. Although it is exceptional in younger people, it is sometimes present in alcoholics or drug addicts or in persons with nerve injuries. The functional goals for young and active people will be higher than those for old and infirm persons.

The other contraindication lies in the complexity of the lesion. Distal humerus fractures are rather rare lesions. As a consequence, only few surgeons are sufficiently experienced to treat them. Surgeons should always have a clear understanding of the fractures they want to operate on and should be aware of the limitations of their own ability. An osteosynthesis with complications, an unstable fixation or an insufficient reconstruction of the articular surface can lead to even worse functional end results than some conservative treatment options. If the complexity of the fracture is such that an acceptable osteosynthesis seems impossible, the surgeon should commit the patient to a colleague's charge or refer them to a more specialized hospital. Finally, the fracture can be comminuted to such an extent that a good reconstruction is not likely, even if performed by an experienced surgeon. In this case, skeletal traction with early and limited active motion under traction may be the best solution.

Complications

Surgery of the distal humerus is a real challenge and complications during surgery or in the postoperative period can occur. The surgeon who wants to operate on the distal humerus must be familiar with all possible complications. Moreover, the operator must know how to prevent or anticipate them or how to deal with them so as to obtain a satisfying functional result.

In recent review articles, Helfet and Schmeling[30] and Morrey[48] summarized the main complications of distal humeral fractures as follows: nerve palsy, arterial injury, failure of fixation or loosening of implants, infection, malunion, non-union and heterotopic ossification.

Although injuries of the three nerves may be seen, the ulnar nerve is the most frequently damaged. This can be explained by its close relationship to the medial condyle[49]. The lesion can be caused by the trauma, but is also seen after percutaneous pinning and open reduction and internal fixation. Its occurrence is described as being between 7% and 15% in the literature. Symptoms are paraesthesia, atrophy and weakness of the muscles innervated by the ulnar nerve[48]. Ulnar nerve palsy even may occur several months to years after elbow injury or operative treatment[50].

A thorough neurological examination must be performed after injury and before treatment. A real or impending compartment syndrome should be excluded. Careful exposure of the ulnar nerve is the best way to prevent any complication after surgery. If a nerve palsy is discovered after surgical treatment of distal humeral fractures, an immediate exploration is mandatory. If present after trauma, a more expectant attitude can be defended. If the ulnar nerve palsy is due to impingement, an anterior transposition is recommended[51].

A lesion of the brachial artery is a rare complication of distal humeral fractures[46,47] but if not recognized, the consequences may be severe. Before and after any treatment, the presence of a radial pulse must be verified. In case the pulse is

absent, an arteriogram is performed. Restoration of arterial continuity is obtained by direct suture or a venous bypass. A compartment syndrome, usually present in young patients and adolescents, must be recognized early and urgently decompressed[45].

Failure of fixation in between 5% and 15% of cases is described in different series in the literature[48]. This is mainly related to the choice of implants, to biomechanically poor constructs[30] or to osteoporosis[52,53]. The best prevention of implant failure is the individualized treatment of distal humeral fractures, based upon a preoperative drawing made for each fracture.

If an olecranon osteotomy is performed, implant failure may also occur[10]. This is prevented by adequate fixation of the olecranon using the classic K-wires and cerclage wiring or spongious screw and cerclage wire.

The incidence of infection is described between 3% and 7%[30]. It is mostly seen in open fractures or fractures with severe soft tissue damage. Keystones in the prevention of infection are early and meticulous debridement, careful handling of soft tissues and the stable fixation of fracture fragments with the correct implants.

Malunion is the healing of fracture fragments in a non-anatomical position. This may have an influence on the function of the elbow joint although sometimes it has only an aesthetic significance[54,55]. Non-union after distal humeral fractures is seen in 1–11%, with a mean ratio of 2%[30]. In a series of 32 patients with non-unions in the distal part of the humerus, Mitsunaga et al.[56] defined infection and comminution as the predisposing factors. Morrey[48] stated that most nonunions occurred following failed internal fixation and that most were seen in the supracondylar region. Others deny the relationship between inadequate internal fixation and non-union[8,57]. The non-union may present as a painful elbow, an unstable elbow or a stiff elbow joint. The treatment of the non-union depends on the complaints of the patients, the type of non-union and the degree of osteoporosis. If the surgeon is familiar with internal fixation of distal humeral fractures, stable fixation together with autologous bone grafting should be performed. Usually, this has to be combined with an arthrolysis of the elbow joint itself, as motion generally occurs in the pseudarthrosis and not in the elbow joint. In the case of patients over the age of 65, with significant osteoporosis, joint replacement may be considered. In the series described by Morrey[58], long-term results were excellent. We do not have any experience with elbow joint arthroplasty after trauma.

Heterotopic bone formation or myositis ossificans is seen in 3–30% after elbow trauma[13,30,48]. Although the cause of this is not clear, some associations are clear. Ectopic bone formation is more often seen after severe elbow trauma with major soft tissue damage, after elbow trauma with closed head injury, after repeated surgical or nonsurgical manipulations of the elbow joint and after passive motion or stretching of the joint[59,60]. To prevent heterotopic bone formation, meticulous care of the soft tissues seems essential. Passive stretching of the elbow joint should be condemned, although some authors recommend immediate postoperative continuous passive motion[43]. The use of anti-inflammatory agents such as indomethacin seems promising when started perioperatively and given for at least 3 weeks, but a statistically significant effect has not been proven[61].

Functional end results

In the past few decades a lot of different series of operatively treated distal humeral fractures have been published in the literature[17–21,23,62,63]. Most emphasis has been on intercondylar fractures, which are the most difficult to treat. The most important problems that interfere with a good or excellent functional recovery are instability, pain, loss of motion and incongruency of the articular surfaces. Frequently, these problems are interrelated. An excellent or good functional result can be defined as a stable elbow joint with only minimal pain, minimal axial or rotational deformity, and with a range of motion between 15° and 130°. Riseborough and Radin[9] defined a 'good' result as a range of motion from a flexion contracture of 30° or less to at least 115° flexion with only minor subjective symptoms, 'fair' a range of motion from a flexion contracture of between 30° and 60°, and at least 115° of flexion with only minor subjective symptoms, and 'poor' a range of motion from a flexion contracture of 60° or more to less than 115° of flexion or with major subjective symptoms. Cassebaum[64] graded flexion from 15° to 130° as 'excellent', flexion from 40° to 120° as 'good' and flexion to less than 110° as 'fair'. In the series by Helfet and Schmeling, an average of 75% good to excellent and 10–15% poor results were seen[30].

It is obvious that, in all methods, elbow motion plays a major role in the estimation of the functional end result. Loss of motion is related to the presence of fibrous fissue and scar tissue around the elbow joint, to intra-articular adhesions, to condylar malunion or articular malalignment and to ectopic bone formation. Morrey[48] subdivides the different factors leading to loss of motion into an 'intrinsic' group and an 'extrinsic' group. We can avoid most problems leading to diminished mobility by treating distal humeral fractures early, achieving anatomical reduction and stable fixation and through careful handling of the soft tissues.

If the diminished mobility of the elbow joint lies within the functional range of motion, nothing need be done. If the mobility is severely limited or flexion is diminished so that the hand cannot reach the face, an operative arthrolysis should be considered. The last is performed through a lateral approach, combined with anti-inflammatory agents given until 3 months after surgery, and followed by a rigorous programme of continuous passive motion, flexion and extension splints and active physiotherapy. During the surgical procedures all intra-articular adhesions must be removed, the olecranon, radial and coronoid fossae liberated from scar tissue, the tip of the olecranon removed and the anterior capsule resected[48,65]. If periarticular ossification is present, it is also removed. Before arthrolysis of an elbow joint with periarticular ossification, a technetium bone scan is performed to make sure that bone formation is inactive.

Instibility after operative treatment of distal humeral fractures is not common, if condylar fragments are removed at the time of operation. This can also occur after radial head removal, but this will be discussed in another chapter. Instability can also be the consequence of ligamentous injury, but this is very uncommon in distal humeral fractures. Ligamentous repair alone is seldom necessary or recommended. Instability as a consequence of dislocation of the elbow joint is discussed below.

Elbow dislocation

After shoulder and finger joint dislocations, dislocations of the elbow are the most frequent in the human skeleton. Generally, dislocation is a consequence of indirect forces through the forearm, such as a fall on the outstretched hand with the arm in extension and abduction. The olecranon

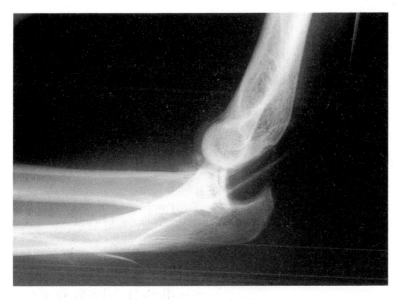

Figure 13.15(a) Perched dislocation of the left elbow joint

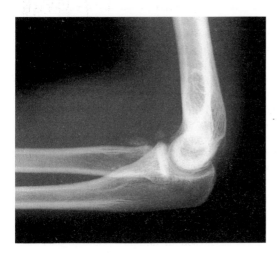

Figure 13.15(b) After reduction, a fracture of the tip of the olecranon and an avulsion fragment of the radial head are clearly visible

acts as a lever in the olecranon fossa and pushes the distal humerus through the anterior capsule[66]. The question whether a fall on the outstretched hand will lead to a dislocation of the elbow, to a distal humeral fracture, to a fracture of the radial head or to a combination of these, depends on the degree of flexion of the elbow joint at the time of injury, on the pro-supination of the forearm and on additional rotational forces. In a minority of cases, the dislocation follows a direct blow on the flexed elbow.

In his classification of adult elbow dislocations, Stimson[67] identified different groups, according to the position of the radius and ulna with respect to the distal humerus. He distinguished dislocations with displacement of radius and ulna, dislocations of the radius alone and dislocations of the ulna alone:

Dislocation of radius and ulna
- posterior-lateral
- posterior-medial
- medial (inward)
- lateral (outward)
- anterior
- divergent antero-posterior
- divergent medio-lateral

Dislocation of radius alone
- anterior
- posterior
- lateral

Dislocation of ulna alone
- anterior
- posterior

Perched dislocation[48]

Morrey[48] adds the category of 'perched dislocation', an incomplete posterior dislocation that does not spontaneously resolve (Figures 13.15a, b).

Posterior dislocations

Posterior dislocations account for about 85% of all elbow dislocations. They can be subdivided into those with posterolateral or those with postero-medial displacement. In a typical dorsal disloca-tion, the elbow joint shows significant swelling, and is very painful, its position fixed in 45–60% of flexion. The forearm seems to be shortened and the tip of the olecranon projects more posteriorly than in intracondylar or supracondylar fractures of the humerus. The anatomical relationship between the olecranon and both epicondyles is disturbed. The neurovascular structures may be torn or even interrupted at the time of injury and a careful examination must be performed before any treat-ment[68–74]. Antero-posterior and lateral X-rays will confirm the diagnosis. They are also indispensable to exclude associated intra-articular or extra-articular lesions (Figure 13.15a, b). These lesions are discussed below. In the case of associated frac-tures, oblique X-rays or tomography may be necessary to obtain a clear view of the origin of all fracture fragments.

The proper management of posterior disloca-tions consists of closed reduction, followed by immobilization. Reduction must be performed as soon as possible, in order to restore the articular anatomy, to preclude extreme swelling and to regain normal function. The reduction is carried out under general anaesthesia or regional block, since the use of tranquillizers may not be sufficient to obtain enough muscle relaxation. We prefer gentle continuous traction with the forearm in a slightly flexed position and the patient supine. At the same time, a careful counter-traction can be used against the distal humerus and a forward pressure put upon the olecranon. During the reduc-tion manoeuvre, the lateral or medial displacement is simultaneously corrected.

Once the elbow is reduced, it must regain its full range of motion. The reduction manoeuvre is carried out by one surgeon with or without an assistant. Although some authors[75] recommend a prone position for the patient, with the elbow flexed at 90° and the forearm hanging down, the author finds this method to be more cumbersome and more dangerous for the patient. Hyperexten-sion of the elbow joint before reduction and flex-ion cannot be recommended, as this can increase the damage to the anterior capsule and the neuro-vascular bundle. It must be repeated that in all reduction manoeuvres, gentle and careful manip-ulation is mandatory in order to minimize soft tissue trauma with the risk of myositis ossificans, or iatrogenic neurovascular damage.

Open reduction is only indicated if several care-ful attempts at reduction have been fruitless. This is seldom the case in acute elbow dislocations. If indicated, it is mainly because of entrapment of fracture fragments, ligaments or neurovascular structures. Some authors[76–78] have compared the long-term results of primary open and closed reduction of acute elbow dislocations and have not found significant differences.

After reduction, stability must be tested and X-rays should confirm the anatomical realignment. A tendency to redislocation or instability may be caused by soft tissue entrapment, by associated fractures or even by incarceration of avulsed frac-ture fragments[79,80].

The arm is temporarily elevated above heart level. The patient must be reviewed at regular intervals for control of the soft tissue swelling, and assessment of the neurovascular status of the arm. If a compartment syndrome develops, urgent fasci-otomy of the flexor compartment with transection of the inelastic lacertus fibrosus is necessary.

The after-care depends on the stability of the elbow joint following reduction. If the joint is free and stable, a dorsal splint is applied, with the elbow in 90° of flexion, until swelling and pain subside. Active motion is allowed, out of the splint, as soon as tolerated by the patient. Like Protzman[81], we believe that the longer the immo-bilization, the higher the risk of a flexion con-tracture of the elbow. If instability persists, a longer period of immobilization will be necessary.

Occasionally patients present with old unre-duced elbow dislocations. If they present within 2 weeks after injury, a closed reduction may still be possible. If not, open reduction may be necessary. After 2 weeks, a closed reduction is not possible. More extensive surgical approaches with excision of the capsule and removal of all intra-articular adhesions are then required[82].

Other dislocations

Medial and lateral dislocations of the radius and ulna account for only 2–3% of all dislocations[66,83]. They are the result of a direct blow to the elbow and almost always are associated with consider-able soft tissue damage. In this type of dislocation, the forearm does not appear shortened, and some degree of motion may be possible. The reduction manoeuvre is similar to that of a posterior disloca-tion, but lateral or medial pressure is more import-ant than traction and counter-traction.

Anterior dislocation is extremely rare[84,85]. It is caused by a direct postero-anterior force on the olecranon of a flexed elbow. Clinical signs are opposite from those of posterior dislocations: the elbow is in extension, the arm seems shortened but the forearm lengthened. The reduction manoeuvre is also the opposite to that for posterior dislocations: first gentle longitudinal traction on the forearm, which is then pushed backwards. As with posterior dislocations, an open reduction for medial, lateral or anterior dislocations is only indicated if closed reduction fails.

Divergent dislocations of the elbow are a rarity. In this type, the ulna and radius dissociate from each other and dislocate in an opposite direction. In the medio-lateral subtype, the ulna displaces medially and the radius laterally. In the antero-posterior subtype, the ulna displaces dorsally and the radius anteriorly[85]. It is obvious that in both subtypes the interosseous membrane and the distal radio-ulnar joint are disrupted. A distal ulnar fracture may also be present. The lesion can only be the result of a high-energy trauma; soft tissue swelling and significant soft tissue damage are always present. The humero-ulnar joint is reduced first and the humero-radial joint thereafter. The after-care is similar to that of other dislocations. If the elbow joint remains unstable and a recurrent humero-radial dislocation occurs, an open reduction with repair of the annular ligament is recommended.

The isolated dislocation of the radial head is also a rarity[48]. It is more frequently seen in children, but in adults it is generally associated with a proximal fracture of the ulna. This entity is known as a Monteggia fracture and will be discussed in relation to the forearm. Because of its rarity, a fracture of the ulna should always be looked for when an isolated fracture of the radial head is diagnosed on an elbow-X-ray. Congenital dislocations must be separated from post-traumatic ones by a clear history of trauma. The reduction is carried out with direct pressure on the radial head. If the reduction is unstable or if it cannot be obtained, an open reduction may be necessary. Repair of the annular ligament is then recommended.

Isolated dislocation of the ulna is also extremely rare. Although Stimson[67] demonstrated how to reproduce isolated ulno-humeral dislocation in 1890, others could not reproduce his experiments and have questioned the existence of this type of dislocation[48]. The author's institution has not had any experience with this dislocation. De Lee *et al.*[38] describes that the patient with a posterior dislocation of the ulna holds his elbow in extension.

The carrying angle is lost, and the forearm seems to be in varus. The patient with an anterior dislocation of the ulna has his elbow flexed. There is an increase of valgus between forearm and arm. The reduction is carried out by pushing the ulna anteriorly or backwards while holding the forearm in valgus or varus, respectively.

Associated lesions

Of all elbow dislocations, 10–50% are associated with fractures or osteochondral lesions[48]. The most common are fracture of the medial epicondyle, fracture of the coronoid process, fracture of the radial head and osteochondral lesions. The avulsion of the medial epicondyle can vary from a minimal displacement to an incarceration within the joint. It can be the reason for an uncomplete reduction or for residual instability. After each reduction manoeuvre, X-rays of good quality must exclude the presence of an intra-articular bone fragment. If the medial epicondyle is incarcerated, it is best removed in an open procedure and the avulsed, medial epicondyle fixed with one or two small fragment screws (see Figures 13.7a and 13.7b).

Fractures of the coronoid process are classified by Regan and Morrey[86] by the size of the fracture fragment. Half of all fractures of the coronoid process are associated with elbow dislocations. The fracture is a result of contracture of the brachialis muscle or of a posterior dislocation of the ulna itself. Larger fragments (types II and III) should be fixed with a small fragment lag screw. Non-union of the coronoid process can be a reason for recurrent elbow dislocation.[87] Radial head and neck fractures and compression lesions of the radial head may be as frequent as 10% in elbow dislocations[73]. Broberg and Morrey[88] classified them as Mason type IV injuries. They will be discussed in relation to radial head injuries. The therapeutic principle is that the radial head fracture is treated after the reduction of the elbow joint as with an isolated radial head fracture[88].

Osteochondral fractures may be much more common than previously suspected. The osteochondral fragments are avulsed from the capitulum, the radial head or other structures. They may interfere with mobility of the elbow joint. If there is any mechanical hindrance or intra-articular bone crepitus after closed reduction, an osteochondral fragment must be looked for. The fragment should be removed if it is small, or reattached if it is large. When the fragment is not recognized and elbow motion started, severe damage of the articular cartilage may occur rapidly.

Complications

Neurovascular problems and compartment syndrome are the most important complications of elbow dislocation. Although rare, elbow dislocations may be combined with stretching of the median nerve[68,69,72,74]. The brachial artery may also be damaged[70,71]. Therefore, it is necessary to perform a thorough neurovascular examination before any attempt at reduction. This reduction must be carried out with care! Gentle manipulation is mandatory, and over-extension of the elbow joint is forbidden! After reduction, the neurovascular examination must be repeated. Median nerve entrapment leads to incomplete reduction and to median nerve palsy. If such entrapment is present, a surgical exposure of the nerve is necessary.

The ulnar nerve is more commonly over-stretched at the time of dislocation than the median nerve. Delayed ulnar nerve palsy may occur as a result of heterotopic bone formation or ossification of the ulnar nerve sulcus. An anterior transposition may then be indicated. The brachial artery may be trapped within the joint after reduction. Clinical examination reveals no radial pulse. As in distal humeral fractures, an arteriogram must be obtained quickly and the lesion repaired if necessary.

In patients with extensive soft tissue damage or intramuscular bleeding, swelling may be so severe that a compartment syndrome develops. Swelling and pain in the whole flexor compartment of the forearm, aggravated by finger or wrist extension, are the first symptoms. They are followed by pallor and paresis or paralysis. Pulselessness is the last symptom of a severe and fully developed syndrome. The treatment is urgent decompression of the flexor compartment, transection of the lacertus fibrosus and opening of the lower brachial fascia[45]. The brachial artery and its branches should be explored in the elbow fossa.

Functional results and sequelae

If an uncomplicated elbow dislocation can be reduced safely and early, a good functional end result, with sufficient stability and a nearly optimal range of motion, may be expected. As in distal humeral injuries, factors influencing the end results are the severity of the soft tissue injury, associated lesions, the time between trauma and reduction, the number of attempts at reduction, and the after-care.

Elbow stiffness is probably the most common sequela of an elbow dislocation. The longer the time of immobilization, the higher the chance of elbow stiffness. We therefore advocate active mobilization of the elbow as early as is acceptable for the patient. Fortunately, the loss of motion is a mild extension deficit and generally does not hinder the activities of daily life. If the loss of motion is severe, other factors such as ectopic bone formation, or associated fractures of the coronoid process, or the radial head, can be found.

Both ectopic bone formation and myositis ossificans are often seen after elbow dislocations. The bone formation may be situated in the capsule or in the collateral ligaments. Myositis ossificans is generally situated in the fleshy brachialis muscle, which is damaged at the time of dislocation. Factors of decisive influence in the development of ectopic bone are the severity of the soft tissue damage at the time of injury and after reduction, the time between trauma and reduction and the type of rehabilitation. It is generally accepted now that stretching, massage and passive motion of the elbow joint favours ectopic bone formation and must be abandoned totally[13,30,38,42,48]. Once ectopic bone is developing, it is impossible to stop its progression. The elbow joint should be left alone until painful motion and local tenderness subside. When the bone has become mature surgical excision can be planned. It usually improves elbow motion, but a full range of motion is never regained. Indomethacin has been advocated for the prevention of heterotopic bone formation, but its final activity is not fully understood or proven[60,61].

Osteochondral fragments which were not recognized after elbow reduction may be responsible for wear of articular surfaces, with development of post-traumatic arthritis. Their presence must be suspected in patients with a mechanical hindrance, bone crepitus or painful movement. Tomography or oblique X-rays may be helpful to localize them. Excision is the only solution in the patient with delayed diagnosis. The removal is carried out by arthroscopy or arthrotomy.

Residual instability resulting in recurrent dislocation is a rare sequel after elbow dislocation[48]. If instability persists immediately after reduction, entrapment of neurovascular structures, osteochondral fragments or associated fractures must be looked for and treated adequately. In cases of recurrent dislocation, an insufficient lateral ligament complex may be the reason. Osborne and Cotterill[89] recommended the repair of the lateral complex and obtained good results. Morrey[48] and O'Driscoll *et al.*[90] more often observed a pivot subluxation of the elbow joint, owing to a deficiency of the lateral collateral ligament.

References

1. Netter, F.H. (ed.). *The Ciba Collection of Medical Illustrations*, Vol. 8: *Musculoskeletal System.* Part I: *Anatomy, Physiology and Metabolic Disorders*, Ciba-Geigy Corporation, Summit, New Jersey (1987), pp. 42–43

2. Sobotta, J. and Becher, H. (eds). *Atlas der Anatomie des Menschen.* 17. Auflage, Band 1, Urban and Schwarzenberg, Munich (1972), (i) pp. 68–69, (ii) p. 112

3. Barnard, L.B. and McCoy, S.M. The supracondyloid process of the humerus. *J. Bone Joint Surg.*, 28, 845–850 (1946)

4. Milch, H. Fractures and fracture-dislocations of the humeral condyles. *J. Trauma*, 4, 592–607 (1964)

5. Kapandji, I.A. and Bewegingsleer Deel, I. *De bovenste extremiteit*, Bohn, Scheltema and Holkema, Utrecht (1986)

6. Magnuson, P.B. and Stack, J.K. *Fractures*, 5th edn, J.B. Lippincott, Philadelphia (1949)

7. Heim, U.F.A. Die Grenzziehung zwischen Diaphyse und Metaphyse mit Hilfe der Viereckmessung. Ein Beitrag zur Klassifizierung und Dokumentierung von Frakturen der langen Röhrenknochen am Beispiel der distalen Tibia. *Unfallchirurg*, 90, 274–280 (1987)

8. Horne, G. Supracondylar fractures of the humerus in adults. *J. Trauma*, 20, 71–74 (1980)

9. Riseborough, E.J. and Radin, E.L. Intercondylar T-fractures of the humerus in the adult (a comparison of operative and non-operative treatment in twenty-nine cases). *J. Bone Joint Surg.*, 51A, 130–141 (1969)

10. Henley, M.B., Bone, L.B. and Parker, B. Operative management of intra-articular fractures of the distal humerus. *J. Orthop. Trauma*, 1, 24–35 (1987)

11. Henley, M.B. Intro-articular distal humeral fractures in adults. *Orthopedic Clinics of North America*, 18, 11–23 (1987)

12. Müller, M.E., Nazarian, S. and Koch, P. *Classification AO des Fractures*, Springer-Verlag, Berlin (1987)

13. Schatzker, J. and Tile, M. *The Rationale of Operative Fracture Care*, Springer-Verlag, Berlin (1987)

14. Conn, J. and Wade, P.A. Injuries of the elbow (a ten year review). *J. Trauma*, 1, 248–268 (1961)

15. Keon-Cohen, B.T. Fractures of the elbow. *J. Bone Joint Surg.*, 48A, 1623–1639 (1966)

16. Bickel, W.E. and Perry, R.E. Comminuted fractures of the distal humerus. *J. Am. Med. Ass.*, 184, 553–557 (1963)

17. Gabel, G.T., Hanson, G., Bennett, J.B., Noble, P.C. and Tullos, H.S. Intraarticular fractures of the distal humerus in the adult. *Clin. Orthop.*, 216, 99–108 (1987)

18. Holdsworth, B.J. and Mossad, M.M. Fractures of the adult distal humerus: elbow function after internal fixation. *J. Bone Joint Surg.*, 72B, 362–365 (1990)

19. Jupiter, J.B., Neff, U., Hozach, P. and Allgöwer, M. Intercondylar fractures of the humerus. *J. Bone Joint Surg.*, 67A, 226–239 (1985)

20. Lansinger, O. and Märe, K. Intercondylar T-fractures of the humerus in adults. *Arch. Orthop. Trauma Surg.*, 100, 37–42 (1982)

21. Letsch, R., Schmit-Neuerburg, K.P., Stürmer, K.M. and Walz, M. Intraarticular fractures of the distal humerus, surgical treatment and results. *Clin. Orthop.*, 241, 238–244 (1989)

22. Müller, M.E., Allgöwer, M., Schneider, R. and Willenegger, H. *Manual of Internal Fixation*, 3rd edn. Springer-Verlag, Berlin (1991)

23. Waddell, J.P., Hatch, J. and Richards, R. Supracondylar fractures of the humerus: results of treatment. *J. Trauma*, 28, 1615–1621 (1988)

24. Smith, F.M. Displacement of the medial epicondyle of the humerus into the elbow joint. *Ann. Surg.*, 124, 410–425 (1946)

25. Wilson, J.N. The treatment of fractures of the medial epicondyle of the humerus. *J. Bone Joint Surg.*, 42B, 778–781 (1960)

26. Roberts, J.B. and Kelly, J.A. *Treatise on Fractures*, 2nd edn, J.B. Lippincott, Philadelphia (1921)

27. Merle D'Aubigne, R., Meary, R. and Carlios, J. Fractures sus- et intercondyliennes récentes de l'adulte. *Revue Chir. Orthop. Répar. Appar. Moteur*, 50, 279–288 (1964)

28. Siris, I.E. Supracondylar fractures of the humerus. *Surg. Gynecol. Obstet.*, 68, 201–222 (1939)

29. Miller, O.L. Blind nailing of the T-fracture of the lower end of the humerus which involves the joint. *J. Bone Joint Surg.*, 21, 933–938 (1939)

30. Helfet, D.L. and Schmeling, G.J. Bicondylar intraarticular fractures of the distal humerus in adults. *Clin. Orthop.*, 292, 26–36 (1993)

31. Heim, U. and Pfeiffer, K.M. The elbow. In *Small Fragment Set Manual Technique Recommended by the ASIF Group.* Second revised and enlarged edn (eds U. Heim and K.M. Pfeiffer), Springer-Verlag, Berlin (1982), pp. 83–94

32. Knight, R.A. Fractures of the humeral condyles in adults. *South. Med. J.*, 48, 1165–1173 (1955)

33. Lee, W.E. and Summey, T.J. Fracture of the capitulum of the humerus. *Ann. Surg.*, 99, 497–509 (1934)

34. Lindem, M.C. Fractures of the capitulum and trochlea. *Ann. Surg.*, 76, 78–82 (1922)

35. Hahn, N.F. Fall von eine besondere Varietät der Frakturen des Ellenbogens. *Z. Wundärzte Geburtshelfe*, 6, 185–189 (1953)

36. Steinthal, D. Die isolierte Fraktur der Eminentia capitata in Ellenbogengelenk. *Zentralbl. Chirurg.*, 15, 17–20 (1898)

37. Lorenz, H. Zur Kenntniss der Fractura humeri (eminentiae capitatae). *Dtsche Z. Chir.*, 78, 531–545 (1905)

38. De Lee, J.C., Green, D.P. and Wilkins, K.E. Fractures and dislocations of the elbow. In *Factures in Adults* (eds C.A.

Rockwood and D.P. Green), J.B. Lippincott, Philadelphia (1984), pp. 572–581

39. Schwarz, B., Schmitt, O. and Mittelmeier, H. Spätschäden des Nervus ulnaris nach Traumen am Ellenbogengelenk. *Unfallchirurg*, **88**, 208–213 (1985)

40. Hansen, S.T. Jr and Swientkowski, M.F. *Orthopaedic Trauma Protocols*, Raven Press, New York (1993), pp. 100–107

41. Helfet, D.L. and Hotchkis, R.N. Internal fixation of the distal humerus: a biochemical comparison of methods. *J. Orthop. Trauma*, **4**, 260–264 (1990)

42. Dowden, J.W. The principle of early active movement in treating fractures of the upper extremity. *Clin. Orthop.*, **4**, 146 (1981)

43. Salter, R.B., Simmonds, D.F., Malcolm, B.W., Ruble, E.J., MacMicheal, D. and Clements, N.D. The biological effect of continuous passive motion on the healing of full thickness defects in articular cartilage. *J. Bone Joint Surg.*, **62A**, 1232 (1980)

44. Feil, J., Burri, C. and Kiefer, H. Offene Frakturen des Ellenbogengelenkes. *Orthopäde*, **17**, 272 (1988)

45. Holden, C.E.A. The pathology and prevention of Volkmann's contracture. *J. Bone Joint Surg.*, **61B**, 296–300 (1979)

46. Ashbell, T.S., Kleinert, H.E. and Kutz, J.E. Vascular injuries about the elbow. *Clin. Orthop.*, **50**, 107–127 (1967)

47. Henderson, R.S. and Robertson, I.M. Open dislocation of the elbow with rupture of the brachial artery. *J. Bone Joint Surg.*, **34B**, 636–637 (1952)

48. Morrey, B.F. Fractures and dislocations of the elbow. In *Fractures and Dislocations* (eds. R.B. Gustilo, R.F. Kyle and D. Templeman), Mosby – Year Book Inc., St. Louis (1993), pp. 387–498

49. Bryan, R.S. Fracture about the elbow in adults. In American Academy of Orthopaedic Surgeons: *Instructional Course Lectures*, Vol. 30, C.V. Mosby Co, St. Louis (1981)

50. Schwarz, B., Schmitt, O. and Mittelmeier, H. Spätschäden des Nervus Ulnaris nach Traumen am Ellenbogengelenk. *Unfallchirurg*, **88**, 208–213 (1985)

51. Schäfer, E.R., Bushe, K.A. and Deftereos, T.H. Probleme der Ulnarisverlagerung bei Verletzungen im Ellenbogenbereich. *Chir. Plast.*, **3**, 64–68 (1967)

52. Södergard, J., Sandelin, J. and Böstman, O. Mechanical failures of internal fixation in T- and Y-fractures of the distal humerus. *J. Trauma*, **33**, 687–690 (1992)

53. Södergard, J., Sandelin, J. and Böstman, O. Postoperative complications of distal humeral fractures. *Acta Orthop. Scand.*, **63**, 85–89 (1992)

54. Campbell, W.C. Malunited fractures and unreduced dislocations about the elbow. *J. Am. Med. Ass.*, **92**, 122–128 (1929)

55. Smith, L. Deformity following supracondylar fracture of the humerus. *J. Bone Joint Surg.*, **42A**, 235–252 (1960)

56. Mitsunaga, M.S., Bryan, R.S. and Lindscheid, R.L. Condylar non-unions of the elbow. *J. Trauma*, **22**, 787–792 (1982)

57. Ackerman, G. and Jupiter, J.B. Nonunion of fractures of

the distal end of the humerus. *J. Bone Joint Surg.*, **75A**, 75–80 (1988)

58. Morrey, B.F. (ed.) *The Elbow and its Disorders*, W.B. Saunders, Philadelphia (1985)

59. Mohan, K. Myositis ossificans traumatica of the elbow. *Int. Surg.*, **57**, 475–478 (1972)

60. Rieger, H., Pennig, D., Grünert, J. and Brug, E. Heterotope Ossifikationen aus Unfallchirurgischer Sicht. *Unfallchirurg*, **94**, 144 (1991)

61. Ritter, M.A. and Gioe, J.J. The effect of indomethacin on para-articular ectopic ossification following total hip arthroplasty. *Clin. Orthop.*, **167**, 113–117 (1982)

62. Burri, C., Henkemeyer, H. and Spier, W. Results of operative treatment of intraarticular fractures of the distal humerus. *Acta Orthop. Belg.*, **41**, 227–234 (1975)

63. Lob, G., Burri, C. and Feil, J. Die operative Behandlung von distalen intraartikulären Humerusfrakturen: Ergebnis von 412 nachkontrollierten Fällen (AO-Sammelstatistik). *Langenbecks Arch. Chir.*, **364**, 359 (1984)

64. Cassebaum, W.H. Open reduction of T and Y fractures of the lower end of the humerus. *J. Trauma*, **9**, 915–919 (1969)

65. Wilson, P.D. Capsulectomy for the relief of flexion contractures of the elbow following fracture. *J. Bone Joint Surg.*, **26**, 71–86 (1944)

66. Lindscheid, R.L. Dislocations of the elbow. In *The Elbow and its Disorders* (ed. B.F. Morrey), W.B. Saunders, Philadelphia (1985)

67. Stimson, L.A. *A Treatise on Fractures*, Henry C. Lea's, Philadelphia (1890)

68. Galbraith, K.A. and McCullough, C.J. Acute nerve injury as a complication of closed fractures or dislocations of the elbow injury, **11**, 159–164 (1979)

69. Hallet, J. Entrapment of the median nerve after dislocation of the elbow. A case report. *J. Bone Joint Surg.*, **63B**, 408–412 (1981)

70. Hennig, K. and Franke, D. Posterior displacement of brachial artery following closed elbow dislocation. *J. Trauma*, **20**, 96–98 (1980)

71. Louis, D.S., Ricciardi, J.E. and Spengler, C.M. Arterial injury: a complication of posterior elbow dislocation: a clinical and anatomical study. *J. Bone Joint Surg.*, **56A**, 1631–1636 (1974)

72. Mannerfelt, L. Median nerve entrapment after dislocation of the elbow (report of a case). *J. Bone Joint Surg.*, **50B**, 152–155 (1968)

73. Neviaser, J.S. and Wickstrom, J.K. Dislocation of the elbow: a retrospective study of 115 patients. *South. Med. J.*, **70–79**, 172–173 (1977)

74. Watson–Jones, R. Primary nerve lesions in injuries of the elbow and wrist. *J. Bone Joint Surg.*, **12**, 121–126 (1930)

75. Meyn, M.A. and Quigley, T.B. Reduction of posterior dislocation of the elbow by traction on the dangling arm. *Clin. Orthop.*, **103**, 106–108 (1974)

76. Durig, M., Muller, W., Ruedi, T.P. and Gauer, E.F. The operative treatment of elbow dislocation in the adult. *J. Bone Joint Surg.*, **61A**, 239–244 (1979)

77. Josefsson, P.L., Johnell, O. and Gentz, C.F. Long-term

sequelae of simple dislocation of the elbow. *J. Bone Joint Surg.*, **66A**, 927 (1984)

78. Mehlhoff, T.L., Noble, M.S., Bennett, J.B. *et al.* Simple dislocations of the elbow in the adult. *J. Bone Joint Surg.*, **70**, 224–249 (1988)

79. Hassmann, G.C., Brunn, F. and Neer, C.S. Recurrent dislocation of the elbow. *J. Bone Joint Surg.*, **57A**, 1080–1084 (1975)

80. Jacobs, R.L. Recurrent dislocation of the elbow joint. A case report and a review of the literature. *Clin. Orthop.*, **74**, 151–154 (1971)

81. Protzman, R.R. Dislocation of the elbow joint. *J. Bone Joint Surg.*, **60A**, 539–541 (1978)

82. Bryan, R.S. and Morrey, B.F. Extensive posterior exposure of the elbow. A triceps-sparing approach. *Clin. Orthop.*, **166**, 188–192 (1982)

83. Exarchou, E.J. Lateral dislocation of the elbow. *Acta Orthop. Scand.*, **48**, 161–163 (1977)

84. Cohn, I. Forward dislocation of both bones of the forearm at the elbow. *Surg. Gynecol. Obstet.*, **35**, 776–788 (1922)

85. Oury, J.H., Roe, R.D. and Laning, R.C. A case of bilateral anterior dislocations of the elbow. *J. Trauma*, **12**, 170–173 (1972)

86. Regan, W. and Morrey, B. Fractures of the coronoid process of the ulna. *J. Bone Joint Surg.*, **71A**, 1348–1354 (1989)

87. Bopp, F., Tielemann, F.W. and Holz, U. Ellenbogenluxation mit Frakturen am Processus Coronoideus und Radiusköpfchentrümmerfraktur. *Unfallchirurg*, **94**, 322–324 (1991)

88. Broberg, M. and Morrey, B.F. Treatment of radial head fracture and elbow dislocation. A long-term follow-up study. *Clin. Orthop.*, **216**, 109–119 (1987)

89. Osborne, G. and Cotterill, P. Recurrent dislocation of the elbow. *J. Bone Joint Surg.*, **48B**, 340–346 (1966)

90. O'Driscoll, S.W., Morrey, B.F. and Bell, D.F. The lateral pivot-shift test of the elbow. *J. Bone Joint Surg.*, **72A**, 440–446 (1990)

14

Fractures of the humerus in children

Lutz von Laer and Christoph Lampert

Growth plate and growth

Proximal end (Figure 14.1)

The proximal growth plate accounts for approximately 80% of humeral growth. At birth there are three ossification centres, one for the head epiphysis and one for each tuberosity. Radiologically only the head ossification centre is visible, the tuberosity centres appearing between five and seven months after birth. The tuberosity ossification centres unite after four or five years and all three of the proximal ossification centres are united by about the age of 12 years. Growth plate closure starts centrally and medially and is complete between 16 and 19 years of age.

Distal end (Figure 14.2)

The distal growth plate accounts for the remaining 20% of humeral growth. Distally there are four different ossification centres, two of these being epiphyseal and two apophyseal. None of these centres are visible on X-ray at birth. The capitellar ossification centre appears by about the third or fourth month followed by the ulnar epicondylar centre between the fourth and fifth year. The trochlear ossification centre usually appears as a number of multi-focal centres at about eight to ten years of age and the radial epicondylar centre can be seen by about 12 years of age. Union of the ossification centres occurs at different times with the trochlear centre uniting between ten and twelve

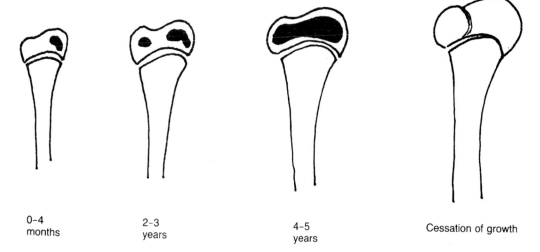

0–4 months   2–3 years   4–5 years   Cessation of growth

Figure 14.1 Development of the proximal humerus (see text)

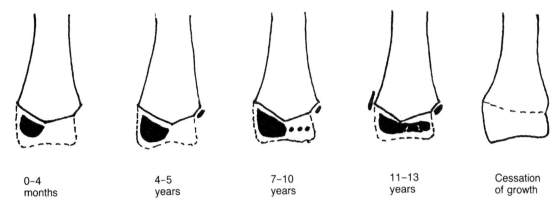

| 0–4 months | 4–5 years | 7–10 years | 11–13 years | Cessation of growth |

Figure 14.2 Development of the distal humerus (see text)

years of age, the capitellar centre at about 14 years and the ulnar epicondylar centre between 15 and 17 years of age.

Growth disturbances

Both proximal and distal growth plates can be partially or totally affected by either stimulative or inhibitive growth disturbances although inhibitive growth disturbances are rarely encountered in the upper extremity[1,2]. In the proximal humerus partial growth plate closure usually leads to early growth arrest at the medial side of the plate. The ensuing growth disturbance produces an increasing varus deformity. Early complete proximal growth plate arrest will result in shortening of the whole humerus. Early partial closure of the distal humeral growth plate is rare and usually iatrogenic.

The most frequent growth disturbance is stimulation of the growth plates following fracture. Increased activity can invariably be detected in adjacent growth plates after fracture. The alternate effects of stimulation and inhibition tend to lead to humeral lengthening in children of less than ten years of age and shortening in older children although the effect is variable. The average discrepancy measures about 1 cm in both cases[2-6]. The classic location for post-traumatic growth plate stimulation is the distal humerus. For example, after fracture of the radial condyle of the distal humerus a partial stimulation of this growth plate will occur. Radial condylar fracture will result in a slight varus deformity and ulnar condylar fracture in a slight valgus deformity. The duration of the stimulus and therefore the overall angle deformity depends on the elapsed time before bone consolidation. Although the fracture line in these

distal humeral condylar fractures crosses the growth plate, growth stimulation rather than inhibition is the result.

'Spontaneous' correction

The apparent spontaneous correction of a residual post-traumatic deformity depends on the relative growth potential of the neighbouring physes and on the functional loading of the surrounding muscles and the adjacent joints.

There is an excellent potential for correction of post-traumatic deformity in all three directions in the proximal humeral metaphysis in children over the age of 12 years because of the proximity to the proximal humeral growth plates and the considerable arc of movement permitted by the glenohumeral joint[7]. Varus deformities will correct better than valgus deformities.

In diaphyseal fractures transverse displacement will be corrected even in the adolescent age groups. However angular deformities are less well corrected. Anterior or posterior angular deformities or varus or valgus deformities are only corrected in children up to five years of age with varus deformities showing more improvement than valgus deformities.

In the distal humeral metaphysis the potential for spontaneous correction decreases markedly. This is partly due to the low activity of the adjacent distal growth plate and partly because the plane of angulation is at right angles to the motion plane of the elbow. Angular deformation in the motion plane of the elbow (anterior or posterior angulation) will correct spontaneously. However, the fact that the distal humeral growth plate grows slowly, contributes only 20% of overall humeral growth and closes early, means that correction will be slow and strongly age dependent. The borderline age limit is assumed to be 5–7 years[8]. The correction of side-to-side displacement at this site is good.

Spontaneous correction of a rotational deformity is complex and needs to be considered separately. As with the femur a spontaneous physiological decrease in retroversion occurs in the proximal humerus during growth. At birth the angle of retroversion is about 50–60°, reducing to 20–30° by the time full skeletal growth is achieved. Therefore post-traumatic rotational deformities will tend to correct spontaneously and the clinical relevance for the shoulder joint can be ignored even when due to a distal supracondylar fracture with marked rotational deformities[9,10]. However, distally the rotational deformity will obviously remain unchanged and is responsible for a poor cosmetic result. In conclusion, post-traumatic rotational deformities of the humerus can be corrected proximally but not distally.

Fractures

Ten per cent of all fractures of the upper extremity are humeral fractures.

Fractures of the proximal humerus

Incidence

About 40% of all humeral fractures are located proximally.

Type of fracture

One third of all fractures are epiphyseal, the remaining two thirds being metaphyseal. The latter are stable compression fractures in 50% of cases and relatively stable transverse fractures in the remaining 50% (Figure 14.3). Epiphyseal fractures with wide open plates (articular fractures) do not occur at this site[2,11,12].

Peri- and post-traumatic problems

The sequelae of growth disturbance are rarely of clinical relevance in this location. In displaced fractures an interposition of the long head of biceps sometimes occurs. This hinders closed reduction and necessitates open surgery.

Diagnosis

An antero-posterior (AP) X-ray is usually sufficient to diagnose fractures of the proximal hum-

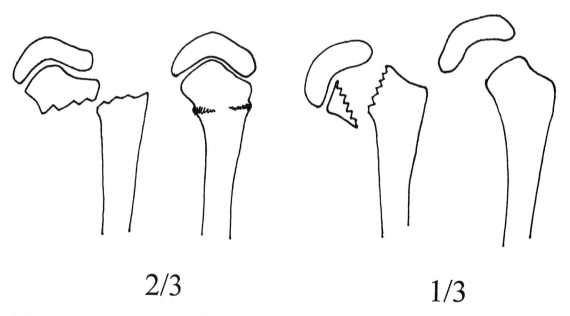

2/3   1/3

Figure 14.3 Fracture types of the proximal humerus: in one-third of all cases there is a lysis of the epiphysis with or without a metaphyseal wedge (right) and in two-thirds there are stable or unstable metaphyseal fractures (left)

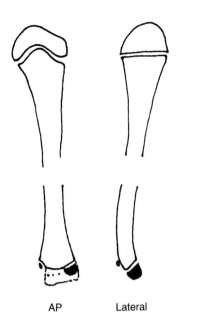

Figure 14.4 AP and lateral views of the proximal humerus (see text)

erus. In addition, the Y-view or supraspinatus outlet view is useful as lateral displacement can be adequately assessed. Oblique radiographs should be avoided as they are difficult to read and growth plates are commonly misinterpreted as fracture lines.

The evaluation of the direction of fracture displacement can be difficult because without the presence of the elbow joint on the radiograph it can be difficult to distinguish between an antero-posterior and lateral view of the humerus. However the surgeon should remember that the orientation of the humerus can be distinguished by the position of the epiphyseal growth plates (Figure 14.4).

Treatment

When considering treatment it is important to assess the degree of fracture displacement. Fractures may be completely displaced with no bone contact or they may be referred to as undisplaced with some bony apposition. In these fractures it is important to distinguish between stable and relatively stable fractures (Figure 14.5). All stable metaphyseal fractures are immobilized in a Gilchrist bandage. Relatively stable fractures are usually immobilized in a plaster of Paris enhanced Desault bandage, this usually being applied using analgesia rather than anaesthesia (Figure 14.6).

Completely displaced fractures should be reduced under general anaesthesia. For children less than 12 years of age a plaster of Paris enhanced Desault bandage is the fixation of choice. In children over 12 years of age we advocate stabilizing the fracture by intramedullary nail-

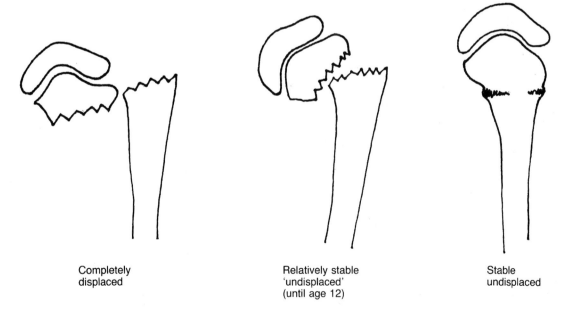

Completely
displaced

Relatively stable
'undisplaced'
(until age 12)

Stable
undisplaced

Figure 14.5 Stable and unstable fractures of the proximal humerus. Almost one-third of these fractures are completely displaced (left), a further one-third are stable fractures (right) and the remaining third are relatively stable, tilted fractures

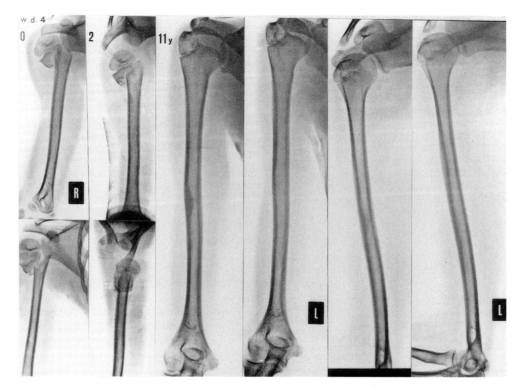

Figure 14.6 The treatment of stable and 'relatively stable' proximal fractures of the humerus. 'Relatively stable' fractures are immobilized in a plaster of Paris enhanced Desault bandage in patients under 12 years of age. This is effective even if there is a tilt in one or two planes as in this four-year-old boy. The follow-up after seven years shows a complete spontaneous correction of the original tilt

ing with Prévot nails or rounded K-wires. These nails will be pushed upwards from the radial epicondyles (Figure 14.7).

Open reduction is only undertaken in cases of irreducible fractures, these usually being epiphyseal fractures with interposition of the biceps tendon[2,4,11,13,14]. The approach is usually through the anterior axillary fold. The interposed soft tissue is removed and the fracture reduced and held by percutaneously inserted Kirschner wires (Figure 14.8). These are removed after fracture union.

Duration of fixation and rehabilitation

The duration of immobilization depends on the age of the patient: until the age of 5–7 years external immobilization should be retained for 14 days and after this age for about three weeks. It is rarely necessary to continue immobilization after this time although the occasional adolescent with a painful callus does require more prolonged support in a Gilchrist sling or Desault cast. Fractures

treated by intramedullary nailing are usually managed without any external support.

Most children spontaneously carry out their own rehabilitation programme of joint mobilization and physiotherapy is only indicated if the patient has not reached a full range of motion within six weeks. Follow-up is usually undertaken on a three-weekly basis until a full range of motion is achieved. Subsequently the patients are asked to attend the follow-up clinic if there is a deterioration in shoulder function or an alteration of humeral length. In the rare case of growth disturbance after epiphyseal fracture longer follow-up is necessary. Should there be a clinically obvious angular deformity in patients less than 13 years of age we suggest a six-monthly follow-up until both parents and patient are satisfied.

Metal removal

Percutaneous K-wires are removed after fracture consolidation usually between three and five weeks after insertion. This is usually done without

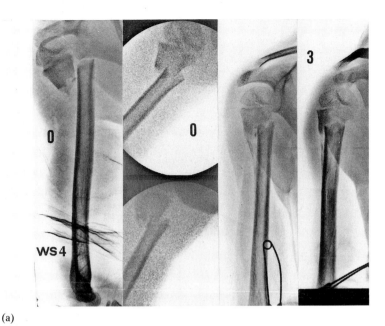

(a)

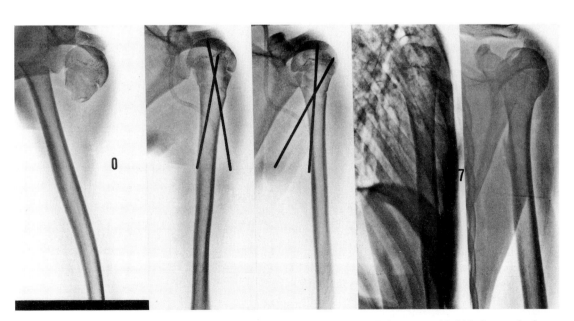

(b)

Figure 14.7   Treatment of unstable proximal fractures of the humerus. (a) Completely displaced fractures are reduced and closed in patients under the age of 12 years. (b) Above 12 years of age, reduction should be held either by intramedullary nailing with curved K-wires or with Prévot nails which are introduced distally at the radial epicondyle and pushed through the epiphyseal plate

Figure 14.8   Treatment of unstable complete fractures with interposed soft tissues. This ten-year-old girl had a completely displaced, closed proximal humeral fracture. Closed reduction was unsuccessful. At open reduction the long head of the biceps tendon was found to be interposed between the bone fragments. Two crossed K-wires were introduced percutaneously. Late follow-up shows a slightly premature closing of the entire epiphyseal plate but a good overall position

anaesthesia. We recommend the removal of intra-medullary nails at the same time using general anaesthesia.

Fractures of the middle third

Incidence

Diaphyseal fractures are rarely seen during growth and comprise only about 10% of humeral fractures.

Type of fracture

There are similarities between the fracture morphology in children and adults, although in children transverse and oblique fractures are encountered more frequently than comminuted fractures. Oblique fractures may be associated with a torsional butterfly fragment.

Peri- and post-traumatic problems

The sequelae of post-traumatic diaphyseal deformity are usually of little clinical importance. Surgeons should, however, remember that fractures between the middle and distal thirds of the humerus may cause damage to the radial nerve.

Diagnosis

Antero-posterior and lateral radiographs are invariably sufficient both for fracture diagnosis and for assessment of deformity and displacement.

Treatment

The treatment of virtually all fractures of the middle third of the humerus is non-operative and, if possible, functional. Initially a plaster of Paris Desault bandage is applied using axial traction on the elbow. Sometimes analgesics are required. After about five to eight days this bandage can be removed and a Sarmiento brace should be applied. At this time X-rays of the fracture should be taken. Lateral displacement of not more than the diameter of the shaft and shortening of less than 3 cm can be tolerated, with the agreement of the parents and the child. Angular deformity of less than 10° in each plane is acceptable. If a general anaesthetic is necessary to obtain a reduction we fix the fracture using either an intramedullary nail or an external fixation device.

Primary operative treatment is only indicated in polytrauma patients, in open fractures where there is considerable soft tissue damage and in other situations where a general anaesthetic is required. Depending on the degree of damage to the soft tissues we advocate an external fixator, intermedullary nails or rounded K-wires. Usually the wires or nails will be inserted distally at the radial epicondyle and only rarely are they inserted in an antegrade manner through the greater tuberosity.

An isolated paresis of the radial nerve is not an indication for operation. The fracture is treated non-operatively and allowed to consolidate. If there is no sign of recovery at the time of fracture union we will undertake a late exploration of the nerve (Figure 14.9).

Duration of fixation in rehabilitation

Depending on the age of the patient and the type of fracture the use of the Sarmiento brace will be continued for between three and six weeks. After it is removed full range of motion is usually achieved and the patient can slowly regain normal activities.

Physiotherapy treatment is rarely required and only in cases with significant reduction of function four weeks after the brace has been discontinued is physiotherapy indicated.

Once there are no more complaints during daily activities follow-up can be stopped. Growth disturbances are rare.

Metal removal

Intramedullary nails, external fixators or K-wires can be removed after consolidation of the fracture about four to six weeks after the operation.

Fractures of the distal third

Incidence

Fractures of the distal third of the humerus comprise about 50% of all humeral fractures. The most common fracture in this location is the supracondylar fracture followed by condylar fractures and epicondylar fractures.

Type of fracture

Unlike fractures of the proximal and middle thirds of the humerus distal humeral fractures must be

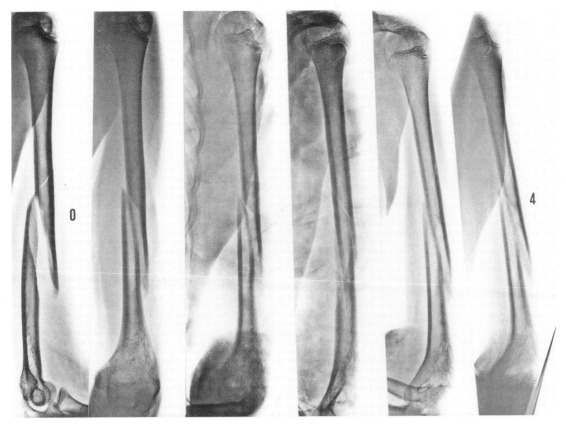

Figure 14.9 Treatment of a diaphyseal fracture of the humerus. A 16-year-old boy with a displaced fracture of the humeral diaphysis complicated by sensory and motor damage to the radial nerve. A plaster of Paris enhanced Desault bandage was applied under slight axial traction and analgesia. After four weeks the fracture had healed clinically and radiologically. At this time there was some recovery of the radial nerve palsy and no exploration was required. Four months after the injury the nerve had completely recovered.

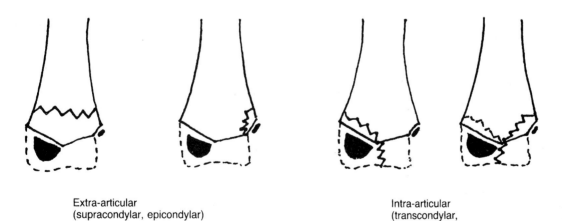

Extra-articular
(supracondylar, epicondylar)

Intra-articular
(transcondylar,
radial, ulnar/Y)

Figure 14.10 Fracture types of the distal humerus. Extra-articular and intra-articular fractures have to be distinguished. Supracondylar and epicondylar fractures are extra-articular fractures, whereas radial and ulnar condylar fractures and the transcondylar Y-fracture are intra-articular fractures

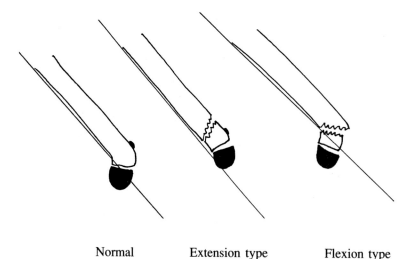

Normal   Extension type   Flexion type

Figure 14.11 A diagrammatic representation of the elbow seen in a lateral view to show the normal appearance, the extension type of supracondylar fracture (90%) and the flexion type (10%)

divided into extra- and intra-articular fractures. Supracondylar and epicondylar fractures are extra-articular whereas radial and ulnar condylar fractures and transcondylar Y-fractures are intra-articular (Figure 14.10).

Supracondylar fractures

Type of fractures. Ninety per cent of supracondylar fractures are extension injuries, the remaining 10% occurring following a flexion injury (Figure 14.11). A number of different classifications have been used such as those of Baumann[15] and Felsenreich[16]. These predominantly classify the fractures based on the extent of displacement. However, the

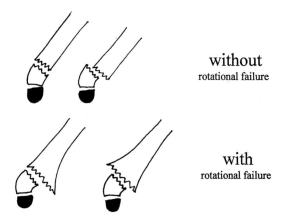

without
rotational failure

with
rotational failure

Figure 14.12 Classification of supracondylar fractures. From the therapeutic and prognostic point of view it is necessary to ascertain whether there is a rotational deformity associated with the fracture

most important factor in supracondylar fractures is the extent of any rotational deformity and we therefore suggest that it is only necessary to differentiate between fractures that present with or without a rotational deformity[1] (Figure 14.12).

Peri- and post-traumatic problems. The worst complication of supracondylar fracture is post-traumatic ischaemia leading to a Volkmann contracture[17–20]. Fortunately this complication is rarely encountered today because of early detection and appropriate treatment. However, if the patient complains of increasing pain the surgeon should always be aware of the possibility of compartment syndrome. If the early clinical signs are not definitive intra-compartmental pressure monitoring should be undertaken. When the pressure continuously exceeds 35 mm it is mandatory to undertake a fasciotomy of the forearm compartments.

Growth disturbances usually involving the radial part of the distal humeral physis may occur but rarely have any clinical relevance. The main problem associated with supracondylar fractures is rotation. To correct a rotational deformity and maintain the correction until consolidation occurs is one of the major problems facing the surgeon. A persistent rotational deformity leads to the following problems:

- instability of the fracture
- ventral spur
- temporary rotational overloading of the shoulder
- persistent distal rotation deformity
- post-traumatic 'iatrogenic' irritation of the ulnar nerve.

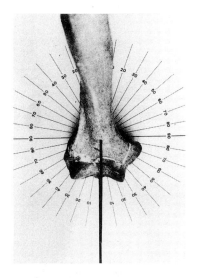

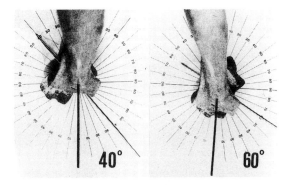

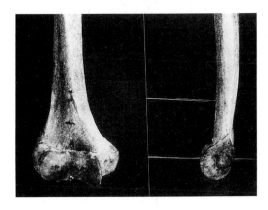

(a)

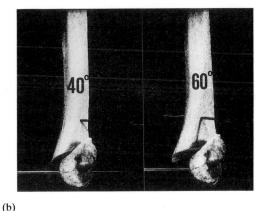

(b)

Figure 14.13 The amount of rotational deformity in supracondylar fractures. (a) The rotational deformity cannot be detected clinically in a fresh fracture. Rotation can only be seen on the lateral radiograph depending on the size of the spur. (b) In the model rotational deformity is between 40–60°

Because of the tone of the shoulder musculature and the position of immobilization with the forearm placed on the chest there is a tendency to torsion of both fragments in supracondylar fractures. The proximal fragment tends to rotate externally and the distal fragment internally. If there is a rotational deformity of more than 30° (Figure 14.13) the fracture will only make contact at one point: the small lamina of the olecranon fossa. Thus the fracture will be unstable and has a high chance of slipping, usually into a varus position[1,9,10].

The rotational deformity cannot be measured clinically before reduction and it therefore cannot be corrected directly during repositioning of the fragments. It can only be seen by visualizing the ventral (or occasional dorsal) spur. If this spur remains it will initially be a hindrance to elbow flexion although as it resolves within two years the

function will return. Because of the range of motion of the shoulder a rotational deformity has little clinical relevance.

The rotational and varus deformities associated with supracondylar fractures remain unchanged during growth. It is the varus deformity which provides most of the cosmetic problem which is associated with this fracture[9,21] (Figure 14.14).

Deformities of the ulnar canal associated with irritation of the ulnar nerve secondary to rotation of the distal humeral fragment are very seldom described in the literature[22].

Diagnosis. Usually standard antero-posterior and lateral X-rays are sufficient to diagnose this fracture. In clinically obvious deformities an X-ray in one plane may be all that is required to confirm the presence of a fracture. Comparison X-rays of

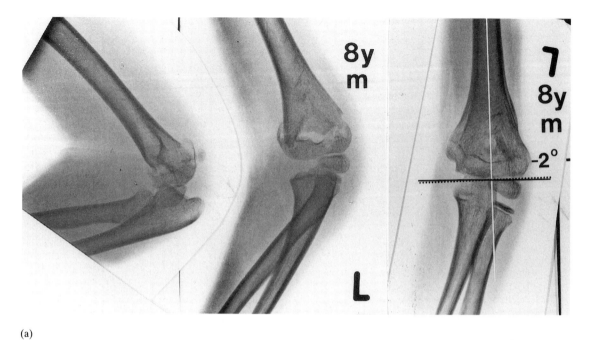

(a)

(b)

(c)

Figure 14.14(a–c)   Distal rotational deformity after a supracondylar fracture. (a) An eight-year-old boy with a displaced fracture with rotational deformity and ulnar tilt. The extent of the rotational deformity was initially misinterpreted and the fracture was treated non-operatively without reduction. The fracture healed in a varus position. (b) A CT scan shows a distal rotational deformity of about 45°. In addition the forward tilt of the radial column is cosmetically unsatisfactory. (c) Nearly two years after the fracture the shoulder demonstrates a free range of motion but the varus is unchanged

the contralateral side are unnecessary. The Rogers line can be helpful[23] although it must not be forgotten that the patient has come for treatment, not just for a correct diagnosis[1].

Treatment. Undisplaced fractures should be immobilized in a collar and cuff or dorsal plaster brace for two to three weeks. Consolidation can be confirmed clinically without the need for further X-rays.

Fractures that show only an anterior angulation without any rotational deformity can be corrected by manipulation and analgesia and immobilized in a collar and cuff. For patients with an anterior angulation of more than 30° a lateral X-ray following the application of the collar and cuff should be undertaken to exclude any secondary rotational deformity. If this is found the ensuing treatment will follow the principles laid down for primary fractures associated with a rotational component[1].

All fractures that present with a primary rotational deformity or with complete displacement should be reduced carefully under general anaesthesia. The most commonly used manoeuvre for reduction was first described by Blount[24]: first, continuous traction of the extended elbow; secondly, reduction by pronation and simultaneous flexion of the elbow. The distal fragment will be manoeuvred anteriorly by the surgeon's thumb.

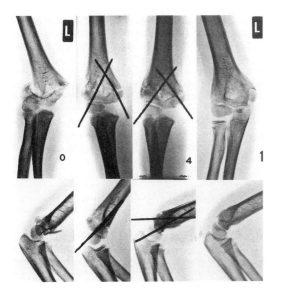

Figure 14.15 Treatment of supracondylar fractures. Percutaneously inserted crossed K-wires are widely used to treat fractures where a good reduction has been achieved. This is illustrated in a 6-year-old girl who also had an undisplaced proximal radial epiphyseal lysis.

The aim of the reduction is to correct all the rotational deformity and more than 3 mm of lateral displacement. This target should be achieved with one reduction. Failure to do so suggests that there is soft tissue impingement which should be treated by open reduction. Multiple attempts at closed reduction may well cause considerable iatrogenic damage. A number of methods have been described to retain the reduced fracture position: the collar and cuff of Blount, the traction treatment of Baumann, percutaneous K-wiring, open K-wiring and many other treatment methods have their proponents[25–35]. In the interests of the patient the treatment should be as straightforward as possible. In addition, the treatment should do no harm – psychologically or physically. This means that multiple re-reductions and changing of treatment methods are obsolete and either signify failure to use the right reduction technique or to appreciate the problems associated with supracondylar fractures. We believe that traction therapy should be abandoned and the surgeon should be careful about using the collar and cuff method under many circumstances. These therapies frequently demand a lengthy hospital stay or are related to multiple re-reductions and changing of treatment methods. However, even the more stable fixation methods utilizing K-wires also give rise to concern. Secondary rotational and lateral malalignment is reported in all methods[25–27]. Follow-up studies using different scoring methods tend to disguise the facts,[34,36] the incidence of complications being as high as 15–30%.

In the past few years we have used the crossed K-wire technique (Figure 14.15). However in a follow-up study we found that 10% of the cases had secondary varus deformities although these produced only cosmetic problems. In addition in 10% of the cases temporary irritations of the ulnar nerve occurred. Although the overall prognosis is good this is an avoidable complication[35,37]. We have therefore changed our approach to use an external fixation device placed on the radial side. This allows control of secondary malalignment of the radial condyle by use of compression if even a slight rotation is noted. In addition the ulnar side is untouched and the nerve is therefore not at risk. The only problem is damage to the radial nerve due to an inappropriate positioning of the proximal wire. This can be prevented by correct pre- and per-operative analysis of the position of the bone fragments. The method cannot be applied to radially comminuted fractures. If comminution is detected it is important that another fixation

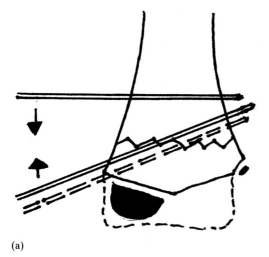

(a)

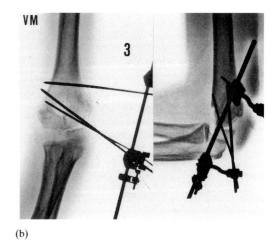

(b)

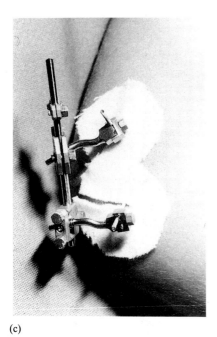

(c)

Figure 14.16(a–c)   The treatment of displaced supracondylar fractures. The radially located external fixator ensures excellent treatment by preventing forward rotation of the radial condyle and ulnar tilt. After perfect reduction of the radial column the fracture will be fixed by one or two percutaneously inserted radial K-wires. The fracture reduction can be maintained by this procedure. Two or three fingers above a K-wire will be inserted into the diaphysis to provide a second point of fixation for the external fixator. A small Hoffmann external fixator is applied and used to compress the fracture. After three weeks the fracture will be stable enough for motion. A rotational deformity of up to 20° is of little clinical or functional significance

method is employed. Thus far our results are encouraging (Figure 14.16). When selecting a treatment method it is particularly important to select one which prevents the formation of a varus deformity. The results of corrective osteotomy for this problem are poor[38–43] and it is just as important to achieve an anatomical reduction as it is to achieve secure bone fixation.

Primary open reduction does not necessarily guarantee a better fracture reduction. Open reduction is only performed if the fracture cannot be reduced at the first attempt. We suggest the posterior approach for cosmetic reasons. Only in cases where we require access to the vessels or the nerves do we use an anterolateral approach. Initially we approach the ulnar column protecting the ulnar nerve and securing the column by a percutaneous K-wire. The radial column is then treated in a similar manner.

Direction of fixation and rehabilitation. The duration of external fixation should not exceed

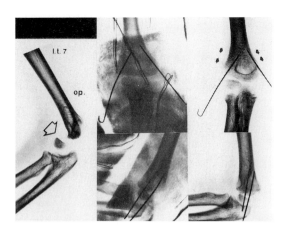

Figure 14.17 Epiphyseolysis of the distal humerus. A seven-year-old boy with an epiphyseolysis of the capitulum and the trochlea. Reduction and fixation was performed as for a displaced supracondylar fracture. This fracture healed after three weeks. (By courtesy of Dr Lusche, Krankenhaus Lörrach)

three weeks. We suggest that any ancillary immobilization is discarded after two weeks in favour of elbow mobilization if X-rays show sufficient callus formation and the patient is not in significant discomfort. No external force should be applied to the child's arm. Depending on the extent of damage to the soft tissues around the elbow joint it may take up to six or eight weeks for a normal range of elbow motion to be achieved. If function does not improve spontaneously and continuously we institute physiotherapy treatment. This is most often required in older children. Even if the patient has not recovered a full range of elbow motion, sports activities may be commenced if the patient is particularly keen to do so. Treatment and follow-up can be stopped when the patient has achieved a full range of motion and the axes of both elbow are equal. This is only possible to judge in full elbow extension.

The most peripheral and rarely seen form of the distal humeral fracture is epiphyseolysis of the trochlea and capitulum (Figure 14.17). The treatment and prognosis for this unusual injury are the same as for supracondylar fractures.

Fractures of the radial condyle

Incidence. This is the second most frequent fracture involving the distant humerus as well as the second most frequent fracture involving the elbow joint.

Type of fracture. We prefer not to classify fractures of the radial condyle by morphological criteria or by the mechanism of trauma[19,44–46], but by the amount of displacement. Undisplaced fractures are stable centrally and therefore represent incomplete articular fractures. Primary or secondary displaced fractures have a displacement of more than 2 mm in the central part and are therefore complete articular fractures (Figure 14.18).

Peri- and post-traumatic problems. All fractures whether or not they are displaced are physeal-crossing fractures of the Salter IV or Aitken III types. The typical growth disturbance is a temporary partial radial stimulation which leads to an variable varus deformation of the elbow[47–50]. The extent of the varus deformity depends on the time to consolidation and this may vary between four weeks and two years. The longer the consolidation time the greater the tendency for a varus deformity to occur.

The second clinically more important problem associated with fractures of the radial condyle relates to the possibility of delayed or non-union. The pressure of the radial head may cause a secondary displacement of the fracture and if this is not noticed by the surgeon it may lead to a pseudarthrosis even when an adequate cast is applied[46,48–50] (Figure 14.19). Such a pseudarthrosis usually produces a noticeable cubitus valgus[19,51]. If there is a cubitus valgus of more than 10°, secondary damage to the ulnar nerve can be expected. Radial condylar non-unions are difficult to treat but fortunately many patients with this condition have a good long-term functional result.

Diagnosis. Antero-posterior and lateral X-rays are usually sufficient to diagnose radial condylar fractures. Displaced fractures are easy to diagnose and rarely missed. The central and peripheral part of the fracture are the key areas in which to look for displacement (Figure 14.18b)[18]. Undisplaced radial condylar fractures may provide diagnostic difficulties. If any swelling of the soft tissues is noted either clinically or on the antero-posterior radiograph the radial cortices must be examined very carefully. Often little more than an interruption of the cortical line can be detected on an antero-posterior X-ray. When such an irregularity is confirmed then a fracture may often be recognized on the lateral X-ray. The fracture line normally starts at the dorsal proximal metaphysis and crosses the epiphyseal plane ventrally and distally (see Figure 14.19). With all undisplaced fractures secondary

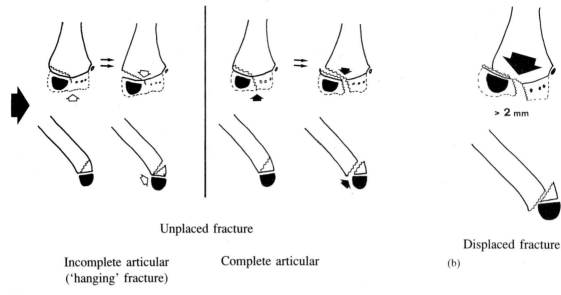

Unplaced fracture

Incomplete articular   Complete articular   (b)
('hanging' fracture)

Displaced fracture

(a)

Figure 14.18   Undisplaced and displaced fractures of the humeral radial condyle. (a) In undisplaced fractures of the radial condyle of the humerus we must distinguish between incomplete and complete articular fractures. Incomplete fractures are stable and can be treated non-operatively. The undisplaced complete articular fractures tend to displace secondarily even in a cast and should be treated like displaced primary fractures. (b) It is important to examine the central part of the joint to assess the amount of articular displacement. It is recommended that an X-ray out of plaster be obtained after four days to differentiate between undisplaced complete intra-articular fractures and incomplete intra-articular fractures. If the central part of the joint remains stable the articular fracture will be incomplete and undisplaced (see also Figure 14.20)

displacement must be excluded because the trochlea cannot be completely visualized radiologically and the X-ray does not allow differentiation between complete and incomplete (the so-called 'hanging') articular fractures.

Undisplaced complete articular fractures tend to undergo displacement centrally and therefore can produce a non-union. Undisplaced but incomplete hanging articular fractures do not displace centrally and unite without delay (Figure 14.20). If there is diagnostic difficulty ordinary antero-posterior and lateral X-rays can be repeated on the fourth or fifth day after fracture. If the fracture gap is widened centrally on the antero-posterior view and in the anterior part of the lateral X-ray by more than 2 mm the fracture is complete and must be fixed operatively[1] (Figure 14.21). If there is difficulty in diagnosing the fracture alternative imaging techniques such as CAT scanning, MRI scanning, arthroscopy or arthrography can be employed[51,52,53]

Treatment. Undisplaced radial condylar fractures

are treated non-operatively and are immobilized using a dorsal plaster of Paris splint. Further X-rays are obtained about the fourth day to distinguish between a complete and incomplete fracture. If the fracture is seen to be incomplete the splint is completed to a full cast. If it is impossible to distinguish between a complete or incomplete fracture at that time the splint is left for a further four days and repeat X-rays taken.

All primary displaced fractures and all fractures that show secondary displacement must be reduced as they are intra-articular fractures. Usually open reduction and internal fixation are performed[49,50]. We usually use a small fragment screw which penetrates the contralateral cortex and thereby compresses the fracture. If the fracture can be closed under compression the consolidation time rarely exceeds four weeks. Should the fragment be too small to allow the use of a bone screw two small K-wires or absorbable pins can be used[6,19,47,48,51,54].

Duration of fixation and rehabilitation. Non-

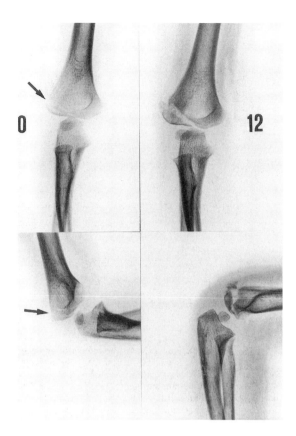

Figure 14.19 Secondary displacement of a primarily undisplaced radial condylar fracture. The patient was a $2\frac{1}{2}$-year-old girl who had an undisplaced fracture of the radial condyle. The fracture was promptly diagnosed and treated in a cast. Unfortunately no X-ray was taken after four days and after six weeks, at the time of cast removal, it was noted that there had been a secondary displacement. Twelve weeks after the fracture there was a non-union which could only be treated by internal fixation. (By courtesy of Dr Bornhauser, Stans)

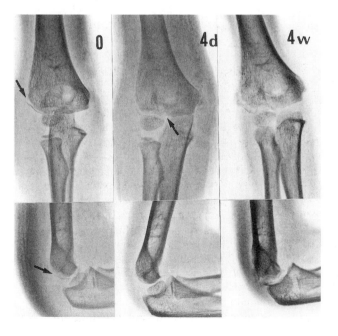

Figure 14.20 Treatment of an undisplaced radial condylar fracture. The patient was a seven-year-old boy who had an undisplaced fracture of the radial condyle. Non-operative management was undertaken. At four days an X-ray out of plaster showed that the fracture and the important central part of the joint were stable and non-operative treatment was continued. The fracture healed after four weeks

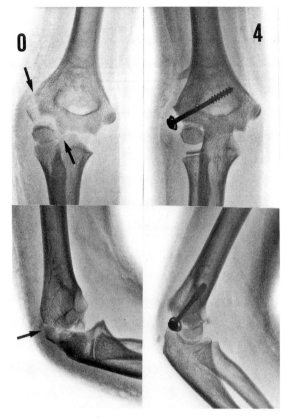

Figure 14.21 Treatment of displaced radial condyle fractures. An 8-year-old girl with a primarily displaced radial condylar. This was treated by open reduction and internal fixation using a metaphyseal screw supplemented with a washer. The fracture was stable four weeks after surgery

operatively treated fractures are immobilized in a cast for four weeks. After union has been demonstrated clinically and radiologically the elbow can be mobilized without the use of physiotherapy. Internally fixed fractures can be treated by early joint mobilization depending on the age and activity level of the patient. If there is any doubt about the stability of fracture after fixation a plaster of Paris cast should be applied. A full range of joint motion can normally be expected within four to six weeks. Once full movement has been achieved the patient can return to normal activities.

As these fractures cross the growth plate it is important that follow-up be continued every six months for at least two years after the fracture. However treatment can be stopped once the patient has achieved both a full range of motion and symmetrical elbow axes. Follow-up can usually be stopped about two years after the accident even when the patient has a varus deformity provided there are no signs of an increase in the deformity.

Fractures of the ulnar condyle

Fractures of the ulnar condyle of the distal humerus are rarely seen during skeletal growth but when they are encountered they present with fewer problems than do fractures of the radial condyle[1,48]. However, as with the radial condylar fracture a partial temporary stimulation of the growth plate often occurs, this usually being associated with a fracture that crosses the growth plate. The result is usually a slight valgus deformation of the elbow. However the fracture heals quickly and therefore does not cause a clinically relevant growth disturbance.

The treatment is the same as for radial condylar fractures. Undisplaced fractures are treated conservatively and displaced fractures will be treated by open reduction and internal fixation. It is suggested that the immobilization is maintained for four weeks and that surgeons follow the same rehabilitation regime as has been suggested for radial condylar fractures.

Transcondylar Y-fractures

These fractures are also very uncommon in children. They are usually undisplaced and such fractures can be treated non-operatively. Where the fracture is displaced it should be operatively reduced through a dorsal approach then internally fixed using percutaneous K-wires. Postoperatively the elbow should be placed in a plaster brace for three to four weeks.

Following this injury a partial radial stimulation with slight radial overgrowth may occur. This can lead to a varus deformity of the elbow axis. The follow-up and rehabilitation are the same as has been described for radial condylar fractures.

Ulnar and radial epicondylar fractures

Incidence. Ulnar epicondylar fractures are the third most frequent injury involving the distal humerus in children.

Type of fracture. The most frequent epicondylar fracture is that on the ulnar side. It is a relatively common accompaniment of an elbow dislocation and although it does occur alone, surgeons should

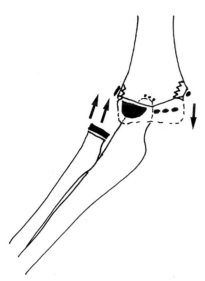

Figure 14.22 Epicondylar fractures. These fractures are usually associated with elbow dislocation. Usually the ulnar epicondyle is involved, the radial epicondyle being rarely fractured

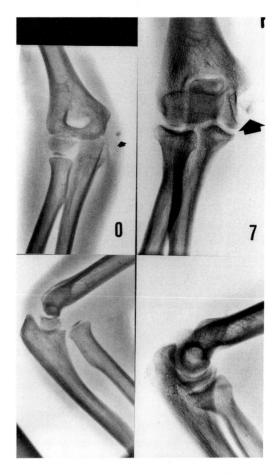

Figure 14.23 An example of a non-union after fracture of the ulnar epicondyle. The patient was an 8-year-old boy who had an isolated fracture of the radial head which was primarily treated by closed reduction. The displaced fracture of the ulnar epicondyle was initially missed and resulted in a non-union. Seven years later the patient was subjectively and objectively asymptomatic with a full range of motion in the elbow and normal arc

always be aware of the possibility of a dislocation and spontaneous reduction when an ulnar epicondylar fracture is seen. The fragment is pulled in a distal and ventral direction by the flexor muscles (Figure 14.22)[22]. Fractures of the radial epicondyle are uncommon but can also occur in association with an elbow dislocation.

Post-traumatic problems. Growth disturbances following epicondylar fractures are rare. Non-operatively managed fractures of the ulnar epicondyle can occasionally result in non-union (Figure 14.23)[1,23,55]. However such non-unions are symptom-free in 90% of cases. In about 10% of cases ulnar nerve irritation can occur secondary to ulnar canal deformation either as a result of the fracture, a subsequent non-union or an epicondylar malunion.

Diagnosis. Normally only antero-posterior and lateral X-rays are required to diagnose epicondylar fractures. If the child is under the age of four or five years and the epicondyle is not radiologically visible the fracture will usually be obvious clinically. However, epicondylar avulsion fractures and dislocations are most frequently encountered in children of at least ten years of age.

Treatment. For the purposes of treatment fracture displacement is defined as more than 5 mm of a fracture gap. Non-displaced fractures should be treated by immobilization in a plaster of Paris cast for about three weeks (Figure 14.24). Should the fracture proceed to a symptomatic non-union this can be successfully treated by operative fixation at a later date. Displacement of more than 5 mm or any displacement of the fragment into the joint is an indication for open reduction and internal fixation. The fragment is usually fixed by a bone screw although smaller fragments can also be attached by K-wires or absorbable pins. In these cases we apply a plaster brace postoperatively; otherwise functional treatment is indicated.

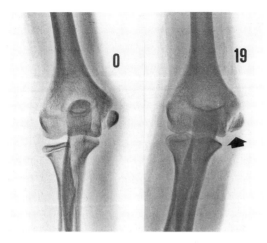

O　19

Figure 14.24　An example of non-operative management of an ulnar epicondylar fracture. The patient was a 15-year-old girl who presented with a moderately displaced fracture of the ulnar epicondyle. Despite her age and the degree of displacement, the fracture was treated non-operatively. The fracture was stable during elbow motion after two and a half weeks. Six weeks after the injury the patient had a full range of motion and was subjectively asymptomatic

Duration of fixation and rehabilitation. Usually the elbow does not have to be immobilized for more than two or occasionally three weeks. If a K-wire has been used it can be removed at three weeks without any anaesthesia and bone screws can be safely taken out under local anaesthesia after three months.

The postoperative treatment follows the same basic principles as for the other elbow fractures. As a rule the child will usually mobilize the joint spontaneously. If there is little progress after four weeks of elbow mobilization a physiotherapy regime should be commenced. Generally the older the patient the earlier the physiotherapy should start, particularly if there has been a previous elbow dislocation. Once the joint has reached a full range of motion the patient can commence sporting activities, this usually being eight to twelve weeks after the accident.

Once the epicondylar fracture has united and a full range of motion is restored to the joint, the treatment can be discontinued. Should a non-union occur we will follow the patient for one year. In cases where there is full asymptomatic function of the joint we discontinue follow-up; otherwise we consider revision surgery depending upon the patient.

References

1. von Laer, L. *Frakturen und Luxationen im Wachstumsalter,* Thieme, Stuttgart (1991).
2. von Laer, L. Fractures around the child's shoulder. In *Shoulder Surgery in Europe* (ed. C. Gerber), Springer, Berlin (1992).
3. von Laer, L. and Gschwend, C. Korrekturmechanismen und Wachstumsstörungen am proximalen Humerusende – primäre und sekundäre. Therapie traumatischer Läsionen. In Chapchal G, ed. *Verletzungen und Erkrankungen der Schulterregion* (ed, C. Chapchal), Tieme, Stuttgart (1984)
4. Frey, C. and Kloti, J. Spätresultate nach subkapitalen Humerusfrakturen bei Kindern. *Z. Kinderchir.,* **44,** 280–282 (1989)
5. Larsen, C.F., Kiaer, T. and Lindequist, S. Fractures of the proximal humerus in children. Nine-year follow-up of 64 unoperated on cases. *Acta Orthop. Scand.,* **61,** 255–257 (1990)
6. Rockwood, C.A.J., Wilkins, K.E. and King, R.E. *Fractures in Children,* Lippincott, Philadelphia (1984)
7. Wahl, D. *Das Wachstumsverhalten der langen Röhrenknochen des Armes nach mechanischer Schädigung,* Habilitationsschrift, DDR (1981)
8. von Laer, L. Die supracondyläre Humerusfraktur im Wachstumsalter. *Arch. Orthop. Trauma Surg.,* **95,** 123 (1979)
9. Kissling, D. *Die supracondyläre Humerusfraktur-Bedeutung und Schicksal des Rotationsfehlers im Rahmen kindlicher supracondylärer Humerusfrakturen.* Diss, Basel (1985)
10. Resch, H. and Helweg, G. Signifikanz von Rotationsfehlstellungen bei suprakondylären Humerusfrakturen in Kindern. *Aktuel. Traumatol.,* **17,** 65–72 (1987)
11. Kohler, R. and Trillaud, J.M. Fracture and fracture separation of the proximal humerus in children: report of 136 cases. *J. Pediatr. Orthop.* **3,** 326–332 (1983)
12 Ritter, G., Verletngen des Schultergürtels und der oberen Extremität. In *Das verletzte Kind* (ed. H. Sauer), Thieme, Stuttgart (1984)
13. Curtiss, R.J.J. Operative management of children's fractures of the shoulder region. *Orthop. Clin. North Am.,* **21,** 315–324 (1990)
14. Siebler, G., Kuner, E.H. and Schmitt, A. Operative Behandlung von proximalen Humerusfrakturen in Kindern und Adoleszenten -Indikationen, Technik, Spätresultate. *Unfallchirugie,* **10,** 237–244 (1984)
15. Baumann, E. Ellbogen. In *Spezielle Frakturen- und Luxationslehre* (ed. H. Nigst), Thieme, Stuttgart (1965)

16. Felsenreich, F. Kindliche supracondyläre Frakturen und posttraumatische Deformitäten des Ellbogengelenkes. *Arch. Orthop. Unfall. Chir.* **29**, 555 (1931)

17. Clement, D.A. Assessment of a treatment plan for managing acute vascular complications associated with supracondylar fractures of the humerus in children. *J. Pediatr. Orthop.*, **10**, 97–100 (1990)

18. Kurer, M.H. and Regan, M.W. Completely displaced supracondylar fracture of the humerus in children. A review of 1708 comparable cases. *Clin. Orthop.*, 205–214 (1990)

19. Ogden, J.A. *Skeletal injury in the child*, Lea and Febiger, Philadelphia (1982)

20. Prone, A.M., Graham, H.K. and Krajbich, J.J. Management of displaced extension-type supracondylar fractures of the humerus in children [published erratum appears in *J. Bone Surg.*, **70-1**, 1114 (1988)] [see comments] *J. Bone Joint Surg.*, **70A**, 641–650 (1988)

21. von Laer, L., Brunner, R. and Lampert, C. Fehlverheite suprakindyläre und kondyläre Humerusfrakturen. *Orthopäde*, **20**, 331–340 (1991)

22. Uchida, Y. and Sugoika, Y. Ulnar nerve palsy after supracondylar humerus fracture. *Acta Orthop. Scand.*, **2**, 118 (1990)

23. Rogers, L.F., Malave, S., White, H. and Tachdijan, M.O. Plastic bowing and greenstick supracondyral fractures of the humerus: radiographic clues to obscure fractures of the elbow in children. *Radiology*, **128**, 145–150 (1978)

24. Blount, W.P. *Knochenbrüche bei Kindern*, Thieme, Stuttgart (1957)

25. Franke, C., Reilmann, H. and Weinreich, M. Langzeitresultate der Behandlung von suprakondylären Humerusfrakturen bei Kindern. *Unfallchirg*, **95**, 401–404 (1992)

26. Celiker, O., Pestilci, F.I. and Tuzuner, M. Supracondylar fractures of the humerus in children: analysis of the results in 142 patients. *J. Orthop. Trauma*, **4**, 265–269 (1990)

27. Furrer, M., Mark, G. and Ruedi, T. Die Behandlung der dislozierten suprakondylären Humerusfraktur bei Kindern. *Z. Unfallchir. Versicherungsmed. Berufskr.*, **82**, 264–265 (1980)

28. Goudarzi, Y.M. Indikationen für verschiedene Behandlungsverfahren bei der Therapie von suprakondylären Humerusfrakturen bei Kindern. *Unfallchirugie*, **13**, 8–13 (1987)

29. Aronson, D.D. and Prager, B.I. Supracondylar fractures of the humerus in children. A modified technique for closed pinning. *Clin. Orthop.*, **219**, 174–184 (1987)

30. Asche, H. Behandlungsmöglichketein mit dem Fixateur externe. In *Operationsindikationen bei Frakturen im Kindeslater* (ed. Hofmann-v. Kapherr), Fischer, Stuttgart (1987)

31. Prevot, J., Lascombes, P., Metaizeau, J.P. and Blanquart, D. [Supracondylar fractures of the humerus in children: treatment by downward nailing.] *Rev. Chir. Orthop. Reparatrice Appar. Mot.*, **76**, 191–197 (1990)

32. Schuck, R., Bartsch, M. and LInk, W. Chirurgische Therapie der distalen Humerusfraktur bei Kindern. *Z. Kinderchir.*, **44**, 283–285 (1989)

33. Taller S. Die Anwendung des Fixateur externe in der Behandlung der suprakondylären Humerusfraktur bei Kindern. *Zentrabl. Chir.*, **111**, 1217–1227 (1986)

34. Morger, R. *Frakturen und Luxationen am kindlichen Ellbogen*, Bibliotheca paediatrica, Fasc.83. Karger, Basel (1965)

35. Mutschler, W. and Suger, G. Die radialseitige Spickdrahtosteosynthese der dislozierten suprakondylären Humerusfraktur beim Kind. *Operat. Orthop. Traumatol.* (in press)

36. Bialik, V., Weiner, A. and Fishman, J. Scoring system for assessing the treatment of suprarcondylar fractures of the humerus. *Isr. J. Med. Sci.*, **19**, 173–175 (1983)

37. Royce, R.O., Dutkowsky, J.P., Kasser, J.R., and Rand, F.R. Neurlogic complications after K-wire fixation of supracondylar humerus fractures in children. *J. Pediatr. Orthop.*, **11**, 191–194 (1991)

38. France, J. and Strong, M. Deformity and function in supracondylar fractures of the humerus in children variously treated by closed reduction and splinting, traction and percutaneous pinning. *J. Pediatr. Orthop.*, **12**, 494–498 (1992)

39. Uchida, Y., Ogata, K. and Sugioka, Y. A new three-dimensional osteotomy for cubitus varus deformity after supracondylar fracture of the humerus in children. *J. Pediatr. Orthop.*, **11**, 327–331 (1991)

40. Ippolito, E., Moneta, M.R. and D'Arrigo, C. Post-traumatic cubitus varus. Long-term follow-up of corrective supracondylar humeral osteotomy in children. *J. Bone Joint Surg.*, **72A**, 757–765 (1990)

41. Oppenheim, W.L., Clader, T.J., Smith, C. and Bayer, M. Supracondylar humeral osteotomy for traumatic childhood cubitus varus deformity. *Clin. Orthop*, **188**, 34–39 (184)

42. Labelle, H., Bunnell, W.P., Duhaime, M. and Poitras, B. Cubitus varus deformity following supracondylar fractures of the humerus in children. *J. Pediatr. Orthop.*, **2**, 539–546 (1982)

43. Bellmore, M.C., Barrett, I.R., Middleton, R.W., Scougall, J.S. and Whiteway, D.S. Supracondylar osteotomy of the humerus for correction of cubitus varus. *J. Bone Joint Surg.*, **66B**, 566–572 (1984)

44. Badelon, O., Vie, P., Mazda, K. and Bensahel, H. [Fracture of the external condyle of the humerus in children. Apropos of a series of 46 cases.] *Rev. Chir. Orthop.*, **72(Suppl.2)**, 66–69 (1986)

45. Jakob, R., Fowles, J.V., Rang, M. and Kassab, M.T. Observations concerning fractures of the lateral humeral condyle in children. *J. Bone Joint. Surg.*, **57B**, 430 (1975)

46. Milch, H. Fractures of the external humeral condyle. *J. Am. Med. Ass.*, **160**, 641 (1956)

47. Jeffery, R.S. Injuries of the lateral humeral condyle in children. *J. R. Coll. Surg. Edinb.*, **34**, 156–159 (1989)

48. Kreusch Brinker, R. and Noack, W. Verletzungen der distalen Humerus-Epiphyse während der Wachstumsphase. *Unfallchirugie*, **12**, 60–67 (1986)

49. van Laer, L., Pagels, P. and Schroeder, L. Die Behandlung der Frakturen des Kondylus radialis humeri während der Wachstumsphase. *Unfallheikunde*, **86**, 503–509 (1983)

50. von Laer, L. Die Fraktur des Condylus radialis humeri im Wachstumsalter. *Arch. Orthop. Trauma. Surg.*, **98**, 275 (1981)

51. Rang, M. *Children's Fractures,* Lippincott, Philadelphia (1983)

52. Hoeffel, J.C., Blanquart, D., Galloy, M.A. *et al.* [Fractures of the lateral condyle of the elbow in children. Radiologic aspects.] *J. Radiol.,* **71,** 407–414 (1990)

53. Drvaric, D.M. and Rooks, M.D. Anterior sleeve fracture of the capitulum. *J. Orthop. Trauma,* **4,** 188–192 (1990)

54. Amgwerd, M., and Sacher, P. Die Behandlung der Fraktur des Condylus radialis humeri bein Kindern. *Z. Unfallchir. Versicherungsmed.,* **83,** 49–53 (1990)

55. Wilson, N.I., Ingram, R., Rymanszewski, L. and Miller, J.H. Treatment of fractures of the medial epicondyle of the humerus. *Injury,* **19,** 342–344 (1988)

Index